Praise for *This Is De*

"Dr. Diane McIntosh has achieved the imp ... with this book: she enables everybody to understand depression in a highly readable way. As someone who has suffered from depression, I empathize deeply with Dr. McIntosh's narrative. She combines real-life stories with academic rigour to bring clarity and insight to this debilitating disease. Whether you're a sufferer or a caregiver, *This Is Depression* will be an indispensable guide to understanding and ultimate healing."

MIKE LIPKIN, motivator and coach, Environics/Lipkin

"This book provides balanced and complete information in an easy-to-understand way. Dr. McIntosh cares so passionately about people living with mental illness and offers clear information and optimism. Mental illness does not discriminate; anyone living with mental illness or who cares for someone living with mental illness should read this book."

ALLISON ROSENTHAL, general manager, Otsuka Canada Pharmaceutical Inc.

"Dr. Diane McIntosh is an outstanding communicator. *This Is Depression* translates the way clinicians and researchers think about many aspects of the most disabling disorder in today's society. Her discussion of the genetic and brain disruptions in people with 'major depression' conveys complex science in plain language and provides the rationale for subsequent discussions of cognitive and other 'talk' therapies as well as the different families of medications and 'device' therapies. I recommend *This Is Depression* to anyone who needs to know more about the current understanding and treatments for depression, particularly persons with lived experience and their families. Anyone reading *This Is Depression* before going to see a mental health specialist will be an informed consumer."

SIDNEY H. KENNEDY, MD, FRCPC, FCAHS, professor of psychiatry, University of Toronto; principal investigator, Canadian Biomarker Integration Network in Depression; director, Centre for Depression and Suicide Studies, St. Michael's Hospital

"Thoroughly up to date, this book is comprehensive yet engaging and easy to read. It describes the illness from both personal and clinical perspectives and successfully weaves case vignettes and valuable summaries of complex research literatures. Although there are many books on depression, this unique volume fills a void and I recommend it to depressed people and their loved ones, those who work with or employ depressed people, and mental health professionals looking to sharpen their psychoeducational skills."

DR. MICHAEL THASE, professor of psychiatry, Perelman School of Medicine, University of Pennsylvania

"*This Is Depression* is unique in that although it's intended for people with depression (or their loved ones), it is comprehensive and head and shoulders above the rest of those slim volumes that don't delve into the details. If anyone wants to become an expert on their own illness, this is the book. Readers will be better informed than most clinicians!"

LESLIE L. CITROME, MD, MPH, clinical professor of psychiatry and behavioural sciences, New York Medical College, Valhalla, New York; and private psychiatry practitioner"

This Is Depression

This Is Depression

A Comprehensive, Compassionate Guide for Anyone Who Wants to Understand Depression

Dr. Diane McIntosh

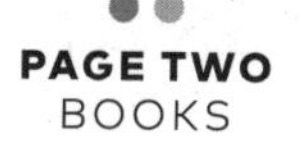

Cataloguing in publication information is available from Library and Archives Canada.

ISBN 978-1-989025-56-7 (paperback)
ISBN 978-1-989025-57-4 (ebook)

Page Two
www.pagetwo.com

Edited by Amanda Lewis
Cover design by Peter Cocking
Cover illustration by Brian Moylan
Interior design by Setareh Ashrafologhalai
Interior illustrations by Michelle Clement
Printed and bound in Canada by Friesens
Distributed in Canada by Raincoast Books
Distributed in the US and internationally by
Publishers Group West, a division of Ingram

19 20 21 22 23 5 4 3 2

drdianemcintosh.com

Some names and identifying details have been changed to protect the privacy of individuals.

This book is not intended as a substitute for the medical advice of physicians. The reader should regularly consult a physician in matters relating to their health and particularly with respect to any symptoms that may require diagnosis or medical attention.

Contents

To my mother, Barbara, and
to my brothers, Martin and Paul

Introduction
Depression affects everyone

Mental illnesses suck.
They are serious, sometimes deadly, isolating, frightening medical disorders that affect the brain and the body.

Every person, at some time in their life, will have a mental illness or love someone who has a mental illness.
Mental illnesses impact our ability to learn and work and play and love. They also cause and worsen physical illnesses, like obesity, heart disease, and **diabetes.**

Stigma regarding mental illness is still a powerful force, provoking shame, promoting isolation, and causing many sufferers to avoid seeking help.

Ignorance drives stigma. By reading this book, you are challenging that stigma head on.
As a psychiatrist, I believe it is a privilege to be invited into a patient's[1] life. Patients share beliefs and experiences that are so

1 In this book, I use the term "patient" because that's how most of the patients I have known prefer to be addressed. However, I want to acknowledge that some people prefer to be addressed as a client or a consumer.

deeply personal, private, and sometimes unsettling that they can hardly bear to think or feel them. Because of the incredible trust my patients place in me, I approach my psychiatric practice seriously and respectfully. For our mutual benefit, I also try to remain light-hearted and maintain my sense of humour—even when confronting **stigma**-laden labels.

Historically, labels like "crazy," "nuts," and "psycho" have been used cruelly to describe someone struggling with a mental illness. However, many of my patients have reclaimed those terms to describe themselves, saying things like, "What do I know? I'm nuts." The truth is you can be "crazy," "nuts," even "mentally ill," and still be smart, funny, and articulate. When you're better, you'll still be a nut. You'll still be you, only well. By discussing depression thoughtfully, with compassion, scientific evidence, and, yes, a bit of humour, I hope to destigmatize mental illness and embolden patients and their families and friends to stand up to ignorance.

In this book, I share my twenty years of psychiatric experience working with patients who have been diagnosed with depression. I also reflect on and interpret what I believe to be the highest quality research evidence regarding depression. My practice is focused on pharmacology, also known as drug therapy, because that has become my area of professional expertise. However, I am also aware of the powerful benefits of psychotherapy, also known as talk therapy, as well as other non-medication approaches, such as faith and exercise.

In these pages, I review the diagnosis of depression and the many possible treatment options. However, psychiatry is much more than simply making a diagnosis and prescribing a pill. For these reasons, I explain the causes of depression, including how life experiences, genetics, **hormones**, and many other factors can provoke its development. Depression is often associated with other mental and physical illnesses, called co-morbid conditions. **Anxiety** is a particularly common symptom associated with depression, and it's important to recognize its powerful influence on depression severity, an individual's functioning, and suicide risk.

I use patient cases throughout the book to illustrate a range of possible depression experiences. I carefully avoided basing these cases on any details I have heard from a real patient, so the names and experiences are entirely fictional. Some of my cases may seem more severe than your personal experience with depression, but that doesn't mean that your symptoms aren't worthy of a careful assessment and possible treatment. I also include some deeply personal stories from my patients who have endured serious depression and found their path to **recovery.** They agreed to share their experiences by writing their own stories because they wish to acknowledge suffering but also inspire readers and instill hope.

While my professional practice is centred on the safe and appropriate prescribing of psychiatric medications, there are other treatments that have sound scientific evidence supporting their use. I discuss *all treatment options* that should be considered when confronting depression. Likewise, because psychiatrists are just one of several professions that have expertise in treating mental illnesses, I describe the work of other mental health professionals and what should be expected from any **therapeutic relationship.**

Many terms you encounter while reading this book may be new, or perhaps used in a context that is new to you. **I have boldfaced these words and concepts in the text, and included definitions for them in a glossary at the back of the book.**

Finally, while treating symptoms is important, **recovery** from depression must include a return to full functioning in all aspects of life. In this book, I address all areas of functioning that are impacted by depression, including family, work, and social relationships.

This book is intended to be a general guide, not an academic review, and so it addresses the questions I am asked every day in my office by patients and their loved ones. I hope that by reading the questions throughout the book, you will recognize that you are not alone. Everyone has many questions, and I endeavour to offer answers and guidance, based on my **clinical experience** and scientific research. One of the most common questions I hear, after meeting a patient for the first time, is "Will I get better?" My answer is always the same, and I say it confidently because I know it is true: "If we work as a team, yes."

Most importantly, through this book I want to encourage readers who are depressed or who love someone who is depressed not to lose hope. Having met hundreds of people who saw only darkness and could not imagine a future without depression, I've learned that it can take time to find the right way; sometimes you will lose your footing or feel like you're running in circles. But there is always a path forward.

1

What is depression?

DEPRESSION IS A highly personal experience. It doesn't just cause miserable emotional and physical symptoms: it also interferes with an individual's ability to function, whether at work, school, home, or in social situations. When you're depressed, just getting out of bed can feel overwhelmingly difficult, so it's little wonder that performing at work, completing school tasks, parenting effectively, or caring for yourself and your family can be difficult or even impossible. Furthermore, depression is a barrier to socializing with friends and participating in previously enjoyed recreational activities, like exercise, hobbies, or going to the movies.

In order to be diagnosed with depression, you must experience functional impairment—the inability to perform normal daily activities that are necessary to meet one's basic needs, fulfill responsibilities, and maintain health and well-being.

How is depression diagnosed?

Sven, a forty-six-year-old professor, unexpectedly submitted a letter of resignation. His boss and colleagues were shocked. Sven had recently been promoted to full professor, he'd won numerous teaching awards, and he was expected to be in the running for department head in the coming years. Sven had always loved his job, but over the past few months, he'd lost interest in going to work or doing just about anything. He was short-tempered with his students, struggled to get his marking done on time, and found it almost impossible to pay attention when his students were presenting or during faculty meetings. He was sleeping very poorly, often lying awake for hours worrying about his health, his family, and his failures at work. As a result, he felt tired and weary all the time. While he confided to a colleague, "I guess I'm just getting old," he was actually worried he was developing **dementia.** After his wife confronted him, asking if his loss of interest in her and their family was due to an affair, Sven tearfully announced that he was certain he had Alzheimer's disease. He apologized for burdening the family and told her they'd all be better off if he were dead.

The ***Diagnostic and Statistical Manual of Mental Disorders*** (**DSM-5**) is the most recent update of the manual that doctors may use to formally diagnose depression. However, past editions of the DSM have had some serious flaws, and the **DSM-5** also has limitations. I consider it a guide that I refer to, along with other tools and my own **clinical experience**, that can help me make a psychiatric diagnosis. Many psychiatrists focus less on the formal diagnosis and more on their patient's symptoms and how those symptoms are impacting their life. It is necessary to have some framework to consider when trying to better understand depression, so below I review the **DSM-5** diagnosis by highlighting the various symptoms that might be part of an individual's experience.

What most of us think of as depression is called major depression in the **DSM-5**. To further complicate the already confusing world of mental illness, mental health professionals may also refer to major depression as a **mood disorder**, an **affective disorder**, or as unipolar depression. Unipolar depression means there is one mood "pole," which differentiates it from **bipolar disorder.** The moods often associated with **bipolar disorder** are polar opposites, including a low (depressed) mood pole and a high (manic) mood pole. For more about the difference between depression and **bipolar disorder**, see page 19.

To meet the **DSM-5** criteria for a diagnosis of major depression, one must have at least five of nine possible symptoms. One of the first two symptoms must be either a depressed mood, or a loss of interest or pleasure in usually enjoyed activities. The other seven symptoms of depression include: alterations in sleep patterns, a change in weight or appetite, restlessness or feeling slowed down, fatigue, feelings of worthlessness or excessive guilt, difficulty concentrating or indecisiveness, and recurrent thoughts of death or suicide. In the following pages, I describe these symptoms in greater depth. Keep in mind that when you consider all the possible combinations of these nine symptoms, there are close to 1,000 different ways depression may be experienced. It's no wonder so many people ask, "What is depression?" Depression can look and feel very different for every individual.

Most people think of depression only in terms of emotions: they think that to be depressed, one must feel sad or down, yet not everyone who is depressed feels that way. Some people will describe feeling "nothing" or "numb." For that reason, a diagnosis of depression might include but doesn't require feelings of sadness or a depressed mood.

A loss of pleasure or interest in usually enjoyed activities, known as **anhedonia**, is probably an even more important indicator of a depression diagnosis than a sad or depressed mood. When depressed, people who usually love to play sports, see their friends, tinker in their woodshop, or play with their children or grandchildren don't seem to care about those things any longer. In fact, nothing (or very little) seems to spark their interest or give them pleasure. If they do feel pleasure, it tends to be very short-lived. This depression-related loss of interest or pleasure can permeate all areas of life, reducing one's enjoyment of work, relationships, sexual activity, hobbies, and anything else that we find enriching or pleasurable.

Depression alters usual patterns of day-to-day life activities, like eating, sleeping, and sexual activity, which are referred to as **vegetative symptoms.** When depressed, most people will experience a reduction in their libido, but the impact on appetite and sleep can be highly variable. Some will experience a noticeable increase in their appetite, craving calorie-laden foods, resulting in significant weight gain, while others lose their appetite completely, resulting in rapid, sometimes alarming, weight loss.

Insomnia is a common sleep disturbance associated with depression. Some will struggle to get to sleep (early **insomnia**), while others can't stay asleep (middle **insomnia**) or awaken too early in the morning and are unable to get back to sleep (terminal **insomnia**). Unfortunately, some will experience all three types of **insomnia** every night and will constantly feel physically and emotionally exhausted.

Others have the opposite issue: they want to sleep 24/7, a symptom known as **hypersomnia.** People who experience **hypersomnia** struggle to function during the day because it feels almost impossible to get out of bed. Despite sleeping many more hours than they usually would, they still feel physically and mentally exhausted. Whether they are sleeping too much or not enough, most people, when they are depressed, never feel refreshed.

A substantially increased appetite and sleeping far too much are referred to as **reversed vegetative symptoms** of depression.

Depression often takes all the joy out of life, which includes stealing your mojo. Depression may greatly reduce interest in sex and the ability to perform sexually or enjoy sexual activity. For many, the loss of sexual interest is wrapped up in their general **anhedonia**, or loss of pleasure in everything they would usually enjoy. Men might experience an inability to get or maintain an erection, while both men and women might find it nearly impossible to have an orgasm. Partners often struggle with their loved one's loss of sexual interest or activity because being rejected sexually feels very personal. However, this reduced sexual desire and activity might have nothing at all to do with an intimate relationship, beyond the fact that one member of the relationship is depressed.

Because some depression treatments can cause changes in appetite, sleep disturbances, and sexual side effects, which might be confused as ongoing depression symptoms, it's important to tell your doctor if you have these symptoms before starting treatment.

Nearly every person struggling with depression will feel that their brain isn't working properly. They might describe feeling like they're in a fog, that they're unable to read even short passages and remember what they've read, or that they're unable to follow conversations or think of words or names quickly. These are **cognitive** symptoms, which may include difficulty with memory, concentration, organization and planning, and slowed thinking speed.

When older people experience depression, they may worry, and can appear to others like they are developing **dementia.** The term **pseudo-dementia** came from the sometimes-severe **cognitive** symptoms associated with depression in elderly patients. However, *people of any age* can experience severe and impairing **cognitive** symptoms, which can profoundly impact their ability to function in their usual manner.

Feeling physically slowed down, fatigued, or a profound lack of energy are very common depression symptoms. However, it's also possible to feel highly agitated or restless when depressed, even while feeling slowed down and exhausted. Agitation and restlessness may also be side effects of medications, so it's important to report these unpleasant symptoms to your doctor so they can be addressed, whether they're related to the illness or the treatment. Additionally, because restlessness and agitation are easily confused with **anxiety**, and may also co-occur with **anxiety**, it's crucial to seek professional help to determine the correct diagnosis.

Feelings of worthlessness or excessive or inappropriate guilt are depression symptoms that loved ones struggle to understand. They wonder how someone who is so well loved can possibly feel unlovable, and how someone who means the world to those who love them can feel unworthy. Unfortunately, that's the reality of depression: it hijacks your brain and tells you lies. The depressed brain thinks, *I'm useless and worthless, and life is hopeless and meaningless.* Truly depressed people believe these thoughts and sometimes act on them.

An important note on suicide

Part of understanding depression is knowing the risks and impacts, and there is no getting around the fact that *depression can carry the risk of suicide*. It's very common for people who are depressed to think about or have fleeting thoughts of suicide as a possible escape from emotional pain. Those with passive **suicidal ideation** wish to die but do not have a specific plan. **Active suicidal ideation** means there is a wish to die as well as a plan to act on that wish. I discuss suicide in greater depth in chapter 16.

If you are having suicidal thoughts, please ask a professional for help. If you don't receive the help you need, please ask someone else. Likewise, urging your loved one to seek help from a professional (e.g., family doctor, psychologist, psychiatrist) and ensuring they attend, or accompanying them to, that appointment is an essential first step. Suicide helplines offer an immediate empathic ear for someone who is suffering. They are also equipped to offer options for urgent community support. Suicide helpline numbers for each province and territory are listed at the end of the book in appendix 1.

What if my symptoms of depression are not captured in the DSM?

One notable limitation of the DSM is its failure to include some other potentially serious symptoms that are commonly associated with depression. Their absence from the depression diagnosis has been hotly debated and, in the case of **anxiety** symptoms particularly, has resulted in the evolution of the diagnosis. As our understanding of psychiatric illnesses grows, mostly thanks to better quality research studies, diagnostic manuals such as the **DSM-5** should become more effective tools, enhancing our ability to make correct diagnoses.

Most people suffering from depression will experience some degree of **anxiety**, which usually means they are worrying excessively about everyday things (e.g., health, work, finances). Additionally, **anxiety** may include constantly feeling like something terrible is about to happen, ruminating about negative thoughts, feeling a loss of control, difficulty concentrating because of focusing on worries, or feeling restless, tense, keyed up, or on edge—all without a clear cause. Most importantly, **anxiety** is an awful experience and dramatically increases the risk of suicide. It's also a common reason for self-medication with alcohol or illicit drugs, which further worsens both the depression and the **anxiety**. (More on the interplay of depression and drugs/alcohol in chapter 5.)

Many people struggling with depression will also experience physical (also called **somatic**) symptoms, such as pain, nausea or diarrhea, dizziness, and an array of other symptoms. For many people, depression hurts. It makes existing pain worse but may also provoke the onset of pain that has no obvious medical cause. **Somatic symptoms** can range from generalized aches and pains to headaches, muscle aches, and tension that can be localized anywhere in the body. **Somatic symptoms** can be especially worrying for someone who is already experiencing **anxiety**, because the mind-body connection is not often emphasized or explained when depression is diagnosed and treated. You can read more about **anxiety** and **somatic symptoms** associated with depression in chapter 5.

Are there different kinds of depression?

The **DSM-5** includes several different *specifiers of depression*, which are groups of depression symptoms that tend to occur together. A few of the more common depression specifiers include: **atypical features, melancholic features, seasonal pattern, psychotic features, peripartum** (pregnancy-related) onset, and **anxious distress.** The **anxious distress specifier** was added to the **DSM-5** to encourage assessors to carefully consider and grade the severity of **anxiety** symptoms when diagnosing depression (for a full discussion of anxious distress, see chapter 5).

Atypical depression features

> Megan first recalled feeling depressed when she was fifteen or sixteen, but she's now twenty-five and she's depressed again. Thinking back, she wonders if she's ever been fully well since her teen years. When she's really feeling down, she tends to eat much more than usual, and she's ashamed to admit she's gained ten pounds over the past few months since she started feeling depressed. She also wants to sleep all the time, preferring staying in bed to almost anything else. She usually sleeps until noon or later, eats all evening, and then sleeps another twelve hours. She's struggling to get to work because she's so tired, emotionally and physically. She feels like she's carrying around a 100-pound weight all day, and her legs feel like lead. Megan and her boyfriend are constantly arguing, because she feels he's short-tempered with her and she's often in tears when they're together. However, recently he surprised her with a lovely bouquet of flowers and they spent a happy, carefree day together. Unfortunately, by the next morning Megan felt very depressed again.

Contrary to what the name suggests, **atypical depression features** are not at all **atypical.** In fact, they're generally considered the most common and the most hereditary group of depression symptoms (for more on the hereditary aspects of depression, see chapter 2). **Atypical** depression tends to start earlier in life, often in the teen years, and is two to three times more common in women than in men. The symptoms can become **chronic** and persistent, especially for those who have had many previous episodes of depression. **Atypical** symptoms are also commonly associated with **bipolar depression.**

Symptoms of an **atypical** depression are like any depression, with respect to sadness or loss of interest, but the mood tends to be reactive. A reactive mood might brighten when something happy or positive happens, but the depressed mood tends to return quickly, soon after the positive event has passed. **Atypical** depression is commonly associated with rejection sensitivity, which means feeling more sensitive to slights and quicker to jump to negative conclusions. **Reversed vegetative symptoms** are also common (e.g., eating too much, with associated weight gain, and sleeping much more than usual without feeling rested). Additionally, people struggling with **atypical** depression tend to feel exhausted and physically weighed down, like their arms and legs are filled with lead.

So why does the DSM refer to this common type of depression as "**atypical**"? Because many of the symptoms are different from, and sometimes the opposite of, what were classically considered "typical" depression symptoms. Those typical depression symptoms are known collectively as **melancholic depression** features.

Melancholic depression features

Jeffrey, seventy-two, had a depression twenty years ago, after his father died unexpectedly, but he sought treatment and recovered. He was well until six months ago and he can't figure out why he's depressed again, because nothing happened to provoke his symptoms. Jeffrey's wife says he is no longer seeing friends and he doesn't seem to care when his beloved grandchildren come over for a visit, which was usually the highlight of his week. In fact, nothing seems to give him any pleasure, even temporarily. To her, he seems agitated but at the same time desperately sad. Jeffrey's worst time of day is in the morning, when he awakens at four o'clock and can't get back to sleep. His wife tells their doctor, "He seems to start the day with a sense of dread. He's also stopped eating and has lost at least twenty pounds. He speaks and moves so slowly now. It's like he's become an old man, almost overnight. He doesn't say much anymore, and when he does, it's mostly to apologize for past mistakes, which I can't even remember."

In contrast to **atypical** depression, **melancholic depression** is more common in older people, tends to be highly impairing, and is the depression type most associated with **psychotic** symptoms. Severe **anhedonia**, or a complete lack of pleasure from nearly every activity that would normally be pleasurable, is typical of **melancholic depression**. Furthermore, the depressed mood does not usually improve, even briefly, when something positive happens. Excessive and inappropriate guilt is a common feature, along with **vegetative symptoms**, such as severe **insomnia**, especially early morning awakening, and loss of appetite, often resulting in weight loss.

Seasonal depression pattern features

Lilly, twenty-six, visited her family doctor in late September because she was worried that her depression was returning. For the past three years, Lilly recalled feeling increasingly withdrawn and anxious "just as the leaves are changing." By Halloween, she felt very depressed and found it nearly impossible to get going in the morning. As a result of her symptoms, she had lost a job and had to drop university courses. She told her doctor, "I can't take another winter like last year. I felt like a groundhog, praying

I would see my shadow, which would mean it was nearly spring." Two years ago, she took a trip to Mexico in late March and felt almost instantly better. When she returned, the days were longer and brighter, and her mood was no longer depressed.

Seasonal depression, previously referred to as seasonal **affective disorder**, refers to recurrent depression episodes that reliably occur and fully resolve at a particular time of the year, usually beginning in the fall or winter and resolving in the spring or summer. The **DSM-5** diagnosis requires that the pattern must be established over two previous years and no non-**seasonal depressions** can have occurred during that same two-year period.

A **seasonal depression** pattern is often associated with **atypical depression features** and is more likely to occur in young women. Seasonality is also common in **bipolar depression.** Because a seasonal pattern of depression is thought to be associated with a lack of light, there is a clear geographical association: it occurs far less often in individuals living in warm, sunny climates.

Research over the last many years has confirmed what those who live with and those who treat severe depression have always known: dark winter months are difficult for just about anyone who has a history of depression. Fortunately, the same treatment used for **seasonal depression** is also helpful for some who experience non-**seasonal depression.** You can read more about **light therapy**, a common treatment for seasonal symptoms, in chapter 13.

Psychotic depression features

Phillip, fifty-two, had been depressed before, but this time his depression started with a belief that his stomach was rotting and needed to be removed. He asked his family doctor to urgently refer him to a surgeon for what he was convinced would be an emergency surgery. When his doctor asked why he was so sure he had a rotting stomach, he responded, "It's because my mother is still angry that I missed her funeral. I should have made it home on time, and I've always felt guilty. I guess it's payback time." Eventually, Phillip began to smell something awful, which he believed was his stomach rotting within him.

Grace, sixty-seven, initially believed her fatigue, poor sleep, and **anxiety** were being caused by the pigeons perching outside her apartment window. Over time, her fears intensified, and she became convinced that the pigeons were carrying a nerve agent and were being employed by Russia to monitor her activities. As a result, she kept her blinds closed and her lights off. She eventually began to hear a voice repeatedly saying, "We're sick now. The Russians sent a nerve agent. We don't tell anyone."

While **psychotic** symptoms are the hallmark of **schizophrenia** or a bipolar manic episode, they may also be associated with severe depression. **Delusions** and **hallucinations** are the most common **psychotic** symptoms. **Delusions** are strongly held false beliefs, like Phillip's belief that his stomach is rotting or Grace's belief that she is being monitored by pigeons. **Hallucinations** are false sensory experiences that can be auditory (e.g., Grace hearing a voice talking about her), olfactory (e.g., the unpleasant odor that only Phillip can smell), or visual (although visual **hallucinations** are an uncommon symptom of **psychotic** depression).

The **delusions** or **hallucinations** associated with depression may be mood-congruent, which means they reflect the sadness and negativity associated with depression. Phillip's belief that his stomach is rotting and his guilt about his mother's death are in keeping with feeling depressed. However, Grace's belief that she is being monitored by Russia-controlled pigeons is mood-incongruent, because her delusion would be considered bizarre, unless she was an ex-KGB operative who defected.

As a point of clarity, it's possible that several specifiers could apply for a single depressive episode. For instance, Philip might have a major depression, with **melancholic** and **psychotic** features.

Peripartum onset features

If depression begins during pregnancy or within four weeks following delivery, the **DSM-5** specifier with **peripartum** onset is used. You'll find more information regarding depression during and after pregnancy in chapter 6, and in chapter 15, I discuss the treatment of pregnancy-related depression.

DSM-5 diagnostic criteria for major depressive episode

To meet the **DSM-5** criteria for major depressive disorder, the following features must be present:

- ☐ Symptoms must be present during the same two-week period.
- ☐ The individual must be experiencing a change from their usual functioning.
- ☐ At least one symptom is either (1) depressed mood or (2) loss of interest or pleasure.

Five or more of the following nine symptoms:

- ☐ 1. Depressed mood most of the day, nearly every day. Patient may report feeling sad, empty, or hopeless or others observe symptoms (e.g., tearfulness). Children and adolescents may have an irritable mood.
- ☐ 2. Markedly diminished interest or pleasure in all, or almost all, activities most of the day, nearly every day.
- ☐ 3. Significant weight loss when not dieting, or weight gain, or decrease or increase in appetite nearly every day.
- ☐ 4. **Insomnia** or sleeping too much nearly every day.
- ☐ 5. Restlessness or feeling slowed down nearly every day, that is observable by others and not merely subjective feelings.
- ☐ 6. Fatigue or loss of energy nearly every day.
- ☐ 7. Feelings of worthlessness or excessive or inappropriate guilt nearly every day. Not merely guilt about being sick.

- [ ] 8. Diminished ability to think or concentrate, or indecisiveness, nearly every day.
- [ ] 9. Recurrent thoughts of death (not just fear of dying), recurrent **suicidal ideation** without a specific plan, or a suicide attempt or a specific plan for committing suicide.
- [ ] The symptoms cause significant distress or impairment in social, occupational, or other important areas of functioning.
- [ ] The episode is not attributable to the effects of a substance (illicit drugs or alcohol) or related to another medical condition.

Adapted from American Psychiatric Association: Diagnostic and Statistical Manual of Mental Disorders, Fifth Edition. *Arlington: VA, American Psychiatric Association, 2013.*

What is bipolar depression?

Adaeze, a twenty-one-year-old university student, went to a walk-in clinic seeking help for "nonstop worry." She told the doctor, "I've been a worrywart for as long as I can remember, but now it's much worse. I'm having **panic attacks** almost every day. When I was in high school, I started to have what I called my 'crash and burn' moods. I'd feel fine and then suddenly I'd feel like dying. These down times used to last a few days, but now they seem to be more severe, lasting weeks at a time. When I'm really down I just want to sleep, but even though I'm sleeping twelve hours or more every night, I never feel rested. I'm missing classes a few times every week because it's so hard to get out of bed. I've also gained twenty pounds, because it seems all I want to do at night is eat. I'm also really irritable with everyone, especially my boyfriend and my mom. I'm sure my boyfriend is going to dump me, because I've gotten so angry, I've thrown things at him. Thankfully, my mom gets it. She told me she was just like me when she was younger, but now she's just depressed and worried all the time."

Major depression is often referred to as a **mood disorder**, because one of its defining symptoms is a depressed mood. It is also called unipolar depression: "unipolar" literally means "one pole" and refers to the low or depressed mood.

Bipolar disorder is also considered a **mood disorder** but is defined by the presence of two "polar opposite" mood types. A diagnosis of **bipolar disorder** requires an elevated mood episode (a high pole known as mania or hypomania, depending on the severity) and often a low pole, which is **bipolar depression.**

While unipolar and **bipolar depression** can look to an observer and feel to the sufferer like the same disorder, they are truly distinct in terms of their causes, their appropriate treatments, and their impact on an individual's physical and mental well-being.

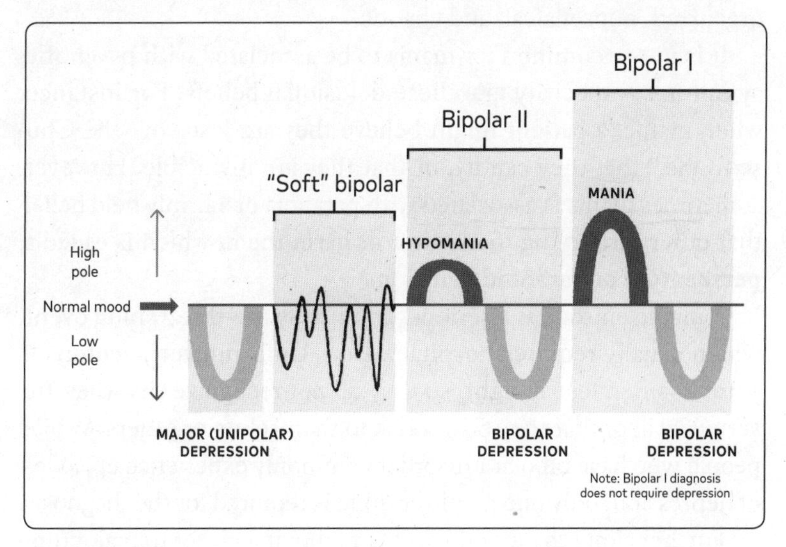

Bipolar disorder is an umbrella term, which includes several unique bipolar subtypes: bipolar I disorder, bipolar II disorder, and what is sometimes called "soft" bipolar (known in the **DSM-5** as "other specified" and "unspecified" **bipolar disorder**).

I tend to think of major depression and **bipolar disorder** as existing on opposite ends of a **mood disorder** spectrum, with major depression at one end and bipolar I disorder at the other. In between are bipolar II and other **mood disorders** that are not quite unipolar and not quite bipolar but are real, serious disorders that are challenging to diagnose. "Soft" **bipolar disorder** is very often undiagnosed or misdiagnosed, which can result in negative long-term consequences.

A **DSM-5** diagnosis of bipolar I disorder requires that a patient has had a manic episode, which is an elevated, high, or irritable mood, agitation, and usually a frenzied and chaotic level of activity. Mania is associated with an extremely high level of excitement or energy, an exaggerated sense of self-worth or self-esteem, little or no need for sleep, racing thoughts, much more social activity, and high-risk behaviours, such as uncharacteristic drug use, spending too much money, or inappropriate or unsafe sexual activity. However, while the person who is manic often views their activities or output as brilliant and perfect, others usually regard them as disorganized, nonsensical, and chaotic.

It is not uncommon for mania to be associated with **psychotic** symptoms, especially grandiose delusional beliefs. For instance, when manic, a patient might believe they are Jesus or "the Chosen One," that they can fly, or that they are invincible. However, sometimes mania is associated with paranoia or a firmly held belief that others are trying to monitor or harm them, which is called a **persecutory or paranoid delusion.**

A manic episode is a serious, potentially life-threatening event, which usually requires hospitalization. Unfortunately, acutely ill patients often lose **insight**, so they do not recognize that they are seriously ill or that they pose a risk to themselves or others. While people who have bipolar I disorder commonly experience episodes of depression, only one manic episode is required for the diagnosis.

Further along the mood spectrum, moving closer to major (unipolar) depression, is bipolar II disorder. Patients diagnosed with bipolar II disorder have had episodes of hypomania, which are like manic episodes but less severe. Hypomania is not associated with **psychosis** and rarely requires hospitalization. In fact, when hypomanic, most people feel smarter, sexier, more creative, more daring, less anxious, and generally more fun-loving, so they're certainly not going to seek out medical assistance to manage their symptoms. They think, *What symptoms? I feel like a million bucks!*

Unlike the bipolar I diagnosis, a bipolar II diagnosis requires a history of depression. Patients with bipolar II spend more than half of their life symptomatic, and most illness episodes are depressed. It's important to remember that bipolar I or II disorder cannot be diagnosed without a current or previous manic or hypomanic episode. However, because an elevated mood is associated with feelings of invincibility, brilliance, sexiness, and charm, folks don't tend to visit with their doctor when they're high.

What many of us call "soft bipolar" is captured in the **DSM-5** under the names "other specified" and "unspecified" bipolar. Other specified refers to those who have met the full **DSM-5** criteria for depression and have met all the criteria for a hypomanic episode, except for the duration. Hypomania must last four days to meet the full criteria. Alternatively, the diagnosis "other specified" also captures those who meet the full criteria for hypomania, but have not met the full depression criteria or have not had a depression episode.

Unspecified bipolar may be used to describe the symptoms of patients who do not meet the full **DSM-5** diagnostic criteria for a bipolar diagnosis, and there is not enough information available to be certain of the correct diagnosis. I use the term to ensure that my patient and their referring doctor understand that I think bipolar might be the correct diagnosis, but I am not certain. Most importantly, I want to be sure all involved are aware of the risks of missing the diagnosis.

Cross-sectionally, depression looks like depression. Without seeing or being told of a manic or hypomanic episode, doctors will often diagnose unipolar depression when faced with bipolar depression.

There are some important indicators that can help to determine when a depression might be associated with **bipolar disorder.** Adaeze has a typical story of likely **bipolar disorder:** she had anxiety symptoms from a very early age, which became progressively worse into her teens and twenties, and her mood symptoms started in her teen years. The first episode of unipolar depression more commonly occurs later in life, often not until age thirty or later. Elevated mood symptoms (mania and hypomania) might not occur until the late teens or early to mid-twenties. This is challenging diagnostically, because Adaeze might not have had an episode of elevated mood, and the diagnosis of bipolar I and II require mood elevation. Depression associated with **bipolar disorder** often has **atypical** features, and Adaeze described sleeping too much, increased appetite, and weight gain. However, **bipolar depression** may also present with **melancholic** features and the usual **vegetative symptoms**, such as **insomnia** and loss of appetite.

Bipolar depression is commonly misdiagnosed as major depression, due to the substantial overlap between the two disorders. However, because they are distinct and unique illnesses, particularly related to how they should be safely and appropriately treated, misdiagnosis can have devastating consequences. One of the most critical reasons that it is essential to correctly differentiate unipolar and **bipolar depression** is because antidepressant medications prescribed to a patient with **bipolar depression** can provoke a manic or hypomanic episode, which carry serious health and safety risks.

Factors that suggest a depression is actually a bipolar depression

- Family history of **bipolar disorder**
- Onset of mood symptoms, especially depression, in teen years (usually before the age of twenty-five)
- Frequent, short episodes of depression (early in the illness, depressive episodes tend to start abruptly, they may last just a day or a few days, and then rapidly resolve), especially during the teens and twenties
- Multiple co-occurring **anxiety disorders**
- A previous diagnosis of **attention deficit hyperactivity disorder (ADHD)**
- **Atypical depression features**
- Antidepressant intolerance, or mania or hypomania provoked by antidepressants

How common is depression?

Very. An estimated 300 million people are affected by depression worldwide. In 2011, the World Mental Health Survey Initiative gathered demographic data from eighteen countries and found that the average lifetime **prevalence** of depression ranged from 11 to 15 percent. This means that up to 15 percent of people will, at some time in their life, experience a depressive episode. The twelve-month **prevalence** of depression, which is the number of people likely to have a depression in a year, was nearly 6 percent.

The Canadian Community Health Survey–Mental Health (CCHS–MH), completed in 2012, found the estimated lifetime **prevalence** of depression was 11.3 percent and the estimated past-year depression **prevalence** was 4.7 percent. In 2016, the US National Survey on Drug Use and Health (NSDUH) found that an estimated 16.2 million adults had at least one depressive episode in the previous year, representing 6.7 percent of all US adults. There are sex differences in depression **prevalence** as well: a US study found the lifetime risk of depression is 21 percent in females and 13 percent in males (read more about the differences in depression risk between the sexes in chapter 6).

Minority groups, especially those who face the greatest burden of discrimination, appear to be more vulnerable to depression than members of the dominant group in a given population. Unfortunately, there is very little research in the area of mental illness among minority groups, but to learn more, see chapter 2.

What is the economic cost of depression?

The World Health Organization uses various measures to determine the overall health of a population. Years of Life Lost (YLL) due to premature death caused by an illness is added to Years Lost Due to Disability (YLD), for people living with an illness or its consequences, to calculate the Disability Adjusted Life Years (DALYs). One DALY can be thought of as one lost year of "healthy" life.

DALYs for all the diseases in a population can be added together to determine the overall burden of disease.

A country's DALYs measure the gap between the current health of a population and the ideal health situation if every person were to live to an advanced age, free of disease and disability.

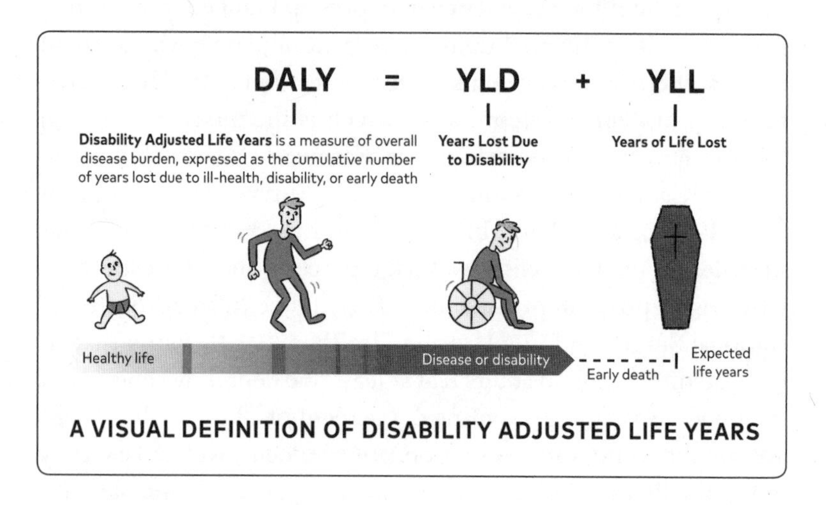

A VISUAL DEFINITION OF DISABILITY ADJUSTED LIFE YEARS

YLDs and DALYs capture the loss of functioning due to an illness (e.g., the ability to earn a living, support yourself and your family, and contribute financially to society), considering an individual's age. If a thirty-year-old is depressed and can't work, their inability to contribute to society is considered costlier than a depressed seventy-year-old who might not be working.

Depression is a crucial contributor of disease burden in developed and developing countries. It is the leading cause of YLDs in fifty-six countries, the second-leading cause in fifty-six countries, and the third in thirty-four countries. Remarkably, researchers have suggested that if depression treatments were widely available and appropriately used, *up to half* of all YLDs could be averted in some countries.

With so many people suffering from depression every year, it's little wonder that the functional decline associated with depression, whether at work, home, or school, costs the economy billions of dollars annually. In the United States alone, the economic burden of depression was estimated to be $83.1 billion in 2000. By 2010, the economic burden increased by 21.5 percent (from $173.2 billion to $210.5 billion, using inflation-adjusted dollars). However, the reasons underlying those costs were unchanged: 45 percent were direct costs (including medical services and prescription drug costs), 5 percent were suicide-related costs (e.g., loss of human capital), and 50 percent were workplace-related costs.

The cost of depression in the workplace can be attributed to absenteeism and **presenteeism. Presenteeism**, which means being at work but not being able to complete your tasks appropriately or in a timely manner, is vastly more common than absenteeism and is estimated to be six times costlier to world economies than being completely absent from work.

Chapter summary

- Depression is a common, serious, sometimes life-threating mental illness.
- The **DSM-5** is a guide to help a healthcare professional make an appropriate diagnosis.
- A depression diagnosis includes a depressed mood and/or **anhedonia** (loss of pleasure or interest in usually enjoyed activities) and an array of other symptoms. Considering all the possible combinations of the nine depression symptoms, there are close to 1,000 different ways depression may be experienced.
- Depression's economic impact is staggering because it causes impairment in social, occupational, and other important areas of functioning.

Recognizing yourself or someone you love in the words and stories describing the depression diagnosis is the first step towards wellness.

A real patient's story

WHEN I AM depressed, my depression is not simply a feeling of sadness or a belief that I am inadequate. In my mind, the negative thoughts and opinions are established facts. I do not "feel" sad in the normal sense of the word. Sadness is what we feel briefly when a good friend moves to a new city or our favourite sports team loses the big game. Similarly, I do not "feel" inadequate in the way most people think of it. Inadequacy is what we feel briefly when we don't achieve a strongly desired goal.

To understand my experience, consider gravity. Gravity is always present even when we are not thinking about it. It was present in the past, it is present now, and it will be present in the future. Everyone agrees that gravity exists and that it will never change. I don't "feel" that gravity exists. I know that it exists and that everyone else knows that it exists. You can't change another person's mind about gravity by saying that it doesn't exist. There is no debate about gravity. Gravity is an established fact.

My experience of depression is the same as my experience of gravity. I don't "feel" that I am worthless. I know that I am worthless. I know that I am a failure and always will be. I know that I am fundamentally and irreparably flawed. I know that people don't want me around. They never did and never will. I know that nobody likes me. Everyone wants me to go away forever. These are not feelings. They are established facts. They are not up for debate. You can't change my mind with logic. When I am depressed, I know that my negative thoughts are true—they were always true, and they always will be.

2

What causes depression?

WHAT CAUSES DEPRESSION? It seems like such a simple question; unfortunately, the answer is complicated because the causes are still not completely known or fully understood.

All mental illnesses have bio-psycho-social origins. "Bio" refers to the biological aspects of these illnesses, such as genetics, **hormones**, and **neurotransmitters.** "Psycho" stands for psychological and can include our personality style or temperament, our innate resilience or vulnerability to **stress**, and our coping style, which refers to our ability to use **cognitive** or emotional skills to manage **stress.** "Social" refers to life circumstances that impact our feelings and functioning, like financial hardship, relationship issues, or legal difficulties.

Note that while I describe some depression risk factors in a particular category, such as including childhood maltreatment as a social risk factor, we know that abuse can provoke serious biological changes and impact an individual's psychological functioning. The three categories I use to describe risk factors overlap and interact extensively.

What are the biological risk factors for depression?

Genetics

Mental illnesses often run in families. Children born into families with a history of mental illnesses that are highly influenced by genetics, like **bipolar disorder**, ADHD, and **schizophrenia**, may have a vulnerability to the illness encoded in their DNA, yet no mental illness is 100 percent genetic. For example, if one identical twin has **schizophrenia**, the other twin has only a 50 percent risk of also developing the disorder, despite having identical DNA.

Scientific research has shown us that depression is influenced to some degree by genetics with twin, family, and adoption studies indicating greater than 40 percent **heritability**. Studies have demonstrated strong evidence for a higher **heritability** risk of depression in women than in men, including a 2018 study that found the **heritability** of depression was 41 percent for men and 49 percent for women.

Those who have an inherited risk for depression:

- are more likely to have had multiple episodes of depression,
- likely had their first depression at a younger age,
- are more likely to have been prescribed antidepressants or another treatment, and
- often have severe anxiety.

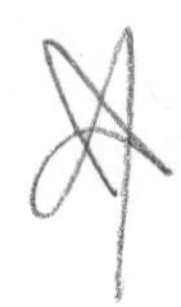

It's important to understand that if the **heritability** of depression is, for example, 45 percent, that does not mean that 45 percent of an individual's depression is due to their **genes** and 55 percent is due to other factors. Nor does it mean that 45 percent of people who have depression are depressed because of their **genes**. This is what **heritability** isn't; what **heritability** is... is complicated!

According to *Merriam-Webster*, **heritability** is the proportion of observed variation in a particular trait (e.g., eye colour, IQ) in a particular population that can be attributed to inherited genetic factors as opposed to environmental factors. Breaking that down into more understandable bits, eye colour varies a great deal in some populations, for instance, among Canadians who might have various shades of blue, green, hazel, or brown eyes. The variation of eye colour in the Canadian population is almost entirely influenced by inherited genetic factors, with little or no influence from environmental factors, such as infectious illnesses, poverty, diet, or other lifestyle factors.

A trait like IQ is also highly variable in any population, and it is also influenced by genetics and environment. Because eye colour is more influenced by genetics than a trait like IQ, which is more susceptible to environmental influences, we say that eye colour is more heritable than IQ. Even the most heritable traits can still be susceptible to environmental influences.

Importantly, the **heritability** of an illness has nothing to do with whether, or to what extent, it is caused by genetics in a particular individual. For instance, **bipolar disorder** is more heritable than major depression, but both disorders are influenced by one's genetics *and* their environment. A person who develops **bipolar disorder** was vulnerable due to their genetics and their environment, and it's impossible to know which was more influential. This is helpful to understand if you have a serious mental illness and you're worried that you might pass the illness on to your children.

Heritability is not an absolute, and mental illnesses are more likely to be influenced by environmental factors than genetics. Unfortunately, many of those environmental factors are not fully understood or even known for certain. For instance, there is high-quality, well-replicated research evidence demonstrating that early (by age fifteen), frequent use of high-potency cannabis can play a role in the onset of **schizophrenia**. However, researchers cannot definitively state, "Cannabis causes **schizophrenia**." It has a role to play in the onset of **schizophrenia** for some individuals, but many cannabis smokers don't develop **schizophrenia**, and many people who develop **schizophrenia** have never smoked cannabis. It is likely that for some vulnerable individuals, cannabis interacts with a genetic vulnerability, resulting in the onset of **schizophrenia**. Perhaps the illness would have occurred anyway, but the evidence suggests it begins many years earlier in association with cannabis use.

Researchers haven't yet figured out precisely which **genes** are responsible for mental illnesses, but many **candidate genes** have been identified. One **gene** that has been associated with an increased risk of depression is the **gene** for the **serotonin transporter**, which has the memorable name SLC6A4. **Serotonin** is a **neurotransmitter** with many functions, but we know it is very important in the development and maintenance of depression (see **neurotransmitters** below). Some individuals carry a variation of the **gene**—called a **gene polymorphism**—that produces the **serotonin transporter.** This variation causes a reduction in the amount of **serotonin** available in the brain. Those with two short variations of the **serotonin transporter gene** (called short/short) have higher rates of **anxiety** and depression.

However, research showing an association between this **gene** and depression is mixed. A 2003 study demonstrated that stressful life events in association with the presence of the short/short variation of the **serotonin transporter gene** were associated with depression. This might explain why it's difficult to consistently demonstrate that the short/short **polymorphism** is an important risk factor for depression. Without a major stressful life event, the **gene** might remain silent, but when a person who has the short/short **gene** is under severe **stress**, the **gene** exerts itself and reduces available **serotonin**, provoking the onset of depression. Interestingly, the risk of depression associated with the **serotonin transporter gene** might be more significant for women than for men.

Neurotransmitters

Our brains are a tangle of billions of brain cells called **neurons**, which send messages to one another at lightning speed. **Neurons** that work together function much like an electrical wire, sending messages around the brain and body that allow us to breathe, walk, and do everything we do as living beings. In fact, **neurons** send messages around the brain in part through actual electrical impulses. However, **neurons** must also rely on chemical messengers, called **neurotransmitters**, to keep the information moving.

Messages are sent within a **neuron** by an electrical impulse, which travels from one end of the cell to the other, but once the impulse reaches the furthest point, the electricity can't just jump to the closest **neuron** and keep moving. There's a gap between the **neurons** called the synaptic cleft. To pass the message on to the next **neuron**, the electrical impulse causes **neurotransmitters** to be released from the end of the first **neuron**. The **neurotransmitters** then move across the synaptic cleft and attach to receptors on the next **neuron**.

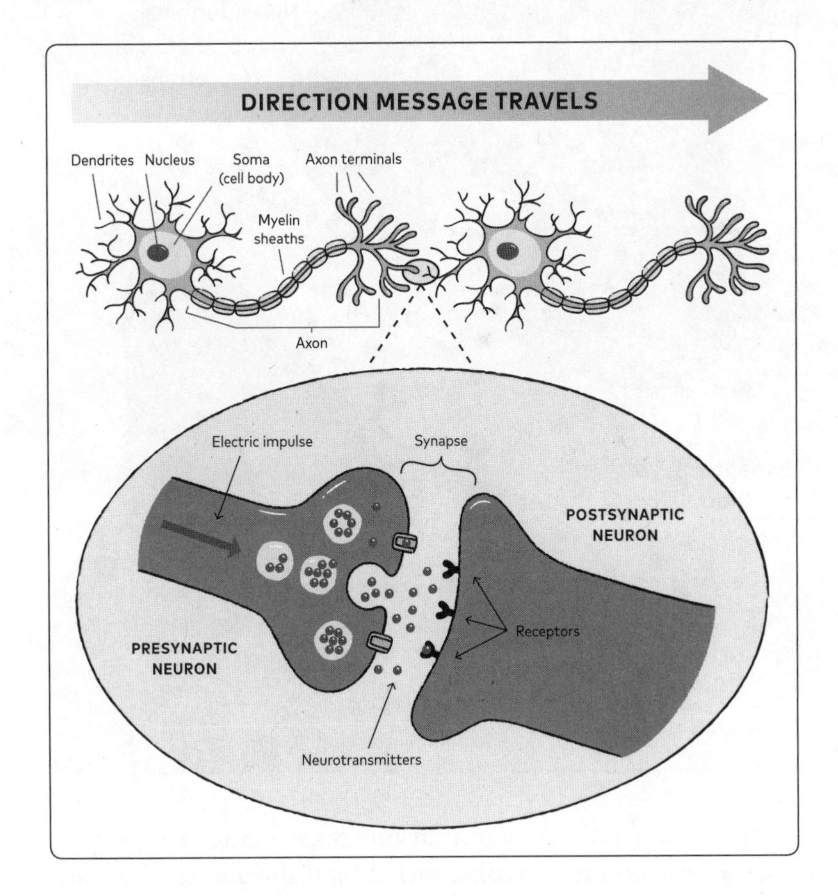

When a **neurotransmitter** attaches to its receptor, it might pass on the message, by provoking another electrical impulse (an excitatory **neurotransmitter**) or terminate the message (an inhibitory **neurotransmitter**). **Neurotransmitters** are necessary for our most basic bodily functions, like breathing, blood pressure, and heart rate, as well as modulating our sleep, appetite, mood, pleasure, and how our brains and bodies react to stressful or frightening events.

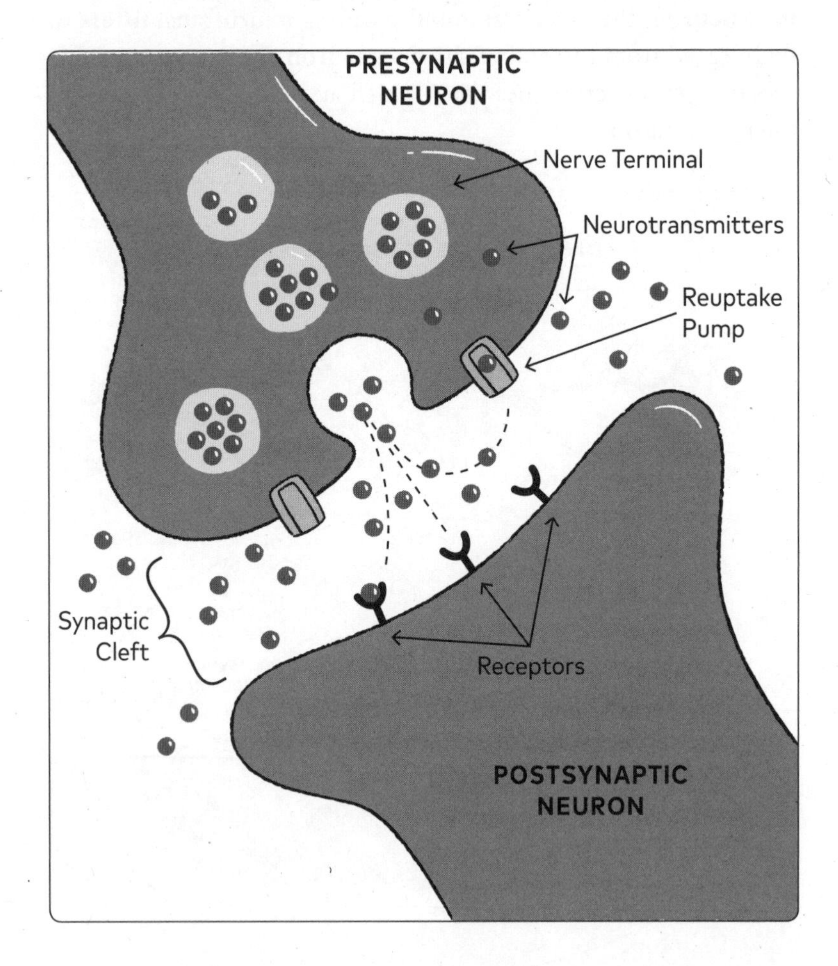

The most important **neurotransmitters** associated with depression are **serotonin**, **norepinephrine**, and **dopamine**. They are also the target of nearly every antidepressant medication. **Glutamate** and GABA are also important depression **neurotransmitters**.

There are medications currently available that target **glutamate** and GABA, but they are also the focus of new drug development, as researchers better understand their importance in the development and severity of depression.

We know that depression is associated with abnormal levels of various **neurotransmitters**, and the amount of these **neurotransmitters** can be altered by various factors, including genetics (as with the **serotonin transporter gene** mentioned earlier), **stress**, diet, and physical activity.

Hormones

Compared to men, women are twice as likely to develop depression, but the differences in depression risk between the sexes isn't apparent until **puberty**. Some research has suggested that girls who enter **puberty** at a younger age might be at greater lifetime risk for depression. However, it's likely that just experiencing **puberty** (which we all endure) might be all that is required to increase a woman's risk, irrespective of age. Women's heightened risk of depression compared to men has been attributed to **estrogen**, because **estrogen** levels increase dramatically at **puberty** and persist until **menopause**. However, despite the equally dramatic drop in **estrogen** that occurs at **menopause**, women's increased risk of depression persists into old age.

Estrogen, likely in association with **serotonin** and **stress hormones** like **cortisol**, affects brain areas that process emotions. While it is considered a sex **hormone, estrogen** has diverse effects that are not generally considered sexy! It protects brain cells and stimulates their growth, and it further promotes brain health by impacting learning, memory, movement, and pain perception. **Estrogen** is also a natural antioxidant and has analgesic (pain-relieving) properties.

Scientific research has clearly demonstrated that the direct effects of **estrogen** on critical brain areas may heighten the risk of depression. However, the indirect effects of the **hormone** might constitute an even greater depression risk. The **estrogen** increase associated with **puberty** dramatically changes a girl's body and behaviour. Girls tend to harshly evaluate themselves and their developing bodies, and this, along with the likelihood of being exposed to adversity at home, school, and within their communities as they make their way through their teen years, **might have a more profound effect on a woman's risk of depression than the direct brain effects of estrogen.** While I have included **hormones** in the "bio" section, it's important to remember that, as described above regarding **estrogen**, the effects of **hormones** may constitute a psycho-social risk for depression as well. For more about sex differences and depression, see chapter 6.

What are the psychological risk factors for depression?

There are many theories regarding our temperament and how our personality develops. Because this book is meant to be a general guide and not an exhaustive academic review, I will focus on what I feel is a helpful way to understand these concepts, especially as they relate to the development and maintenance of depression.

Children are born with innate or baked-in characteristics, known as temperament, which is biologically or genetically determined and independent of learning, values, or life experience. Because temperament reflects our unique personal level of intensity or excitability, it strongly influences how we interact with others and react emotionally to the world around us. Temperament is apparent during infancy, so parents often get a sense of their child's temperament as soon as their bundle of joy pops out of the womb, and those same characteristics remain virtually unchanged throughout life.

There are three classic infant temperaments described in the psychological literature: *difficult*, *easy*, and *slow to warm up*. Difficult babies are fussier, more irritable, and harder to settle, especially when they have a need, such as when they're hungry. Easy babies are thought of as happy and easy-going. They tend to be more relaxed, calmer, and far more flexible with schedules. Finally, some babies are slow to warm up and dislike change or new situations, which can make them fussy, irritable, or unsettled. However, after some time in the new environment, slow to warm up babies usually become more comfortable and, as a result, more easy-going.

Personality is influenced by, but distinctive from, temperament. Unlike temperament, which is hard-wired, one's personality develops over many years and is greatly influenced by our environment. Factors that shape our personality include how we are parented, the education we receive, the culture we grow up in, and other life experiences. Temperament is also an important factor in personality development, which means that our personality is influenced by genetics, as well as being shaped by the world we live in. Our personality plays an essential role in our ability to develop, maintain, reflect upon, and participate in relationships, and healthy relationships are critical for mental and physical wellness.

There has been a great deal of research over many decades exploring how our personality characteristics might influence the development of depression, whether by heightening our risk or by providing protection. As you read about the following personality traits, it's important to think of each as a spectrum of characteristics. Most of us are not at the highest or lowest end of any of these traits but fall somewhere on the spectrum.

Those on the higher end of the *openness to new experiences* personality spectrum are more creative, curious, intense, and seek new challenges and opportunities. Those at the lower end are more cautious, logical, strict, assertive, and inflexible, but they also display perseverance and drive and tend to be more consistent. **Individuals who are avoidant of new experiences may have a greater risk for depression.**

Those high on the *conscientiousness* spectrum tend to be more organized, disciplined, and dependable but also less spontaneous and more stubborn and rigid. While those on the low end of the conscientiousness spectrum tend to be carefree and flexible, they can also be impulsive, unreliable, and disorganized. **Individuals who are on the lower end of the conscientiousness spectrum appear to have a heightened risk for depression.**

The world apparently belongs to extroverts: they're energetic, outgoing, social, and assertive. However, they can also seem pushy, attention-seeking, controlling, and bossy. Introverts may seem shy and stand-offish, which can be misinterpreted as being arrogant or aloof. However, introverts tend to be more **insightful** and thoughtful in their interactions with others, so perhaps the world should be run by more introverts! Unfortunately, **being higher on the *introversion* spectrum has been correlated with depression risk.**

People with a high level of agreeableness are friendly, compassionate, cooperative, and helpful but may also be socially passive and naive. Those on the low end of the *agreeableness* spectrum tend to be more competitive, suspicious, argumentative, and even untrustworthy. Research suggests that **low levels of agreeableness is a risk factor for depression.**

A high degree of neuroticism is the personality characteristic most highly correlated with depression. Those who are high on the *neuroticism* spectrum are more sensitive to emotional **stress** and are considered less "emotionally stable." They are often more dynamic, excitable people, but they also tend to be more vulnerable to **anxiety**, depression, and irritability. Those on the low end of the neuroticism spectrum usually have more calm and stable personalities, but they can also come across as aloof or uncaring. **Many studies have documented the correlation between neuroticism and the onset of depression, as well as a heightened risk of depression recurrence.**

Our temperament is a scaffold upon which we build our personality. Our personality becomes, when we are adults, who we are. Our behaviour is what we do. We can't change our temperament, because it is inherited, but we can change how we think, feel, and behave, so our personality and our behaviour can change. It's certainly more difficult to change once we are adults, but it is absolutely possible to change—for the worse or for the better.

Our level of resiliency or vulnerability to **stress** is related to our temperament and our personality. Some of us are more able to roll with the punches and don't get tied up in knots if things

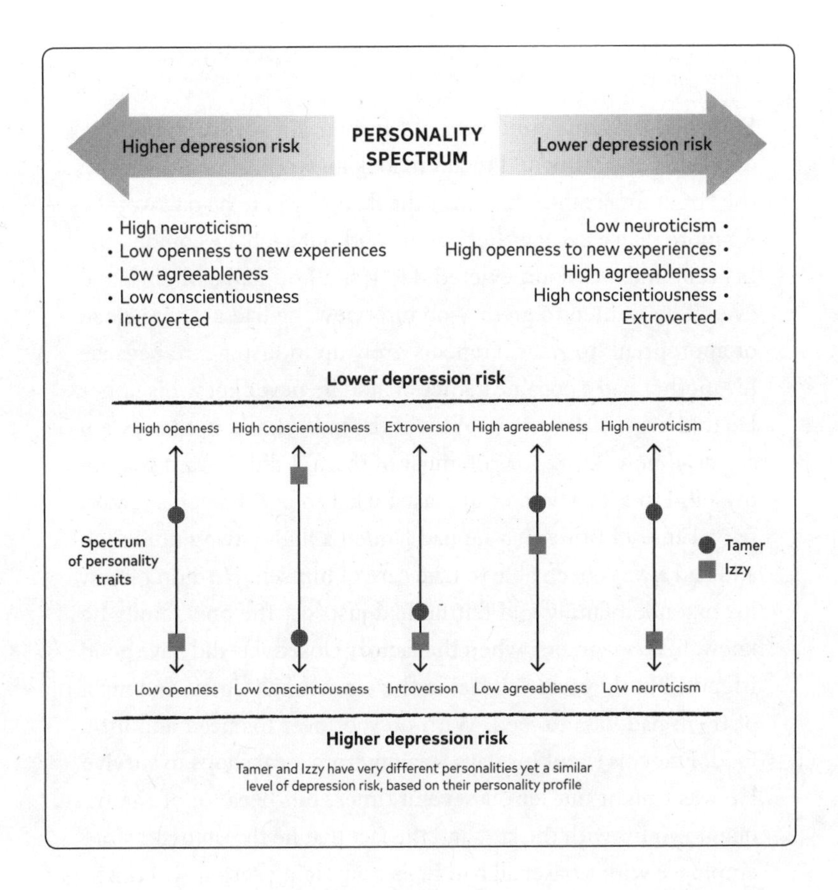

Tamer and Izzy have very different personalities yet a similar level of depression risk, based on their personality profile

aren't going our way. The rest of us seem more vulnerable to **stress**, feeling ill at ease much more often and feeling **distressed** with less provocation. The good news: research clearly demonstrates that it's possible to learn to be more resilient.

Likewise, some of us feel better equipped to manage **stress** because we're more able to implement our coping skills when we need them. It is possible to learn new skills to cope with **stress**, which is the main tenet of **cognitive-behavioural therapy** (**CBT**), a form of psychotherapy. We can learn to identify our **dysfunctional** or unhealthy thinking and change how we react and respond when facing adversity. You can learn more about CBT and other forms of talk therapy in chapter 13.

What are the social risk factors for depression?

> Francois, a twenty-nine-year-old former auto-worker, became depressed and found it difficult to look for work. He was living on the street for six months, since the factory where he had worked for more than a decade shut down. Without a job, he couldn't pay his rent and was soon evicted. He lost all of his belongings, so even if he wanted to go to a job interview, he had nothing clean or appropriate to wear. Francois grew up in foster care because his mother had a cocaine addiction and he never knew his father. He told his social worker, "A lot of the kids I knew in the system are dead now. Drugs or jail, most of them. I didn't want that for myself. I'm a survivor, or at least I used to be." Francois always felt a sense of pride that he had landed a high-paying union job and had always been able to take care of himself. He didn't know his extended family and felt he had just lost the only family he knew, his co-workers, when the factory closed. He did have good friends, but they were all facing the same tough times, and most of them had kids to feed. With no roof over his head and little food, Francois spent his days stealing from local shops to survive. He was caught but let off several times, but because of the frequent run-ins with the law, and the fact that he threatened a store employee with a baseball bat, he is now facing serious jail time.

I use the bio-psycho-social framework to illustrate the many risk factors associated with depression, but it's important to recognize that the three groups are truly fluid and impact one another. For instance, our ability to learn strong coping skills and build resiliency is highly dependent on our social environment. Our social resources (e.g., financial security), human support (e.g., friends, family, co-workers), and safety heavily impact whether our personal coping skills are sufficient. If not and we become overwhelmed, depression may be the result.

Developing resiliency often occurs when we are forced to face **stress** and work to overcome the challenge. However, overwhelming **stress**, especially in situations where there are little or no resources, makes skill-building and personal growth extremely difficult. Without shelter, food, supporters, or a sense of security, Francois is focused only on survival. Even if he was born with the most protective **genes**, a high level of resiliency, and all the right personality traits that should protect him from depression, he could still develop the illness. Poverty, hunger, loneliness, and fear can make the greatest personal strengths difficult to access.

Social support is our emotional safety net. It's the caring, empathic help and support that we believe will be accessible when we need it. That support can come from many sources: family, friends, co-workers, and health professionals. Low social support is strongly associated with depression, while consistent, positive social support appears to protect from depression. Likewise, negative or toxic relationships, especially those that we expect to be supportive—for instance, with partners, parents, and siblings—also increase the risk for depression.

Family conflicts have been shown to trigger the onset and increase the risk for depression **recurrences** in young people. However, the most important factor regarding the quality of support is not who is providing the support (e.g., friend, family member, or caregiver) or the number of supportive relationships we have, but our belief that our supporters are there for us and will respond to a call for help if we need them. If we need to call on our supporters and they do not rise to the challenge, the experience can be devastating.

Some life stressors are obvious: the death of a loved one, facing a life-threatening illness, an unexpected job loss, the family home burning down, a troubled child, criminal prosecution, or a serious accident or assault. All of these social stressors can play a role in provoking depression. However, there are other stressors that might not seem as serious, perhaps because we chose to face them, but they can still be highly stressful and even feel overwhelming. For instance, it seems I am constantly talking to patients about the **stress** associated with moving, whether across the street or across the country (although distance does make it much worse). Yes, you might have decided you want or need to move, but that does not make it a fun or relaxing experience. Likewise, starting a new career, working on a university degree, or trying out for an elite sports team are self-inflicted stressors. The outcome might be fantastic, but the process can be highly stressful. This is important to know not because you shouldn't take the risk, but because having an awareness of the power of **stress**, and planning as best you can to lessen the load, can increase the likelihood that your personal resources aren't overwhelmed.

One of the most powerful social risk factors for depression is childhood maltreatment. While we know that childhood physical or sexual abuse is a very important risk factor for provoking mental illness, research has demonstrated that chaos, neglect, and other types of poor parenting during childhood are also powerful risk factors for depression and **anxiety** later in life. Parents who are physically or emotionally absent and those who use humiliation and other personal attacks to discipline their children contribute to a potent, long-lasting negative impact on a developing brain, as does a lack of loving emotional and physical contact. In fact, early life abuse, neglect, and chaos can have an impact on our biology by changing how our **genes** are transcribed. This biological process is called **epigenetics**, which you can read more about in chapter 3.

Finally, a word about the social challenges faced by racial and sexual minorities and how discrimination might impact mental well-being. The *minority stress model* considers the relationship between minority values and the dominant values in a society and helps to explain why some minority groups are more vulnerable to depression. Because their values are often in conflict with the majority, the minority group suffers alienation and becomes more vulnerable to mental and physical illness.

The health issues suffered by minorities might be explained by the **chronic stress** of living in a hostile racist or homophobic culture. For instance, in some cultures, members of a racial, religious, or sexual minority group might endure a lifetime of prejudice, discrimination, harassment, physical or emotional abuse, and victimization. As a result, those individuals might work to conceal their true identity and expect rejection from those they live and work with, which provokes a chronically high level of **stress** and may result in physical and mental illness.

The **stress** of racism or sexism is uniquely demoralizing and damaging because it tends to be **chronic**, it may be reinforced by societal institutions that are meant to protect vulnerable members (e.g., police, judiciary, legislators), and it is outside an individual's control. One cannot change the fact that they are born gay or Black, nor should they need to. Yet, rather than provoking a sense of pride and belonging, too often our differences result in personal denial and isolation.

In the United States, researchers have found that racial discrimination is a **chronic** stressor among African Americans, which appears to be a risk factor for reduced brain health and mental well-being. Studies of racial minorities suggest that the lifetime risk for depression is significantly higher for Whites compared to Black or Hispanic individuals. However, depression among Black Americans is often more **chronic**, severe, and disabling and is less likely to be appropriately treated, or treated at all, compared with White Americans. Thus, while depression is less common in the Black community, the burden of depression may be greater.

Additionally, while very few Americans receive adequate and appropriate depression therapy, the lowest rates of care are among Hispanic and African American individuals. There are also ethnic or racial differences in the type of care offered, despite similar needs. Those from a minority group are less likely to be offered any form of treatment, and the treatment they receive is less likely to meet the level outlined in current depression treatment guidelines.

A US surgeon general's report detailed that compared to White Americans, African Americans, Latinx, Asian Americans, and Native Americans receive poorer mental healthcare. The authors strongly endorsed mental healthcare that considers and respects culture and affirms patient differences, increasing the likelihood that patients will be comfortable enough to share their concerns and receive appropriate treatment.

In Canada, Indigenous communities suffer from alarming rates of mental illness, substance abuse, and suicide. However, there is little research examining the relationship between racism and depression among Indigenous individuals, particularly those who live on-reserve. Recent studies, from Canadian and US rural Indigenous communities, have found a positive correlation between racial discrimination and life **stress** among adults and depression symptoms among Indigenous adolescents.

The disparity between the physical health of Indigenous peoples and the non-Indigenous population is well known and clearly extends to mental health. A Canadian study found that whether they live on- or off-reserve, Indigenous people continue to have higher rates of physical and mental illness. Some authors have concluded that this disparity is related to "racism and social exclusion." However, there are also biological differences between ethnic communities related to their risk for physical and mental illnesses; for instance, some groups have a greater risk of obesity, heart disease, and depression that are, at least in part, related to genetic factors. Undoubtedly, poverty, insecure or inadequate food and shelter, and a lack of personal safety are also central issues that greatly heighten the risk of serious mental illnesses.

As I noted in chapter 1, historically the DSM has contained some seriously flawed diagnoses. There is no better example than the inclusion of homosexuality as a mental illness, which was not completely removed from the DSM until 1987. The *International Statistical Classification of Diseases and Related Health Problems* (ICD), the diagnostic manual developed by the World Health Organization, only removed homosexuality from its classification with the publication of ICD-10 in 1992.

Historically, marginalization and social exclusion has disadvantaged sexual minorities, including those sometimes self-identified as lesbian, gay, bisexual, transgender, or queer (LGBTQ). The mental health of sexual- and gender-minority groups is adversely impacted by anti-LGBTQ legislation in countries around the world. However, in some countries, the tide is slowly turning. While same-sex behaviour and gender non-conformity was severely stigmatized and even criminalized in North America, the legalization of same-sex marriage and the growing acceptance of gender non-conformity has helped to reduce **stigma** for many individuals. However, sexual minorities continue to face discrimination and victimization, which is strongly associated with heightened psychological **stress** and mental and physical illness. Scientific evidence also suggests that poor mental health may be associated with heightened high-risk behaviours among sexual minorities.

The US National Institutes of Health (NIH) has recognized there is limited research data guiding our understanding of the needs of gender minorities. US surveys suggest that 20 percent of LGBTQ individuals don't tell their healthcare provider about their sexual practices. An even larger percentage of transgender individuals (30 percent) reported they avoid seeking **acute** or preventive healthcare of any kind due to discrimination and disrespect. Many from the LGBTQ community report they have been denied necessary healthcare outright due to their sexuality.

Importantly, how we rate the value of our identity is a central factor in promoting wellness and a sense of belonging. How members of the LGBTQ community perceive the value of their sexual identity is highly dependent on their environment and life experiences. Those with a positive identity have greater mental and physical well-being. They experience greater life satisfaction, feel more socially connected, and have lower rates of depression. As with other minority groups, mental healthcare that considers and respects a patient's sexual or gender differences will increase their comfort, help them to share their health concerns, and ultimately increase the likelihood that they will receive appropriate treatment.

Chapter summary

- All mental illnesses are caused by biological, psychological, and social factors, but it's important to recognize that the three groups are truly fluid and impact one another.
- You are born with your temperament, but your personality, while influenced by your temperament, is mostly developed based on your environment and life experiences.
- There are many important risk factors for depression, but a strong social support network plays a powerfully protective role in reducing the risk of developing depression.
- The **stress** of racism or sexism is uniquely demoralizing and damaging, and has been associated with higher rates or greater severity of mental and physical illnesses.

One might never know *exactly* why an individual developed depression, but by understanding what factors we can control, and those factors we cannot control, we can shift our focus away from assigning blame towards finding solutions.

A real patient's story

I WAS SEXUALLY ABUSED by my stepfather. For years, I thought it was my fault. I still can't think about all the reasons I believed that was the case, but I knew I was to blame. When I told my mother, she chose him over me. That led to years of feeling dirty, unlovable, and worthless. I chose bad boyfriends and two bad husbands because I didn't think I deserved better. Then I got depressed. I know this will sound ridiculous, but getting depressed was both the best and the worst thing that ever happened to me. Don't get me wrong: it was horrible. I felt hopeless and I knew I would never recover. But once I found the right doctor and accepted that I needed treatment, I was finally able to face my past and how sexual and emotional abuse made me vulnerable to depression. Most importantly, I learned it wasn't my fault. It took me years to accept that I was a child and he was 100 percent responsible, and once I did accept that, I was finally free. I still find it hard to trust people, and I am still working on myself, but I don't see myself as hopelessly broken anymore.

3

How do early life experiences impact mental health later in life?

THE MAIN TOPIC in this chapter is **epigenetics**, which helps to explain how the biological, psychological, and social factors discussed in chapter 2 interact to make you the person you are. Unless you happen to be a geneticist, it's necessary to take you back to high school biology class to make sense of this chapter. Welcome to Genetics 101!

What is epigenetics?

Humans are made with a built-in instructions book called **deoxyribonucleic acid**, or **DNA**, which is found in every cell in your body. Your DNA contains your genetic code, which provides the instructions necessary to grow, develop, reproduce, and stay alive. We keep our DNA wrapped around proteins and coiled into X shapes called **chromosomes**. We have twenty-three pairs of **chromosomes** (forty-six **chromosomes** in total). Twenty-two of those pairs look identical, whether we are male or female, but the twenty-third pair are sex **chromosomes.** Males have an X and a Y sex **chromosome,** while females have two X sex **chromosomes.**

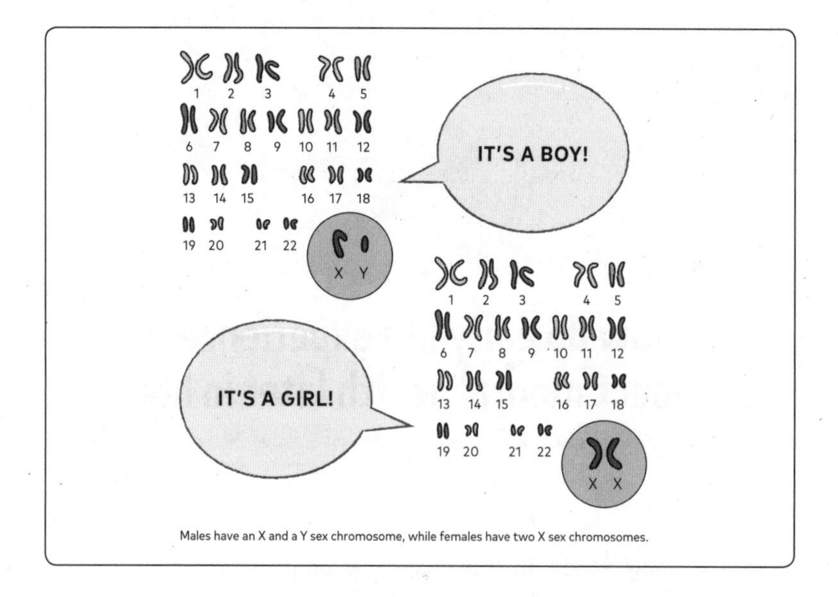

Males have an X and a Y sex chromosome, while females have two X sex chromosomes.

A human being is created by the union of a single egg and a single sperm. The egg and sperm each contain a single copy of its owner's DNA (twenty-three **chromosomes** from each), which means the offspring receives one-half of their DNA from Mom and one-half from Dad. This explains why siblings may not look or behave like they're made by the same parents. Identical twins have exactly the same DNA, but otherwise every sibling receives a different mix of DNA from their parents. It truly is a genetic lottery. One sibling might be short with striking blue eyes, while the other is six feet tall with stinky feet.

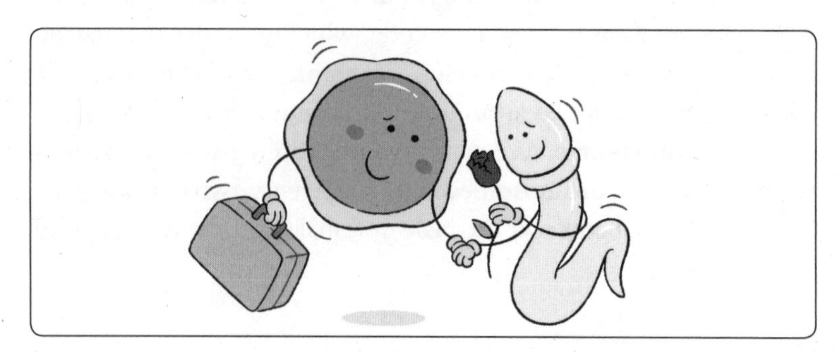

Every cell in your body contains the same DNA. So, how does a cell know to become a brain cell or a liver cell or a skin cell?

I think of DNA as being like a piano keyboard. Every person has their own unique keyboard (except identical twins—they have identical keyboards). Each key on your keyboard represents a section of DNA known as a **gene. Genes** hold the information needed for cellular differentiation: when specific **genes** are turned on (expressed) or turned off (suppressed) they direct what a cell will become. Specific **genes** make proteins and control traits like eye colour or height, and other **genes** direct cells to become heart, brain, or skin cells.

While DNA is responsible for the creation and survival of all living things, it is surprisingly simple—it's made up of just four chemicals: adenine (A), cytosine (C), guanine (G), and thymine (T). **Genes** are composed of sequences of these four chemicals, which hold the instructions that direct a cell to produce specific proteins. For instance, a **gene** might be made of a sequence like A-C-C-T-G-A-A-G-A-T-T-G, which makes a protein necessary to grow hair.

If our DNA is like a piano keyboard, the way the keys are played (the way **genes** are expressed) makes you who you are. Some keys are not played at all and others are always played. Some are played softly while others are played harshly. If, how, and when your **genes** are expressed ultimately makes you the unique individual you are. Think of it as "your song" or "the music of you." Interestingly, your tune can change, and what causes that change is **epigenetics.**

Epigenetics is the science of **gene expression.** Your DNA is written in permanent marker—it can't be changed or erased. **Epigenetics** is written in pencil: how our **genes** are expressed can change, thus we change our tune throughout our life. **Epigenetics** is the interface between nature (the **genes** you inherited from your parents) and nurture (your life experiences). How your **genes** are expressed, whether they are turned off or on, or played softly or harshly depends on the type of **genes** you inherited from your parents, your developmental stage (e.g., **puberty, menopause**), and your environment.

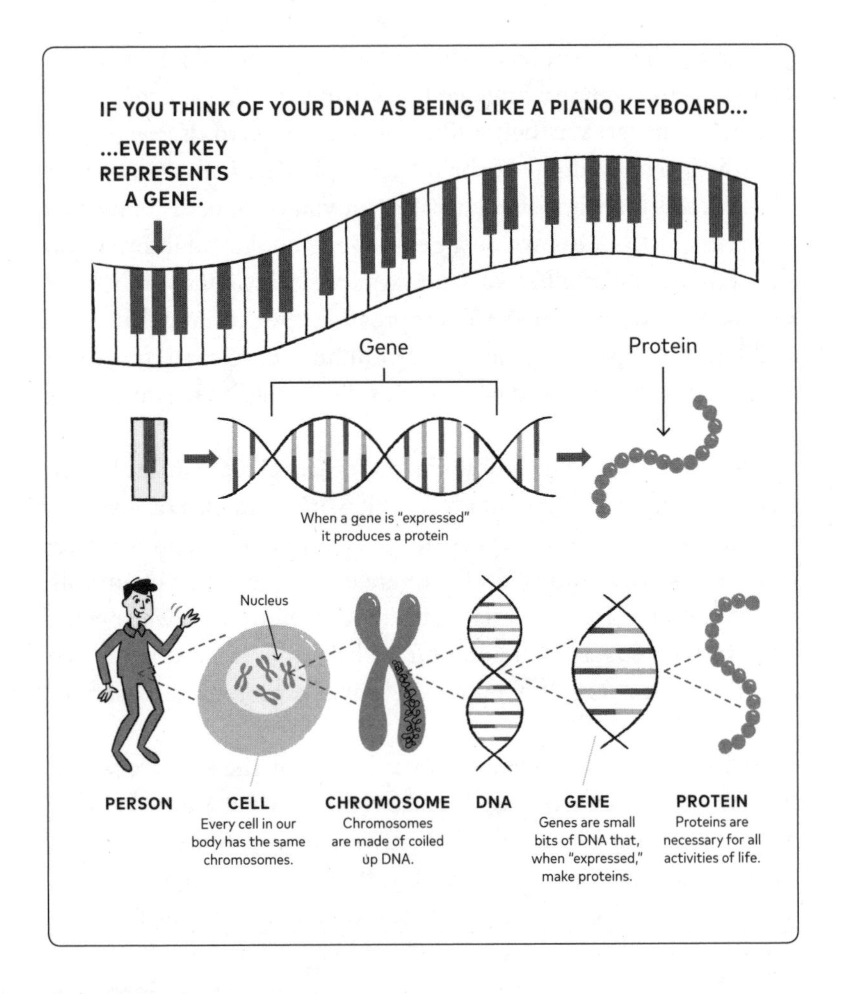

Do epigenetic changes occur during normal development?

Have you ever wondered how, when you were maybe ten, eleven, or twelve, your body knew it was time to develop breasts, pubic hair, or a lower voice? The changes that occur during **puberty** are part of a normal **epigenetic** cascade, caused when some **genes** turn on and others turn off. For instance, during **puberty**, the **genes** that cause breasts to grow would be expressed in females but would be suppressed in males. Of course, this is a very complicated process involving **hormones** and other brain chemicals, but it's all laid out in our instruction booklet—our DNA—and the **genes** that our DNA is composed of. The body changes that take place during **menopause** or pregnancy are other examples of normal **epigenetic** cascades that happen at specific times during our life. When these changes occur can be influenced by **heritability** (inherited biological factors) as well as by our environment. For instance, one girl might start her period at age ten and her girlfriend might not until she's fourteen.

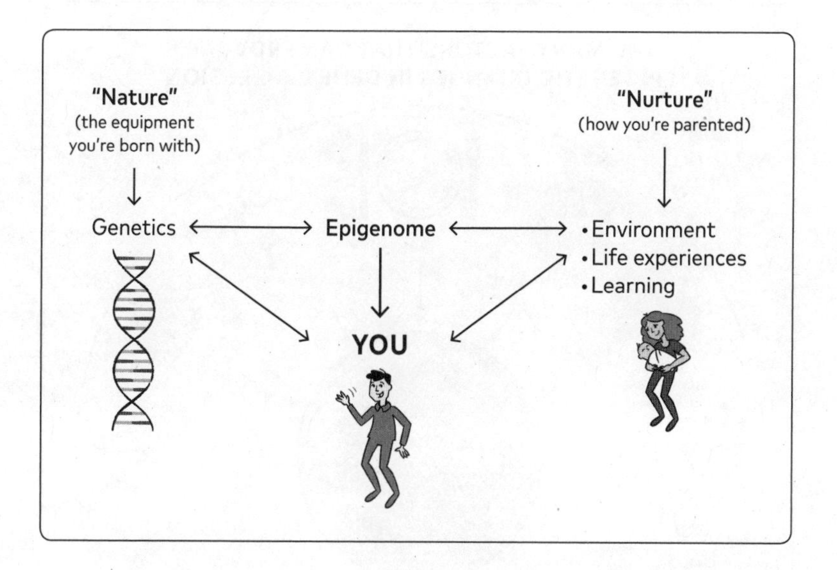

How do epigenetic changes result in illness?

We now know that our inherited genetic code, as well as life events and our environment, can affect how our **genes** are expressed. Toxin-related **epigenetic** changes are an example of our environment impacting **gene expression**. The truly scary part of this story is that research has demonstrated that **epigenetic** changes related to toxins can be inherited by our offspring. For example, we know that toxins found in cigarette smoke are associated with lung cancer and many other forms of cancer. Toxins in the smoke can trigger the expression of cancer-causing **genes** or the suppression of **genes** that protect against cancer. If a father smokes and the toxins in the smoke provoke an **epigenetic** alteration in his genome, that altered **gene** can be passed on to his child. If the **gene**'s **epigenetic** change is activated in his child, it can provoke the development of lung cancer, even if the child is an otherwise healthy non-smoker who has never been exposed to any lung cancer risk factors.

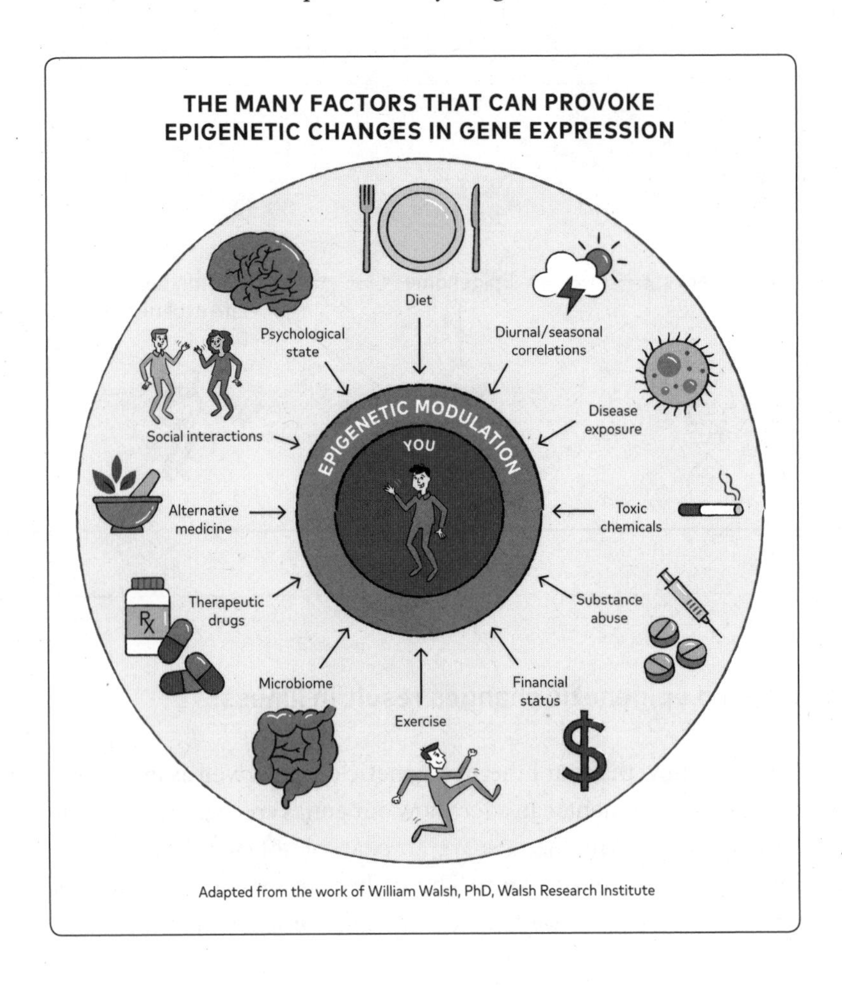

Adapted from the work of William Walsh, PhD, Walsh Research Institute

Research on **schizophrenia** provides several examples of **gene**-environmental interactions that may trigger the development of the illness. Examples of potential triggers that can alter **gene expression** and might provoke the development of **schizophrenia** include infections during pregnancy, abnormal bowel flora (micro-organisms that live in the gut), and smoking cannabis. These and likely other environmental exposures are of greatest concern in vulnerable individuals, like those who have a family history of the disorder. The family history suggests that there are **genes** in those families that constitute a risk for the disorder, and with exposure to a specific infection or cannabis, a **gene** that promotes **schizophrenia** might be activated, resulting in the onset of the disorder. See page 290 for more on the connection between cannabis and **schizophrenia**, and chapter 5 for more on the connection between illicit drugs and depression.

A real patient's story

I DREW GREAT COMFORT from learning about **epigenetics.** It made me understand that I am not inherently flawed. I do not have abnormal DNA. Instead, I experienced things that allowed a **gene** to be expressed. I can now see that my DNA is as good as anyone else's. I am not inherently flawed. The illness truly is not my fault.

How might childhood maltreatment contribute to the risk of depression later in life?

Just like cigarette toxins can cause cancer, there is growing evidence that serious stressors, especially early in life, can alter **gene expression** and contribute to the onset of mental illness later in life.

Most of the scientific research conducted to understand the power of early life nurturing has been done with rats.[2] Rat dads are generally deadbeats, while rat moms tend to be the caring nurturers. Therefore, most rat studies are conducted on rat moms and their pups. Researchers create rat models of **stress**, exposing rat moms to stressful environments that simulate the **stress** a human parent might experience, and then assess the impact on their offspring.

Rat moms who are loving and nurturing will lick their pups a great deal, thus they are called "high lickers." This is a stable trait, meaning that the pups of high-licking moms become high-licking parents themselves. Licking is not just a feel-good experience for the mom and her babies—it actually provokes critical brain development, impacting learning and memory, as well as helping to develop mature metabolic functions and healthy reproduction. The size, strength, intelligence, reproductive capabilities, and physical and mental health of the pups is strongly influenced by the amount of licking. Every rat pup wants a mom who's a "high licker."[3]

A rat mom's licking appears to, among other things, provoke **epigenetic** changes in **genes** that help to manage how a pup responds to **stress**. The most important **stress hormone** for mammals is called **cortisol**, and the level of **cortisol** in our bodies is regulated by glucocorticoid receptors. The **gene** for the glucocorticoid

---

2 Because human babies are not appropriate study subjects, since they should never be exposed to serious **stress**, we are still at the stage of drawing inferences from rat and other animal studies, but the massive quantity of research in this area is building confidence about the findings and their applicability to human beings. It seems obvious, but parenting of human babies should be done by loving and nurturing caregivers.

3 After reading this, please do not ask your child if you were a "high licker," unless you're prepared to fund their psychological **recovery**. After hearing my mother utter that statement, I'm still looking for the right support group!

receptor is greatly influenced by maternal care. Highly licked rat pups have lots of those receptors, so they can manage their body's **stress** response rapidly and get back to normal quickly. Pups from low-licking moms have fewer glucocorticoid receptors, resulting in a less effective response to stressful events. Their response tends to be greatly exaggerated and it takes them much longer to recover and feel calm and safe again.

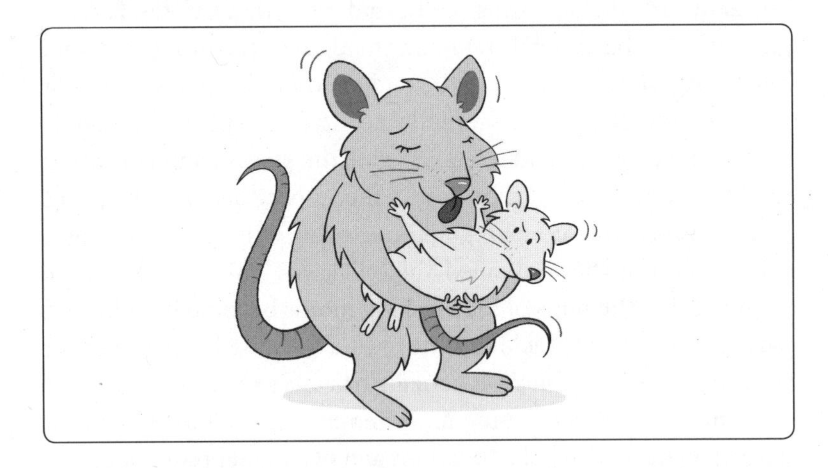

The **heritability** of the licking trait is so important because it suggests that the **epigenetic** changes related to loving and nurturing parenting can be passed down to our children, helping them to be loving and nurturing parents themselves. Unfortunately, the inverse is also true: growing up in an abusive, chaotic, non-nurturing environment can provoke changes to a child's genome that can be passed on to their offspring, heightening the risk of generational abuse, neglect, and family chaos.

There is some good news: rat pups from low-licking moms can be adopted by high-licking moms, and the pup's **stress** response can be normalized. However, what we don't know is how long a pup can be exposed to a stressful, non-nurturing, or abusive environment before the harmful **epigenetic** changes become irreversible. Unfortunately, low-licking rat moms don't become high-licking rat moms, perhaps because they don't have access to high-quality psychotherapy. That said, most human parents have a great ability to change, if that is their wish, especially if they have access to a supportive environment.

Other research has demonstrated the long-term impact of a stressful childhood on **cognitive** functioning, such as memory, concentration, and **executive functioning**, which includes organizing, planning, forward thinking, and critical thinking. When researchers limited mother rat's nesting material, thereby provoking **stress**, their maternal behaviour became less loving and nurturing. The moms would also lick their pups less, resulting in emotional and physical deprivation. The longer the mom was influenced by **stress**, the more anhedonic the pups became, no longer enjoying activities that are usually fun for rat pups.

When the researchers assessed the adolescent pups of **stressed**-out moms, the pups seemed to have normal **cognitive** functioning. Once they reached middle age, however, the rats that experienced maternal deprivation began to show **cognitive** symptoms that were more significant than expected for their age. This implies that their brain functions were prematurely declining and were consistent with what would be expected from a much older rat. More concerning, when researchers then tested the **cognitive** functioning of the adolescent pups in stressful situations, **cognitive** decline was already apparent.

Research has also demonstrated that there are not just emotional implications, such as depression and **anxiety**, resulting from childhood maltreatment. Children who are exposed to severe childhood adversity—such as abuse (physical, sexual, emotional, including unrelenting bullying or racism), the loss of a close loved one, a life-threatening illness, poverty, or a nasty divorce—are at greater risk for physical illnesses as well, including heart disease, obesity, **diabetes**, and other inflammatory illnesses.

Physical, sexual, and emotional abuse is tremendously harmful to developing brains and bodies. Neglect, chaos, and unpredictable, fragmented parenting can also result in enduring harm and impairment in our children. The **epigenetic** changes these stressful exposures provoke might also be heritable. This means that children who have been harmed by a difficult childhood, resulting

CHILDHOOD ADVERSITY REPRESENTS A RISK FOR ADULTHOOD DISEASE

32-year prospective study demonstrating the mental and physical health risks associated with adverse childhood experiences

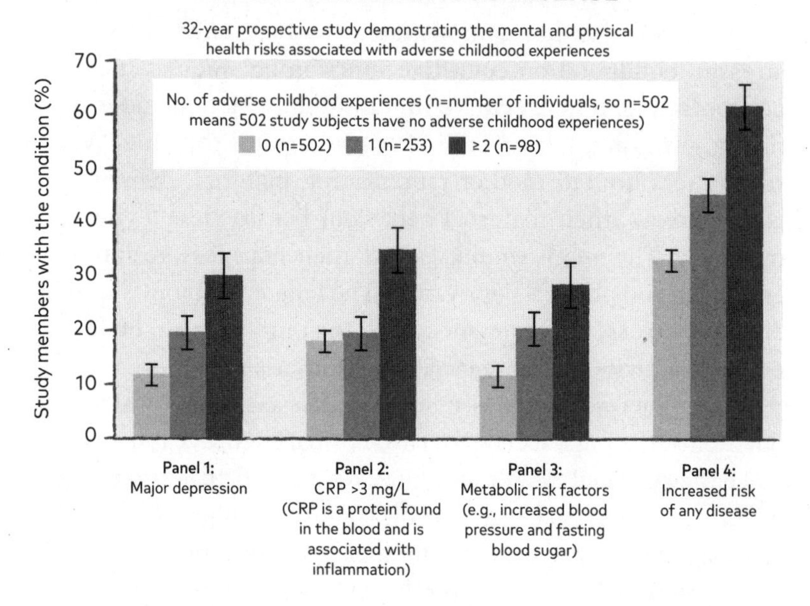

Source: Danese, A., et al. "Adverse childhood experiences and adult risk factors for age-related disease: depression, inflammation, and clustering of metabolic risk markers." *Archives of Pediatrics & Adolescent Medicine* 163 12 (2009 Dec): 1135–43.

in **epigenetic** changes to their genome, can pass those genetic alterations down to their offspring. As a result, their children might also have an abnormal, excessive **stress** response and a heightened risk for depression and **anxiety**.

If something distressing, traumatic, and unfair happened to you as a child, that does not define you. Many people have crappy childhoods, enduring abuse, neglect, chaos, and loss, and become happy, fulfilled, generous, loving adults. They also become great parents, partners, siblings, and members of the community.

No one chooses to be burdened with trauma as a child. One of the reasons traumatic experiences can have such serious impact on children is because they have so little control over what happens to them. However, as adults, we do have control. In fact, the only person on earth we can control is ourselves. If you have taken care of a child, you'll know this only too well: they pop out of the womb and scream, poop, and generally disrupt, and we have absolutely no control over what they do. You can't control your mother, partner, boss, or friends either. You can only control you. This sense of agency is truly one of the most essential concepts to integrate into your adult brain. Why? Because many adults spend way too much time trying to control the people around them, and that just doesn't work.

Chapter summary

- **Epigenetics** represents the interplay between nature (the **genes** you were born with) and nurture (your environment).
- **Genes** are turned on and off at different developmental stages, such as **puberty** and during pregnancy, but can also be influenced by toxins (e.g., smoking) and **chronic**, severe **stress**.
- **Epigenetics** can help to explain why severe childhood adversity may make an individual more vulnerable to developing a mental illness later in life.
- Exposure to severe childhood adversity doesn't make later-life mental illness inevitable.

We have an enormous capacity to change if we wish to, simply by deciding to take control of the one person we can change: ourselves.

A real patient's story

AFTER BEING OFFICIALLY diagnosed with major depressive disorder, I soon began to lose all hope for my future. In hindsight, I wish that I had viewed my diagnosis as the starting point to a medically treatable illness. The problem with depression is that you can't see past your suffering.

When you're depressed, having a positive outcome like other people experience just doesn't feel possible. In that sense, depression requires one to have faith that life can improve despite feeling that it never will. I felt that I had nothing left to lose, so I started to live my life based on the advice that action precedes motivation. I have achieved many of the milestones that I never thought possible, but I also try to celebrate the daily successes. Living with depression is not easy but it can be managed and goals can not only be met but surpassed.

4

Is depression a brain disorder?

CHRONIC DEPRESSION IS an inflammatory illness that causes changes in brain structure and functioning, but the science supporting this concept is not well known outside the world of psychiatric research. I believe it's critically important for anyone who has been depressed to be aware of and understand this information. Knowing that depression is a brain illness that can progress to a **chronic** inflammatory disease, and that the illness tends to worsen over time, can help to make sense of why finding the right treatment, and sticking with it, is essential for getting better and staying well.

How does a healthy brain respond to stress?

To truly understand depression, it's necessary to understand what **stress** is and how severe and prolonged **stress** is an important risk factor for depression.

When you are out for a walk, everything your senses experience is transmitted to your **thalamus**, the brain structure that gathers information from everything you see, hear, taste, or touch. The **thalamus** then sends that information to other relevant brain structures for further analysis. For instance, along your path you might see a beautiful flower. The flower image is sent from the retina in your eye to the **thalamus** and on to the occipital cortex, which, by analyzing the information sent from the retina, understands: *flower*.

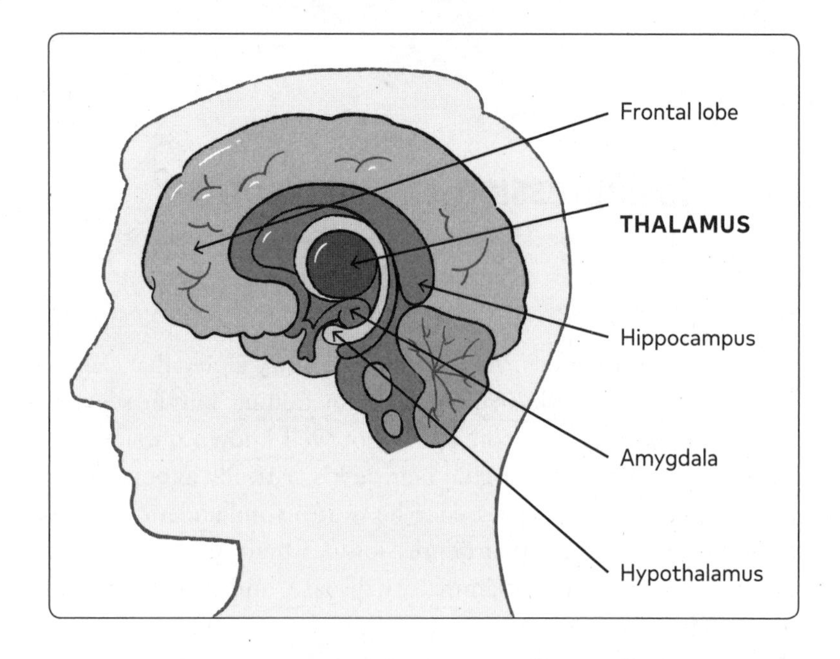

However, if during the walk you are suddenly confronted by a growling dog with its teeth bared, the instant you see and hear the dog, that sensory information will go directly from your **thalamus** to your **amygdala**. The **amygdala** is the brain structure that receives sensory information related to threatening situations at lightning speed, instantly considers the information, and develops a plan: flee, freeze, or fight.

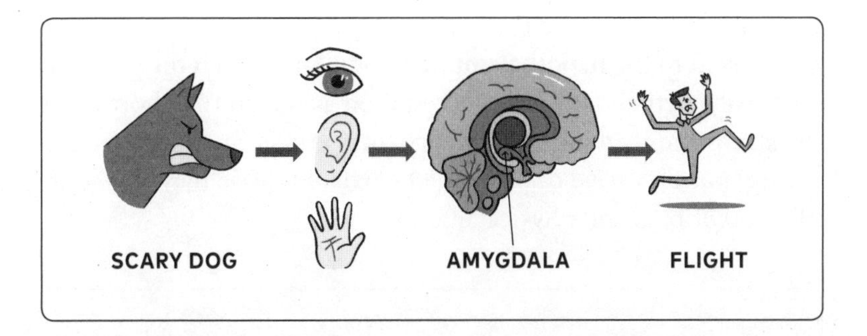

In response to a threatening event, the **amygdala** forwards fear-related messages to the brain's **stress** response command centre, called the **hypothalamic-pituitary-adrenal** (HPA) **axis.** The **hypothalamus** is a brain structure that controls many essential functions necessary for life, including maintaining our **circadian rhythm** (normal sleep and wake cycles) and regulating **hormone** levels, appetite, body temperature, sexual behaviour, and emotions. The **hypothalamus** is located close to and works directly with the **pituitary gland,** which produces essential **hormones** that regulate the thyroid, sexual functioning, and **stress** responses.

The message sent from the **amygdala** in response to that aggressive dog would also request a burst of the **neurotransmitter norepinephrine,** which increases your heart and breathing rate and blood pressure, allowing you to run or take other evasive measures. The **amygdala** would also ask the **hypothalamus** to release **corticotropin-releasing hormone** (CRH), which initiates a cascade of effects when we are exposed to an **anxiety**-provoking situation. CRH prompts the **pituitary gland** to release **adrenocorticotropic hormone** (ACTH), and ACTH triggers the release of **cortisol,** our most important **stress hormone.**

Cortisol is a potent **anti-inflammatory hormone.** Its job is to manage our body's response to **stress** and calm us down as quickly as possible, to prevent widespread tissue and nerve damage associated with **stress** and **inflammation.** In response to a threat, a boost of **cortisol** is necessary to provide the energy needed to mount an effective response that keeps us alive and well. Once there is enough **cortisol** to calm the brain and the body, an "all clear" message is sent to the **hypothalamus** and pituitary, which turns off the HPA axis **cortisol** tap until it's required again. In the short term, the **stress**-induced increase in **cortisol** is crucial and might be lifesaving, but excessive or prolonged **cortisol** release may have crippling emotional and physical effects.

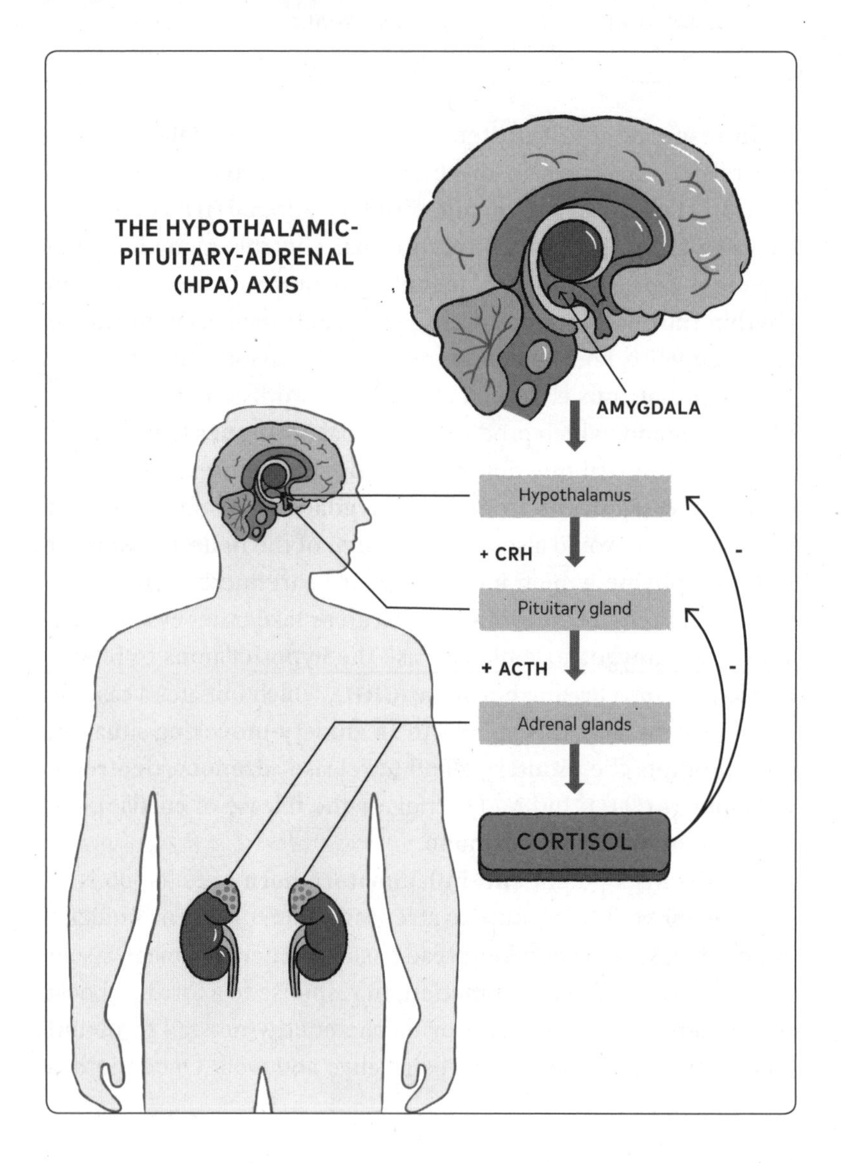

The **amygdala** of a chronically depressed or anxious brain is always screaming at the **hypothalamus**, "This is an emergency!" because it constantly feels under attack, even if there isn't an obvious threat. As a result, the HPA axis is constantly in overdrive, desperately trying to get the **stressed**-out brain to calm down. **Cortisol** levels stay high and don't settle back to normal because the threat never fully resolves, leaving the brain swimming in a high level of **cortisol** for extended periods.

How is the stress response different in a depressed or anxious brain?

Chronically high levels of **cortisol** can have devastating effects on a depressed brain because eventually, in situations of prolonged and severe **stress**, the brain starts to ignore **cortisol**. Much like the boy who cried wolf, the brain stops reacting to the **amygdala**'s cries for help as brain cells become increasingly insensitive to **cortisol**, much like how chronically high levels of insulin lead to insulin insensitivity in type II diabetics. Over time, **cortisol** becomes less effective at preventing **inflammation** and may in fact start to *cause* or *worsen* **inflammation**.

To understand the impact of the brain becoming less sensitive to **cortisol**, which can provoke **inflammation** that damages the brain, it's important to know about some key brain components: **neurons** and **glial cells**.

The human brain is made up of more than 100 billion **neurons**, specialized brain cells that almost instantly send and receive messages between the brain and the body. **Neurons** are responsible for everything you feel, experience, and know. Working alongside the **neurons** are the **glial cells**, which make up 90 percent of the cells in the brain and outnumber **neurons** by a ratio of 10:1. This ratio drops to 1:1 in rodents, which suggests that more **glial cells** are associated with higher-brain functions. After Albert Einstein's death, scientists examined his brain and found it contained more cells than the average brain; however, he didn't have more

neurons—he had more **glial cells.** There are several types of **glial cells,** each with distinctive functions. For this discussion, I focus on two types: **microglia** and **astrocytes.**

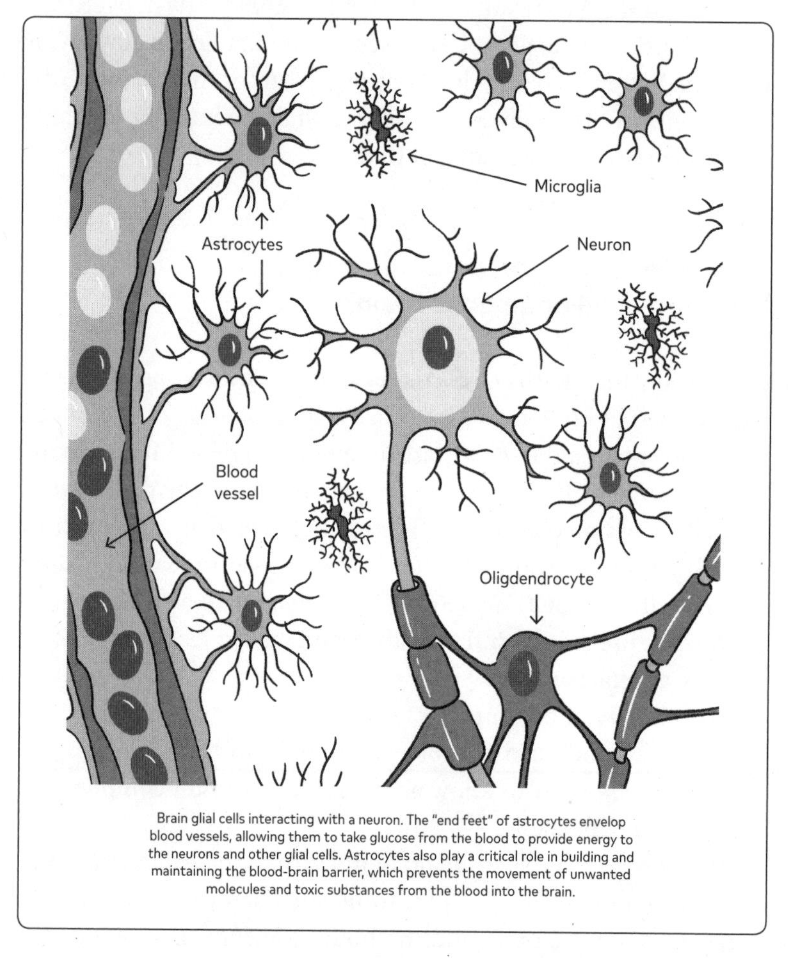

Brain glial cells interacting with a neuron. The "end feet" of astrocytes envelop blood vessels, allowing them to take glucose from the blood to provide energy to the neurons and other glial cells. Astrocytes also play a critical role in building and maintaining the blood-brain barrier, which prevents the movement of unwanted molecules and toxic substances from the blood into the brain.

Microglia are the type of glial cell that I think of as brain vacuum cleaners. They suck up debris and help to keep the brain environment clean and tidy, gobbling up infections and problem proteins and preventing **neurotransmitters** from accumulating and causing harm to the brain. They are also the brain's main line of defence from infections that enter across the mighty, highly protective, **blood-brain barrier**.

When a brain is seriously and chronically depressed and is being bathed in an abnormally high level of **cortisol**, that can cause the **microglia** to revolt. Much like unionized workers when they go on strike, **microglia** stop their vacuum cleaning and become "activated." Activated **microglia** begin releasing immune proteins called **pro-inflammatory cytokines** (**PICs**), which provoke **inflammation**. That causes other **glial cells**, called **astrocytes**, to stop doing their job.

Astrocytes are **neuron**-nurturing **glial cells** that provide nutrition and produce growth factors that keep **neurons** healthy and strong. They also regulate the levels of **neurotransmitters** in the brain, help support the **blood-brain barrier**, and provide many other essential functions that keep the brain healthy and operating normally. However, when **astrocytes** are exposed to rising levels of PICs, they stop nurturing **neurons**, and that's when depression's serious brain effects become apparent.

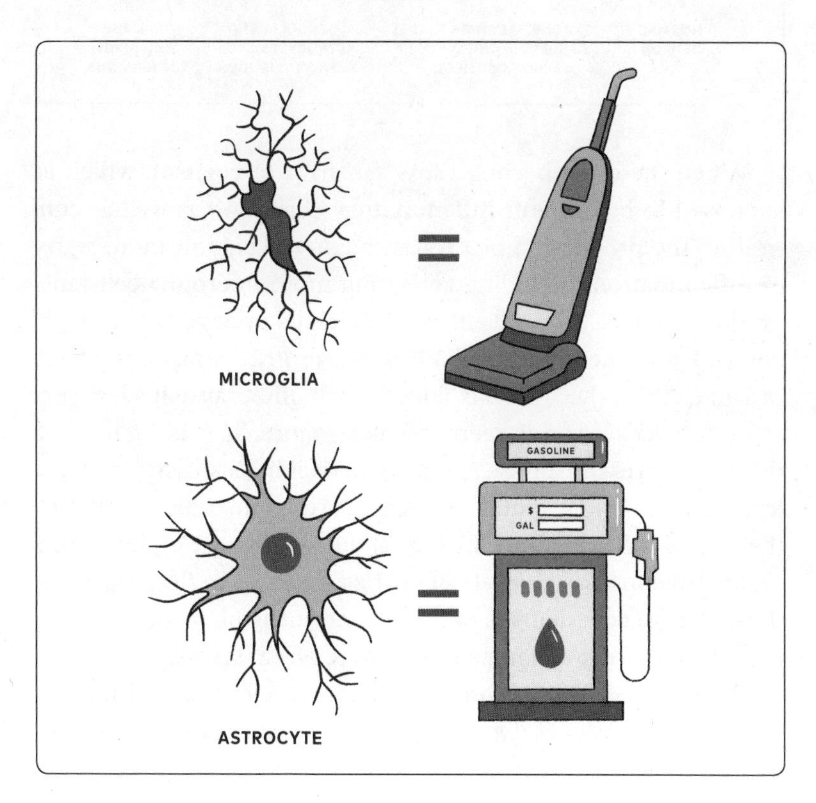

When **astrocytes** aren't working properly, toxins accumulate and begin to damage and even kill **neurons. Astrocytes** also produce a protein called **brain-derived neurotrophic factor** (BDNF), which is essentially brain cell fertilizer. Accumulating PICs can cut the production of BDNF and prevent what little is available from working effectively to support **neurons.**

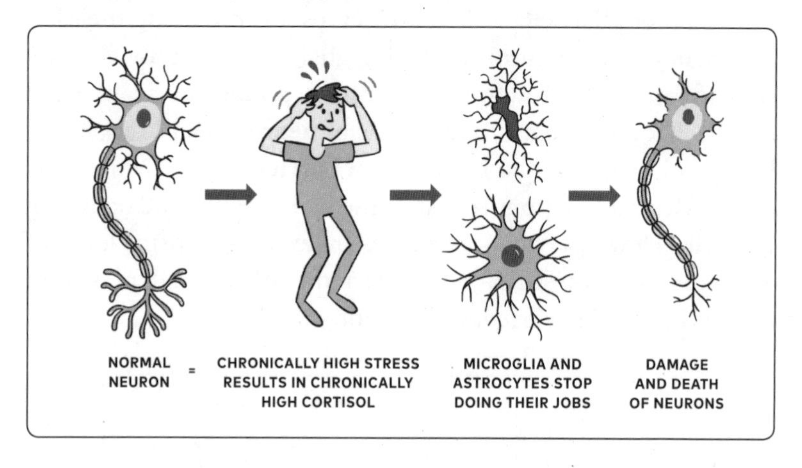

When the brain becomes less sensitive to **cortisol**, which is supposed to be our **anti-inflammatory** champion as well as controlling the production of PICs, it begins to exhibit more signs of **inflammation**, including activating more **microglia** cells and producing more PICs. Eventually, a vicious cycle is set up: high **cortisol** provokes increased PICs, those PICs worsen **cortisol** resistance, and the HPA axis doesn't turn off because it's less sensitive to **cortisol** and it keeps releasing more. This is a failure of the entire **stress**-response system. **Cortisol** insensitivity and high levels of PICs were found in most depression studies assessing the role of **inflammation.** In fact, about 50 percent of depressed brains have increased levels of **cortisol**, and up to 80 percent of those with severe depression have abnormally high **cortisol, cortisol** insensitivity, and impaired **recovery** from **stress.**

What is the fallout from this vicious cycle in actual human beings struggling with depression? Research suggests that **chronic** depression leads to altered brain structure and function. The brain structure most affected by the **neuron** injury and death associated with depression is called the **hippocampus.** Using specialized brain-imaging techniques, researchers have found that the size of the **hippocampus** is reduced in depressed brains, which is especially pronounced in those with the most serious symptoms, those with a longer period of untreated illness, and those with severe **cognitive** symptoms.

Another remarkable research discovery is the loss of **glial cells** in depressed brains. In fact, a reduction in **glial cells** is the most prominent and reproducible finding that researchers report when examining the brain cells of patients who have been depressed. Taken together, damaged and lost **neurons** and reduced glial cell numbers result in serious brain structure and functional changes that lead to both emotional and physical symptoms of depression, which may eventually become **chronic** and sometimes unresponsive to treatment.

A reproduction of microscopic images of glial cells in depressed and non-depressed brains. These pictures show a reduced amount of glial fibrillary acidic protein (GFAP), a critical part of an astrocyte, in a depressed individual's brain.*

CONTROL (27 YEARS OLD)

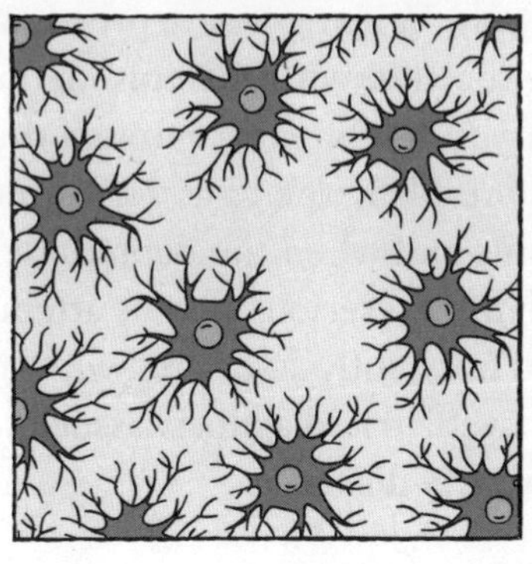

MDD (32 YEARS OLD)

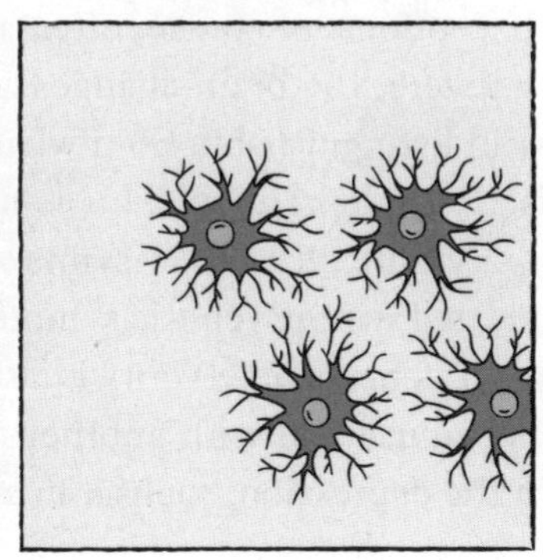

*Reduction in glial cell density and number is the most prominent feature of cell pathology in depression

Source: Rajkowska, G., and Miguel-Hidalgo, J.J. "Gliogenesis and glial pathology in depression." *CNS & Neurological Disorders—Drug Targets* 6 (2007): 219–33.

Once you've been depressed, do you have an increased risk of getting depressed again?

Research suggests that a first depression is associated with mild brain changes and **cognitive** symptoms, but for most people these symptoms are likely to fully resolve with treatment and no **residual symptoms** are likely to remain. However, at least 50 percent of those who recover from a first episode of depression will eventually have another episode in their lifetime, and approximately 80 percent of those who have had two episodes of depression will have another **recurrence.** Nearly 100 percent of those who have had three episodes of depression will get depressed again.

What happens between a first depression and a third depression that makes it more likely for another episode to occur? For most people, once they have had three episodes, depression changes from an **acute** illness to a **chronic** inflammatory illness. Once **inflammation** is established, depression becomes more difficult to treat and is less likely to get better with talk therapy or even one medication treatment. Changes in brain structure and functioning are more likely, and **cognitive** symptoms are often more severe and **chronic.** Once there have been three or more episodes, depression is almost certain to recur unless there is ongoing treatment.

Exceptions, of course, often apply. When a first depression is very severe, the brain changes associated with the episode may look indistinguishable from what you might expect from a third episode of depression. This is more likely the case when there are very difficult to treat symptoms and when the depression is associated with **psychotic** symptoms or a serious suicide attempt. Greater depression severity is also frequently associated with substance abuse and with another psychiatric diagnosis associated with the depression, such as an **anxiety disorder.**

Never, never, never give up

I have learned from my patients that depression is like a brain mutiny. They feel betrayed by their own brain and hopeless to take back control. *Why?* some demand to know. *Why me? Why am I feeling like this?* I don't worry about those who are demanding answers, because they remember what it feels like to be well. They remember their old life, when they felt joy and interest and pleasure, and want it back. The patients who provoke my feelings of fear for their safety and well-being are those who are resigned to depression—they believe they are hopeless and worthless and useless. They *know* the battle is lost. But they're in my office, so I believe there is still some hope lurking inside them. My job is to help them take back control of their brain and their life, but when they're not sure what they're fighting for, just getting started is a battle.

It takes time to get depressed, and it takes time to get better, but every step you take towards wellness, even if it's not a perfect step, is part of the slow journey towards **recovery**.

Does the brain recover when the depression resolves?

Because depression is a brain injury and may eventually become a **chronic** inflammatory illness, it stands to reason that recovering from depression should result in reduced **inflammation** and actual structural brain changes. Happily, this is what occurs, because the brain is a dynamic structure. Human beings can grow new **neurons** throughout their life, although it happens more slowly and less effectively as we move out of our twenties. Growing new **neurons** is called **neurogenesis,** which occurs in a few brain regions but especially in the **hippocampus**, which is also the area where **neurons** are damaged and killed by **chronic** depression.

NEUROGENESIS IN THE BRAIN REGION CALLED THE HIPPOCAMPUS

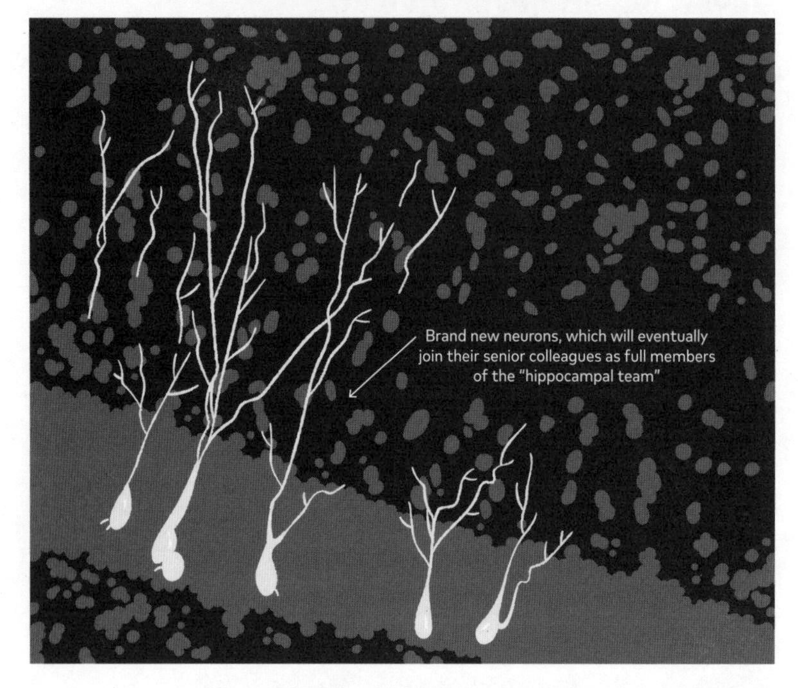

Source: van Praag, H., et al. "Functional neurogenesis in the adult hippocampus." *Nature* 415 6875 (2002): 1030–4.

Not only can we grow new brain cells, we can also change our brain in another remarkable way. The human brain is constantly wiring and rewiring in response to influences like learning new information and developing new skills, engaging social interactions, and other enriching life experiences. The brain's ability to remodel itself is called **neuroplasticity.** Importantly, as discussed, sustained levels of elevated **cortisol**, the **stress hormone** that has been associated with severe and **chronic** depression, can reduce **neurogenesis** and impair **neuroplasticity.**

While there is good **neuroplasticity**, there is also bad **neuroplasticity.** An example of good **neuroplasticity** would occur if you decided to learn to dance. Every time you went to a class and learned a few steps, your brain would be wiring and rewiring to help you to learn and remember those new steps. With each class, the wiring would get stronger and work better, and before long, you wouldn't need to think about the first steps you learned. They'd come naturally. While **neuroplasticity** occurs throughout life, the brain is most plastic during childhood and adolescence, which is why it's faster and easier to learn to dance, or learn just about anything else, when we're young.

There is a saying, "**Neurons** that fire together, wire together." The more you use a specialized group of **neurons**—like the ones you would use when learning a new, complex activity—the more they are firing off electrical messages to each other and eventually they will form a neuronal highway of new wiring. This explains why you can ride a bike or drive a standard-shift car, both complicated brain activities, without having to think about it once you've learned to do it well. When you learned to do these activities, your brain created wiring that is strong, effective, and long-lasting. If you haven't driven a standard-shift car for a while, you'll notice it might take a short time to feel comfortable again, but before long, your brain's "standard-shift-car wiring" will be working like you're an expert again.

A compelling example of bad **neuroplasticity** is the repetitive behaviour associated with **obsessive-compulsive disorder (OCD).** People who struggle with OCD commonly have compulsive behaviours; for instance, they might feel compelled to check the stove to be sure that it's turned off. Unfortunately, they can't just check the stove once, feel reassured, and get on with their day; they might need to check the stove hundreds of times every day. While they might feel momentarily reassured when they check the stove, within moments the intrusive thought, *The stove might be on*, creeps back into their head, and they feel they must check the stove again.

As a quick but important aside, most people with OCD have **insight**, which means they know (a) checking the stove hundreds of times a day makes no sense, and (b) once they check the stove, they'll feel momentarily relieved but then they'll need to check it again. No matter how hard they try not to check the stove, the pressure to check builds up and will not be relieved until the stove is checked again. They get no pleasure or personal benefit from checking the stove, so why do it? Because OCD is a brain disorder, provoking thoughts and behaviours that make absolutely no sense to the brain's owner. They certainly didn't choose to have a brain that makes them waste their valuable time checking the stove.

Compulsions are examples of bad **neuroplasticity** because OCD establishes very strong and long-lasting wiring, resulting from **neurons** firing together repeatedly, which keeps driving compulsive behaviour. The person's brain wiring provokes a thought, *The stove might be on*, and that thought provokes a behaviour, which is to check the stove. By checking the stove, the wiring is further reinforced and strengthened. In fact, every time the person yields to the compulsion and checks the stove, the likelihood that they'll have the thought and check the stove again increases.

The treatment that has the most research evidence supporting its effectiveness for OCD is a type of **cognitive-behavioural therapy (CBT)** called exposure and response prevention (ERP). If our stove-checking friend was working with an excellent ERP therapist, they would be taught to be by the stove (exposure) but to try their best not to check the stove (response-prevention). As you might imagine, this is extremely difficult to do if they've been checking the stove hundreds of times every day. However, every time they don't check the stove, even though their brain is screaming, *CHECK THE STOVE!!!*, they are rewiring their brain to say, *You don't need to check the stove.* The rewiring associated with ERP is an example of good **neuroplasticity**.

Bad **neuroplasticity** also happens in depression. Repetitive negative thoughts, like *You are worthless and useless*, can become hard-wired. The more we think those negative thoughts, the more likely we are to think and believe them. Depression is associated with many negative, repetitive, and **dysfunctional** thoughts, and CBT can be extremely helpful to overcome negative, distorted thinking. You can read more about CBT in chapter 13.

What is BDNF and why is it important in depression?

For **neurogenesis** and **neuroplasticity** to occur, the brain must have a healthy supply of growth factors, which are proteins produced by the **glial cells** called **astrocytes.** One critical growth factor is called **brain-derived neurotrophic factor** (**BDNF**), which is essentially brain cell fertilizer, necessary to grow new and healthy **neurons.** BDNF is brain cell fertilizer that is necessary to grow new and healthy **neurons** and protect them from harm and premature death.

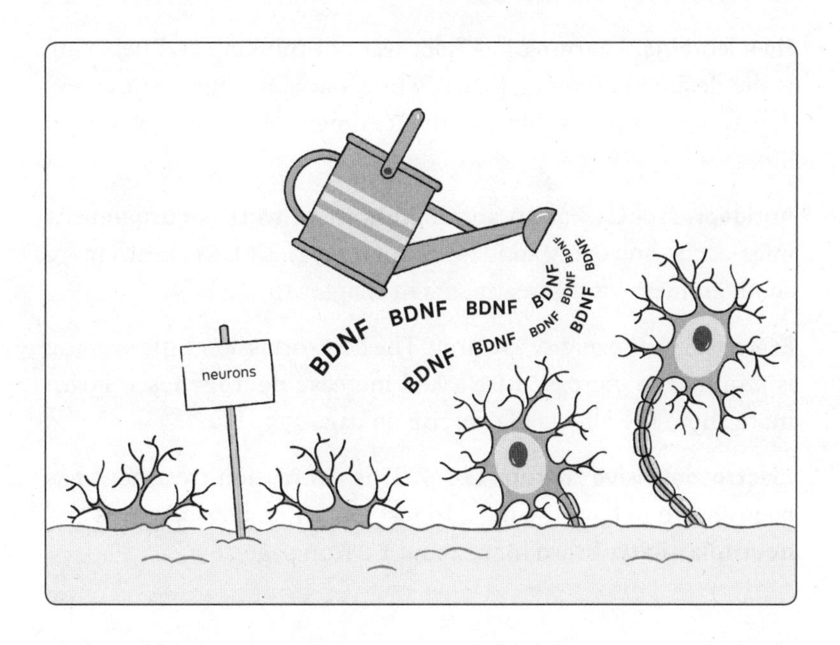

Low levels of BDNF have been found in the brains with depression as well as many other neurological and psychiatric conditions, including Alzheimer's disease, **anxiety**, **schizophrenia**, epilepsy, anorexia nervosa, and OCD. Low BDNF levels have also been associated with certain personality characteristics and reduced **stress** resilience, which heightens the vulnerability for depression. Researchers have demonstrated that BDNF is reduced in people facing chronically high levels of **stress.**

While low BDNF might not be the cause of depression, it is clearly connected to the illness and the progression of depression to a **chronic** inflammatory disorder. Many studies have demonstrated that there are low levels of BDNF in the blood of people suffering from depression. Additionally, there is reduced BDNF in the brains of people who were depressed and committed suicide.

BDNF also plays a critical role in **recovery** from depression, from sources that might come as a surprise. **Recovery** from depression is associated with **neurogenesis**, and **neurogenesis** requires BDNF, so what increases BDNF?

New learning. Learning healthier ways of thinking and behaving is the desired outcome of CBT, which has abundant research evidence supporting its value for the treatment of a variety of mental illnesses.

Antidepressants. For an antidepressant to work, **neurogenesis** must occur, and every antidepressant increases BDNF. Learn more about antidepressant treatments in chapter 10.

Exercise. I view exercise as a drug. The best part is how little exercise is required to increase BDNF and increase **neurogenesis.** Learn more about the effects of exercise on page 275.

Electroconvulsive therapy (ECT). This depression treatment has been shown to have the most robust impact on **neurogenesis** and **neuroplasticity**. Learn more about ECT on page 267.

Chapter summary

- **Chronic** and severe depression is associated with **inflammation** and changes in brain structure and function.
- **Neurogenesis**, or new brain cell growth, happens throughout our lives. Cells lost as a result of depression can be replaced through effective depression treatment, which increases BDNF, our natural brain cell fertilizer.
- Antidepressants, exercise, learning new skills, and other depression treatments increase BDNF, which grows brain cells and contributes to the **recovery** from depression.

We have the ability to grow new brain cells and rewire our brain every day of our lives. In fact, recovery from depression depends on it.

It's not in your stomach; it's in your head

I HAVE FOND MEMORIES of many lovely patients, but most especially I remember those who have taught me an important life lesson. One such patient, I'll call her Mrs. Gupta, helped me greatly in my relationships with many other patients. She was in her eighties when I met her, and when I asked her how she would like to be addressed, she looked taken aback and said, "As Mrs. Gupta, of course."

When we first met, I was not sure why she was referred; she didn't really seem to know and she denied feeling depressed or anxious. Once I had asked every usual question I could think of, I asked her, "Is there anything that's bothering you that perhaps I could help you with?" Mrs. Gupta said, "Well, not really. I suppose I'd be happy if you could take away my upset stomach." Aha!

I learned that Mrs. Gupta had a chronically upset stomach that was fully investigated by her caring family doctor and there was no discernible medical cause. Ultimately, we figured out that she experienced her sadness, which started after the death of her husband, and worry about the future, through her stomach. Mrs. Gupta never uttered the words "depressed," "anxious," "sad," or even "worried" with me. She told me how she was feeling physically, and we used that as a barometer of her mental health.

Mrs. Gupta was a very strong woman, but she also had a difficult illness to manage. She required a high dose of one antidepressant medication because other medications were not helpful or upset her stomach further. She was quite elderly and had a number of medical issues as well, which made her other caregivers anxious, but she soldiered on and ultimately her stomach problem was resolved.

“Of course it’s happening inside your head, Harry, but why on earth should that mean that it is not real?”

J.K. ROWLING

Harry Potter and the Deathly Hallows

5

Does depression co-occur with other illnesses?

As if depression isn't enough to deal with, too often it is accompanied by another psychiatric or physical illness. This is a challenging aspect of diagnosis and treatment because there may be overlap between the symptoms of mental and physical illnesses—for instance, fatigue and pain. Additionally, mental illnesses can heighten the risk of some physical illnesses, and physical illnesses may provoke mental illnesses. Further complicating matters, the treatments used to manage mental or physical illnesses can in some cases provoke side effects that are mental (e.g., provoking depression) or physical (e.g., provoking headaches or diarrhea). Unraveling the underlying causes of symptoms and determining the best course of treatment is challenging, often time-consuming, and can be very frustrating for patients.

What are co-morbidities?

When two or more disorders are present at the same time, the co-occurring disorders are called **co-morbidities.** Frankly, "**co-morbidity**" isn't a word that comfortably rolls off the tongue, but when broken down, it does make sense. The term "morbidity" means illness or disease, so **co-morbidity** refers to having two or more illnesses that occur at the same time. The most common psychiatric **co-morbidity** associated with depression is **anxiety**. As described in chapter 1, most people suffering from depression will experience some symptoms of **anxiety**.

Living with severe **anxiety** is an awful experience. The presence of **anxiety** heightens the risk of suicide, makes depression more difficult to treat, often requires higher doses of antidepressants to manage, and is slower to respond to treatment. **Anxiety** might include excessive worry about everyday things (e.g., health, work, finances, or the future), constantly feeling like something terrible is about to happen, ruminating about negative thoughts, feeling a loss of control, having trouble concentrating, or feeling restless, tense, keyed up, or on edge, all without a clear cause.

The DSM-5 recognized the importance of assessing and grading the severity of **anxiety** symptoms when diagnosing depression by adding a diagnostic specifier, called "with anxious distress." This specifier encourages mental health professionals to consider not only the depression symptoms but also the presence and severity of **anxiety** symptoms. When making a diagnosis of depression, anxious distress should be graded as mild, moderate, or severe. Thus a typical DSM-5 diagnosis would be "major depressive episode with severe anxious distress."

Panic attacks, sometimes referred to as **anxiety** attacks, are sudden, intense, and usually terrifying experiences of **anxiety** that may occur in association with depression. **Panic attacks** are commonly associated with frightening thoughts like, *I'm going to die*, *I'm having a heart attack/stroke*, *I need to escape*, or *I'm going crazy*. The fear of imminent death or the belief that a heart attack or stroke is occurring during a **panic attack** is not surprising: the episodes are usually accompanied by physical symptoms that mimic heart problems, such as a racing heart rate; pressure or pain in the chest; feeling faint, weak, or dizzy; and shortness of breath. Other associated symptoms include shakiness, stomach upset or nausea, and sweating or feeling cold and clammy.

Anxiety symptoms should be differentiated from an **anxiety disorder**. When the **anxiety** symptoms described above occur in association with depression, they will usually get better when the depression resolves, although **anxiety** symptoms are often more difficult to manage than the depression symptoms. **Anxiety disorders** are psychiatric illnesses that often co-occur with depression but are separate illnesses that have distinct **DSM-5** criteria. Unless an **anxiety disorder** is specifically addressed with treatment, it may persist even when the depression symptoms resolve, which increases the risk of depression **relapse** and **recurrence**.

Examples of **anxiety disorders** include **panic disorder** (**PD**), **generalized anxiety disorder** (**GAD**), **post-traumatic stress disorder** (**PTSD**), and **social anxiety disorder** (**SAD**). Historically, **obsessive-compulsive disorder** (**OCD**) and post-traumatic **stress** disorder (PTSD) were included in the **anxiety disorders** group, but now they are in a separate categories in the **DSM-5**. However, just like the other **anxiety disorders**, depression commonly co-occurs with OCD and PTSD, and when they co-occur, they are more difficult to treat than either disorder alone. Furthermore, depression with co-morbid **anxiety**, whether just **anxiety** symptoms or an **anxiety disorder**, is commonly associated with self-medication, whether alcohol or illicit drugs, which further worsens both the depression and the **anxiety**.

Substance abuse and dependence, whether associated with illicit drugs or alcohol, are psychiatric disorders that are frequently associated with depression. When depression occurs co-morbidly with substance abuse or dependence, ideally both disorders should be treated at the same time. There was a time when many psychiatrists believed that depression or any other psychiatric disorder should not be treated until the patient stopped abusing drugs or alcohol. This myth has been debunked. If the patient refuses to stop abusing drugs or alcohol, but they are willing to accept treatment for their depression, treatment should be offered. Once they are engaged, they might be willing to consider addressing the substance abuse as well. Actively abusing substances will no doubt reduce the success of the depression treatment, but it is still better than no treatment at all.

Depression may also occur co-morbidly with any other psychiatric disorder: patients who have **schizophrenia, bipolar disorder**, an eating disorder, **attention deficit hyperactivity disorder (ADHD)**, or a **personality disorder** can also meet the **DSM-5** criteria for depression. Unfortunately, depression may be missed when other symptoms are more obvious to caregivers, sometimes leading to disastrous consequences. The potential for a serious, negative outcome highlights the importance of having a thorough psychiatric assessment. If we think of psychiatric illnesses as being on a spectrum with a great deal of overlap, rather than as a bunch of separate, independent illnesses, it's more likely that all symptoms and disorders will be identified and properly managed, benefitting patients, families, and society.

What is the mind-body connection?

Ricardo, a primary school teacher, says he's had an upset stomach and diarrhea "forever." The symptoms are especially unpleasant when he must talk to parents or his principal, but they can also happen suddenly, with no provocation or warning. He has seen his family doctor repeatedly, yet his many medical investigations have been negative. He's tried treatments from his GP, a naturopath, and even his elderly next-door neighbour's home remedy, and nothing has helped. He told his doctor he's terrified of being more than a few steps away from a bathroom, so he doesn't go out with friends or attend family gatherings anymore. When his doctor asked if he was experiencing anxiety, Ricardo barked, "Of course I'm anxious! Wouldn't you be if you had explosive diarrhea for no reason?"

Ariana has complained to her family doctor about debilitating **chronic** pain and fatigue for the last eighteen months. No medical cause was found, despite many examinations and tests. She attempted to fix the problem herself, changing her mattress, exercising, and restricting caffeine, alcohol, gluten, and lactose, but nothing helped. When her doctor asked her to complete a questionnaire that assessed her mood, she became enraged and felt betrayed. "You don't believe me!" she cried. "Do you think this is all in my head?"

Depression hurts? Need to rush to the toilet before a big presentation? How can your mood or **anxiety** cause such monumental, undeniable effects on your body? Is it all in your head? Well, yes. Pain is all in your head. Even if you have a broken arm, the pain is produced with the help of your brain. But just because physical symptoms aren't caused by an injury or an infection doesn't mean they're not real.

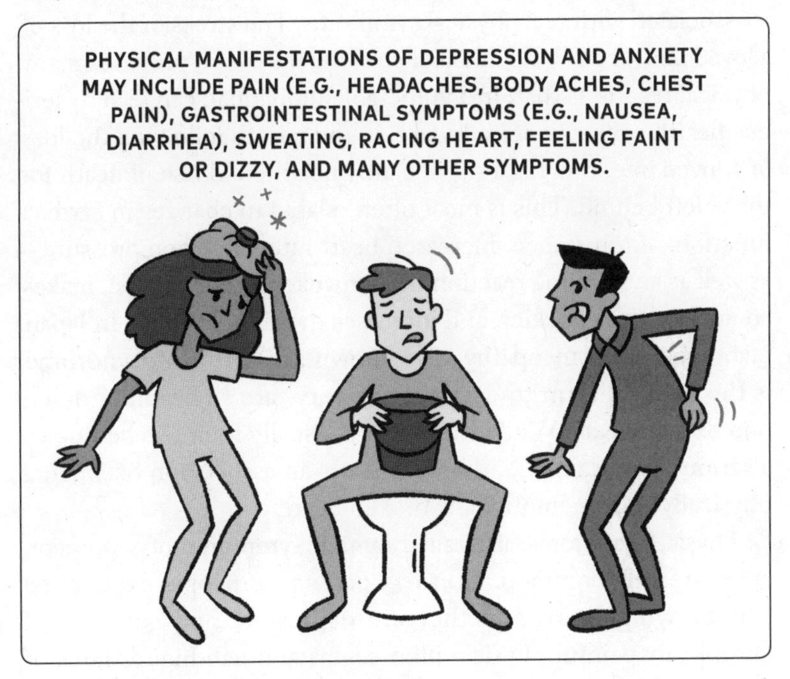

PHYSICAL MANIFESTATIONS OF DEPRESSION AND ANXIETY MAY INCLUDE PAIN (E.G., HEADACHES, BODY ACHES, CHEST PAIN), GASTROINTESTINAL SYMPTOMS (E.G., NAUSEA, DIARRHEA), SWEATING, RACING HEART, FEELING FAINT OR DIZZY, AND MANY OTHER SYMPTOMS.

Pain hurts, whether it's caused by arthritis or depression. Diarrhea is uncomfortable, unpleasant, and at times embarrassing, whether it's due to a virus or **anxiety**. The proof is in the toilet. The diarrhea is real. People living with depression or **anxiety** may experience an array of physical symptoms.

Why is depression associated with physical pain?

A depressed brain can't be disconnected from the rest of the body because the brain controls the body: each breath, every movement, every sensation occurs due to the coordinated activity of various brain structures. The brain sends information to and gathers information from the rest of the body via **neurons**, and that information is used to create what we see, hear, feel, think, and do. Pain is a psychological experience and does not require a physical injury, so pain truly is "all in your head," no matter the cause.

There's a reason we reflect on a serious loss as painful or heart-breaking: the emotional experience of being broken-hearted is associated with real physical symptoms. The **stress** of the loss of a loved one, or any kind of major stressful life event, provokes many physical reactions that, in a vulnerable individual, can lead to serious health consequences. In fact, in the month following the loss of a loved one, there is a significantly heightened risk of death for those left behind. This is most often related to changes in cardiac function—for instance, increased heart rate and blood pressure—as well as an immune reaction that provokes **inflammation**, makes your blood cells stickier, and increases the risk of stroke. In Japan, takotsubo cardiomyopathy, also known as heartbreak syndrome, is the medical term to describe the very rare situation of dying of a broken heart. While the death is usually found to be due to a serious physical issue, there is clearly an association between a physically and an emotionally broken heart.

Physical symptoms, also called **somatic symptoms**, of depression are extremely common. Up to 75 percent of people experience painful symptoms when they are depressed, and sufferers of chronically painful physical illnesses have much higher rates of depression. Because pain is such a profoundly distressing experience, the possibility that the cause of pain could be depression often isn't considered, so for at least half of those struggling with both depression and pain, the depression diagnosis is missed.

When accompanied by painful symptoms, depression is often more severe, more difficult to treat, more **chronic** (on average lasting six months longer), and more likely to recur. Furthermore, there is a clear correlation between the intensity of pain and the severity of depression symptoms. In my **clinical experience**, when someone is struggling with both **chronic** pain and depression, unless both are treated, neither will get better.

Much like depression has bio-psycho-social origins, so does pain. There are several biological reasons that might explain why pain and depression co-occur so frequently. Research has shown that depression is associated with an impaired ability to modulate pain, which means that *pain literally hurts more when you're depressed.*

Recall that the **amygdala**, which you learned about in chapter 4, is the brain region responsible for our rapid response to threatening or frightening experiences. It provokes a flight, fight, or freeze response when trying to keep us safe. We also know that the **amygdala** is over-activated in depressed and anxious brains, and an over-active **amygdala** can heighten pain intensity.

Furthermore, some of the same **neurotransmitters** implicated in depression are also essential for experiencing pain, especially **norepinephrine**. Chronically low levels of **norepinephrine** are associated with depression and **anxiety** symptoms. Some of the antidepressants that increase **norepinephrine** are very helpful for managing pain, even in the absence of depression.

Why is depression associated with an upset stomach and other bowel symptoms?

Gastrointestinal symptoms, sometimes called gut or bowel symptoms, refer to a variety of unpleasant physical experiences. Ricardo's diarrhea would be described as a functional gastrointestinal disorder (FGID). These are **chronic** or recurrent gut symptoms that are not explained by any medical cause. People who have a FGID have a hypersensitive gut and experience a range of symptoms that might include nausea, vomiting, bloating, diarrhea, constipation, and abdominal pain. Irritable bowel syndrome (IBS) is a well-known FGID, and more than 90 percent of people who struggle with IBS also have mood and **anxiety** symptoms.

Like depression and pain, the causes of FGIDs are also bio-psycho-social. Biologically, FGIDs are associated with **chronic stress**, and you will recall that **chronic stress** can provoke **inflammation.** However, in the case of FGIDs, the **inflammation** is in the gut and associated with immune cells, called **mast cells.** In situations of **chronic stress, mast cells** in the gut become activated, much like the activation of **microglia** in the brain associated with **chronic** depression and **anxiety.**

Activated **mast cells** release histamine, which has several functions in the gut. Histamine causes the release of stomach acid, but it also affects how the gut moves, which is called **gut motility.** Excessively increased **gut motility** causes diarrhea, and significantly reduced motility results in constipation. Histamine also causes the pain that is often associated with changes in **gut motility.** Anyone who has ever been **stressed** out before a major competition or career-impacting presentation doesn't need to be told that a high level of **stress** can cause changes in **gut motility.** But when under **chronic stress**, activated **mast cells** can cause unrelenting misery by provoking not only pain but alternating constipation and diarrhea.

Why are physical illnesses, such as obesity, diabetes, and heart disease, associated with depression?

A large body of research has demonstrated that depression is associated with a heightened risk of a variety of serious physical illnesses, such as obesity, **diabetes**, heart diseases, and other inflammatory illnesses. Moreover, people suffering from serious physical illnesses have higher rates of depression. Those who have multiple serious physical illnesses have a correspondingly greater risk of depression.

This mind-body association could be related to several factors, for instance, a treatment used to manage one illness could provoke the onset of another illness. This has been the case for some patients prescribed **atypical antipsychotics**, which are a type of medication sometimes used to treat severe depression. Older drugs of this type are known to increase the risk of obesity and **diabetes.** Additionally, dexamethasone, a steroid drug used to treat **acute** inflammatory illnesses, can provoke depression symptoms.

Another potential explanation for why mental and physical illness so commonly co-occur could be that the symptoms of one illness might provoke the onset of another illness. For instance, the apathy, disinterest, and fatigue associated with depression can result in reduced activity and a sedentary lifestyle, which might lead to weight gain and, ultimately, obesity and **diabetes.** Similarly, the fatigue and inactivity associated with a **chronic** medical condition, such as arthritis, may promote depression.

However, likely the most important common thread tying together mental and physical illnesses is **inflammation.** Major long-term studies of people who are not depressed, across a range of ages, have demonstrated that those with laboratory evidence of an inflammatory physical illness were at far greater risk for developing depression. A very large 2016 study compared the impact of **chronic** medical conditions, with and without **inflammation**, on the incidence of depression and found that there was an increased risk of depression only for those people suffering from illnesses that have an inflammatory component.

Our developing knowledge regarding the relationship between **inflammation** and depression might lead to new treatment options, especially for people suffering from medical illnesses. Some studies have found that the long-term use of **anti-inflammatory** medications, such as statins (used for high cholesterol) and aspirin, might provide some degree of protection against depression. Another large study found that nonsteroidal **anti-inflammatory** drugs (NSAIDs), which are used to treat inflammatory illnesses like arthritis, can improve depressive symptoms and promote **remission** of a depressive episode. Unfortunately, there is very little evidence that **anti-inflammatory** treatments help to reduce depression symptoms and promote **remission** in individuals who do not have a physical illness.

Depression and obesity

While most of us are aware that obesity is a risk factor for many serious medical illnesses such as **diabetes**, cancer, and heart disease, most are unaware of the association between obesity and many psychiatric illnesses, including depression, **bipolar disorder**, and **schizophrenia.**

Obesity rates in developed countries, like the United States and Canada, have skyrocketed over the past thirty years. At present, the diagnosis of obesity is based on body-mass index (BMI), which is calculated by dividing weight, measured in kilograms, by height, measured in metres squared. Obesity in adults is defined as a BMI of greater than or equal to 30. Seventy percent of American adults are now considered overweight (BMI score above 25). In 2017, the Centers for Disease Control and Prevention (CDC) released updated obesity rates. Overall, the **prevalence** of obesity (BMI > 30) was 39.8 percent in adults and 18.5 percent in those under age eighteen. Canadian data from 2014 showed that 40 percent of men and 27.5 percent of women were considered overweight, and 20.2 percent, roughly 5.3 million adults, were obese. Among women, the rate of obesity rose dramatically from 14.5 percent in 2013 to 18.7 percent in 2014.

TRENDS IN OBESITY PREVALENCE AMONG ADULTS AGED 20 AND OVER (AGE ADJUSTED) AND YOUTH AGED 2–19 YEARS

United States, 1999–2000 through 2015–2016

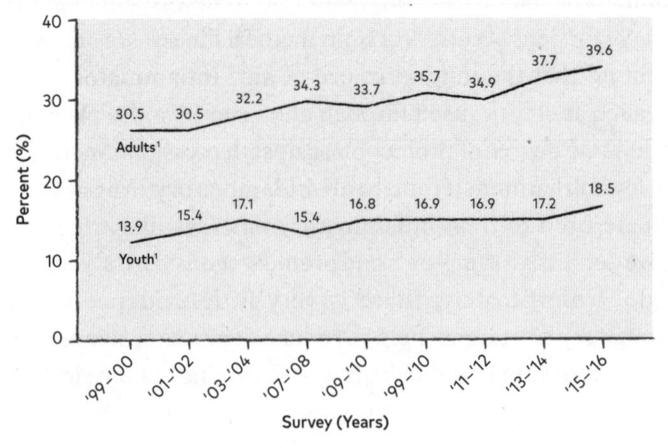

Source: Hales, C.M, et al. "Prevalence of obesity among adults and youth: United States, 2015–2016." *NCHS Data Brief* 288 (2017 Oct). cdc.gov/nchs/data/databriefs/db288.pdf.

Researchers have demonstrated that inflammatory processes underlie both depression and obesity in adults. A major population survey, published in 2014, found that 33 percent of US adults were obese, but that number increased to 43 percent for adults who were depressed. Depression severity was also clearly correlated with obesity risk, whether or not the person was taking antidepressant medication. However, the highest **prevalence** of obesity (54.6 percent) was found in people who had moderate to severe depression and were prescribed antidepressant medication, although the study did not make clear which came first, obesity or depression.

Depression and diabetes

Remarkably, the association between **diabetes** and depression was considered in the seventeenth century, when the English physician Thomas Willis suggested that those suffering from "significant life **stress**, sadness, or long sorrow" were more likely to suffer from **diabetes**. Patients with **diabetes** have approximately twice the risk of depression compared to non-diabetics, and many more diabetics will experience depression symptoms that might not reach the **DSM-5** threshold for a diagnosis but still cause them distress and worsen their **diabetes** control.

There are several reasons that might explain the heightened risk of depression and **diabetes co-morbidity**, but research suggests that childhood adversity, lifestyle choices, and obesity might be important risk factors for both disorders. Additionally, the complications associated with **chronic** depression and **diabetes** seem to heighten the risk of the other disorder.

When depression and **diabetes** co-occur, the prognosis is worse for both disorders, and their co-occurrence is associated with a higher risk of premature death. Diabetics who are depressed have higher rates of **diabetes** complications, poorer blood sugar control, reduced self-care (e.g., less exercise, poor diet, and reduced treatment compliance), and suffer from greater disability.

Disability refers to an individual's inability to perform normal daily activities that are necessary to meet their basic needs, fulfill their usual roles, and to maintain their health and well-being. One major study found that the degree of disability associated with **diabetes** was nearly 2.5 times higher than that of non-diabetics, and the disability associated with depression was three times higher than for non-depressed individuals. However, when depression and **diabetes** are both present, the level of disability soars to more than seven times higher than the disability experienced by people with neither disorder. Additionally, the treatment costs associated with **diabetes** and co-morbid depression are 4.5 times higher than the treatment of **diabetes** alone.

Depression and cardiovascular (heart) disease

Up to 50 percent of patients with **cardiovascular** disease have depression symptoms and up to 30 percent meet the **DSM-5** criteria for a major depressive episode. Large volumes of research have established a strong association between depression and increased disability and death after an **acute** cardiac event, such as a heart attack (also called a **myocardial infarction** or **MI**). The risk of death for patients with heart disease is further increased when depression is associated with **anxiety**, which is considered a risk factor for disability and death following a MI and other forms of heart disease. This heightened risk is perhaps because **anxiety** has been associated with increases in heart rate and abnormal heart rhythms. Interestingly, **anxiety** might cause cardiac patients to seek help for their symptoms, perhaps leading to an earlier diagnosis and lifesaving treatment.

As was discussed for both obesity and **diabetes**, the biology underlying the association between depression and heart disease suggests **inflammation** plays a key role. As an example, patients with heart disease commonly have an increase in a type of protein called natriuretic peptides (NPs), produced by the heart when it is stretched, which occurs in association with heart failure and other cardiac disorders. NPs cause reduced blood pressure and make the heart work harder, which is why high levels of NPs are correlated with the severity of heart disease. Researchers have also found that NPs are associated with emotional regulation and impact the activity of the HPA axis, which, as I discussed in chapter 4, plays a key role in the body's response to **stress** and the management of **inflammation.**

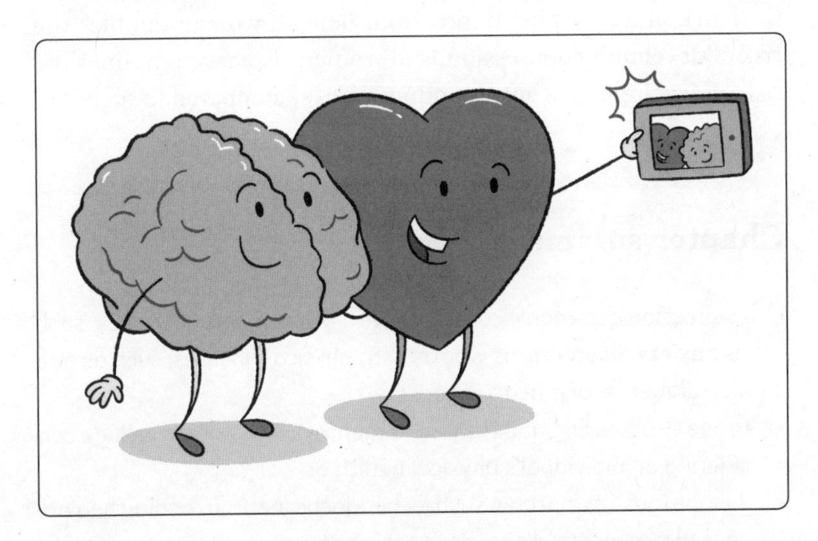

Cardiology research has firmly established the common co-occurrence of depression and heart disease, leading to a shift in the specialty, which has now recognized the importance of diagnosing and treating mental illnesses to improve **recovery** rates and maintain wellness among cardiac rehabilitation patients. Additionally, depression significantly increases the risk for rehospitalizations and death following cardiac bypass surgery. Accordingly, the American Heart Association (AHA) and the US Preventive Services Task Force recommend depression screening for all patients with heart disease. While screening doesn't appear to improve outcomes in people following heart surgery, offering treatment and support to cardiac patients with depression symptoms may improve their quality of life and reduce suffering.

Depression and autoimmune disorders

There is growing research evidence demonstrating the importance of the immune system in the development of depression. Having an autoimmune disorder, such as rheumatoid arthritis, significantly increases the risk of developing depression. Patients with rheumatoid arthritis or multiple sclerosis have a 50 percent lifetime risk of developing depression. Being a woman doubles the risk of developing depression, and women also have ten times the risk of developing an autoimmune disease, compared to men.

Chapter summary

- Depression commonly co-occurs with other mental illnesses, such as **anxiety disorders**, as well as with physical illnesses, such as obesity, **diabetes**, and heart disease.
- Properly assessing and treating a mental illness should include considering an individual's physical health as well.
- Just because symptoms such as headache, nausea, or diarrhea are caused by a mental illness does not mean the symptoms are not real.

If you or someone you love has physical symptoms that are not explained by a medical cause, it's important to consider whether depression or another mental illness could be the possible cause or a contributor.

A real patient's story

PEOPLE DON'T "GET" anxiety. By that, I mean they don't understand it. The general public, some of our friends and family, and even many in the medical profession fail to appreciate what those of us with anxiety are experiencing. We are labelled as "neurotic" and told we worry too much, the undertone being that we have a personality flaw. We are told that our thoughts are irrational—well, duh! Of course they are—that's what makes it a mental illness. If our thoughts were rational, we could just reason our way out of them—"put them in perspective" or "reframe" them. They would just be worry or **stress. Stress** and anxiety are not the same thing. It's been my experience that the amount of suffering that comes with an **anxiety disorder** is grossly underappreciated. Instead of being treated with compassion, we are often seen as an annoyance or even ridiculed. They just don't get it.

6

Are there sex differences when it comes to depression?

THIS WON'T BE a revelation: men and women are different. Sometimes it feels as though we're from different planets! Genetically, males are more like other males (99.9 percent) than they are similar to females (98.5 percent), which is the same percentage similarity males share with chimpanzees (98.5 percent). This figure explains the challenges we have understanding the opposite sex, but it also offers biological **insights** regarding our mental and physical differences.

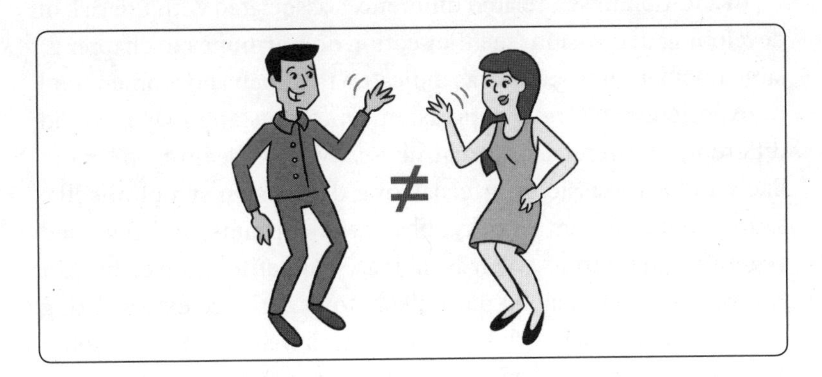

Writing about science, it can sometimes feel as though I'm making sweeping generalizations based on gender. In fact, considerations of sex and gender are relatively new in scientific research and the consideration of those who are gender non-conforming is virtually non-existent. But whether you're a woman who is more in touch with your masculine side or a man with a more feminine identity likely has nothing to do with your depression. Every person is a unique individual; their depression symptoms and response to treatment are unique to them, regardless of their sex or gender. However, based on massive population studies, our sex does impact the frequency of the disorder and may also affect how we experience depression.

Are there differences regarding how men and women experience depression?

You might recall from chapter 3 that we have twenty-three **chromosome** pairs and one of those pairs is made up of sex **chromosomes.** Because every cell has the same DNA, every cell in a woman's body has two X sex **chromosomes** and every cell in a man's body has an X and a Y. The Y **chromosome** contains a **gene** called SRY, which causes a fetus to become a male by developing testicles. But those sex **chromosomes** don't just work on the sexy body parts; they exert their effects throughout the body.

In addition to sex-related differences associated with the risk of developing depression (see the section on **hormones** in chapter 2), large population research has indicated that men and women tend to experience different depression symptoms and may respond differently to depression treatments. Women seem to be more likely to have classic or internalizing depression symptoms like sadness, **anhedonia, anxiety**, physical symptoms, and **reversed vegetative symptoms**, such as increased appetite and weight gain. Conversely, men may be more likely to experience externalizing symptoms, such as irritability and anger, as well as substance abuse and other addictive behaviours. In general, men tend to react more strongly to **stress** associated with failure and a lack of expected achievement, while women tend to react more strongly to **stress** associated with rejection or conflict. Additionally, women are also more likely to experience marital/relationship discord when depressed, while men may report more problems at work.

Interestingly, research has demonstrated that men tend to have a stronger physiological response to **stress** than women. This means that their brains and bodies react more powerfully to **stress**, by releasing higher levels of **stress hormones**, experiencing greater increases in heart rate and blood pressure, and by feeling more negative emotions or more feelings of aggression. While depression-related disability is similar regardless of one's sex, mortality associated with depression is higher in males, likely related in part to a higher incidence of completed suicide as well as greater health-related mortality in general. However, research has shown that higher mortality rates in men who are depressed are not completely attributable to suicide, higher rates of physical illness, or more substance abuse.

Much like how **puberty** heightens depression risk for women, the difference between the sexes regarding **stress** responses starts at **puberty** as well. Intriguingly, men's heightened response to **stress** might actually protect them from depression. As I described in chapter 4, **cortisol**, our major **stress hormone**, acutely buffers the brain from **stress** and promotes rapid brain **recovery** after a major emotional upset. Our body's most important **stress**-response system, the **hypothalamic-pituitary-adrenal (HPA) axis**, is responsible for regulating **cortisol** levels and tends to be under-reactive in people who are experiencing **chronic stress.**

Studies of the HPA axis in depression have revealed both over- and under-active responses to **stress**, and some researchers have also found possible sex differences in how the HPA axis responds during depression. For instance, women are at greater risk for **atypical** depression (see chapter 1), which is characterized by profound fatigue and **reversed vegetative symptoms**, such as increased appetite and sleeping excessively. **Atypical** depression is characterized by reduced HPA axis activity.

Do men and women respond differently to antidepressant treatments?

There have been many studies considering how men and women may respond to depression treatments differently. However, there is no consensus about whether certain antidepressants work better for men or for women. Several studies suggest that between **puberty** and **menopause**, women might respond better to treatments that preferentially target the **neurotransmitter serotonin**, while men and post-menopausal women might respond better to drugs that target **norepinephrine** and **serotonin** or **norepinephrine** alone. Additionally, post-menopausal women seem to respond less robustly to all antidepressants when compared with younger women.

Men absorb, distribute, metabolize, and eliminate medications differently than women do, which helps to explain why men and women also respond differently to many treatments. Studies evaluating new medications were historically limited to males, but with the recognition that male and female bodies manage medications quite differently, researchers now understand the need to assess drug response in both sexes carefully.

The following table demonstrates how male and female bodies manage drugs differently. After a drug is swallowed, it must then be absorbed. Absorption refers to moving a drug into the body: for instance, absorbing a drug from the stomach into the bloodstream, which is called gastric absorption. Drugs may also be absorbed through the skin or through a number of different routes. A drug that is given intravenously does not need to be absorbed, because it is injected directly into the blood.

Once a drug is absorbed, it then must be distributed around the body in order to have an effect where it is needed. Distribution refers to the movement of a drug around the body, to and from the blood and to tissues, such as the brain or to fat or muscle cells.

Some drugs cause an immediate impact when they reach their site of action, while other drugs need to be metabolized, which means they must be broken down into other compounds before they are effective. We have a system of enzymes that are necessary for drug **metabolism**, called the **cytochrome P450 enzymes** (CYP). While most people's CYP system works in a pretty standard manner, some of us have CYP enzymes that are much more active than usual (called rapid or extensive metabolizers), while others might have enzymes that function more slowly than usual (slow or incomplete metabolizers). CYP activity may be influenced by many factors, including sex, age, ethnicity, illness, drugs, and genetics. Most CYP enzyme occurs in the liver, the epicentre of drug **metabolism**, but these enzymes are also active in other areas of the body.

Finally, once you're finished with a drug, it should be eliminated from your body. Some drugs require further **metabolism** before they are eliminated, and most often, we get rid of them through two routes: through the urine or feces. This is why some drugs require a reduced dose or should be avoided in patients that have reduced renal (kidney) or hepatic (liver) function. If your kidneys are not working optimally, you might not be able to get rid of a drug that is usually eliminated via the urine. Likewise, if your liver isn't in top form, you might not be metabolizing medications adequately. Both situations can lead to an accumulation of the drug, which may in turn lead to serious side effects. To learn more about how you can determine your CYP enzyme activity, and how that might influence medication choices, see **pharmacogenomics** in chapter 12.

Activity	Gender difference	Impact on drug level in
Absorption		
Gastric absorption	Lower in women	Reduced
Gastric acidity	Lower in women	Increased
Intestinal transit time	Lower in women	Reduced
Distribution		
Body weight	Lower in women	Increased in women
Body fat	Higher in women	Reduced in women
Metabolism		
CYP450 enzyme activity	Some more active and others less active	Depends on the drug
Elimination		
Renal (kidney) elimination	Slower in women	Increased in women

Adapted from: Crawford, M.B., and DeLisi, L.E. "Issues related to sex differences in antipsychotic treatment." *Current Opinion in Psychiatry* 29 3 (2016): 211–7; Lange, B., et al. "How gender affects the pharmacotherapeutic approach to treating psychosis–a systematic review." *Expert Opinion on Pharmacotherapy* 18 4 (2017): 351–62; Marazziti, D., et al. "Pharmacokinetics and pharmacodynamics of psychotropic drugs: effect of sex." *CNS Spectrums* 18 3 (2013): 118–27.

Despite the sex differences with respect to depression risk, typical depression symptoms, and specific drug responses, men and women are similar regarding the likelihood that depression will become **chronic**, whether their symptoms are likely to resolve (**remission**), and whether they are likely to get sick again (**recurrence**).

Overall, there might be more differences than similarities for depression between the sexes, and these sex-related differences suggest that we should stop viewing depression in men and women as a single homogeneous disorder. While depression treatment must always be personalized for every individual, evidence suggests that a patient's sex should be a more important consideration than it has been historically.

Does pregnancy protect women from depression?

As any new parent will know, given the sleep deprivation, hormonal changes, breastfeeding challenges, and the need to recover from the physical aftermath of childbirth, it's little wonder some studies find that depression **prevalence** rates are slightly higher in the months following delivery. In fact, new mothers commonly report feeling joyful and exhilarated one moment and sad and tearful the next. Commonly referred to as baby blues, for most women this **postpartum** roller coaster quickly resolves in the first week or two following childbirth.

Unfortunately, some women do not experience a resolution of those early mood symptoms. **Peripartum** means "around the time of childbirth" and according to the **DSM-5**, **peripartum**-onset depression occurs during pregnancy or in the four weeks following delivery. However, doctors and researchers commonly extend the time, called **postpartum** onset, to up to twelve months after delivery. About 50 percent of what is called **postpartum** depression actually begins during the pregnancy, and one year after birth about 30 percent of women are still depressed. Pregnancy-related depression also carries a high risk of **relapse**.

Approximately 12 percent of women will experience a depression during their pregnancy, and up to 15 percent will experience depression in the **postpartum** period. These rates are similar to the rates for women who are not pregnant. If the rates of depression are not significantly higher for pregnant and **postpartum** women, it might provoke the question: why include **peripartum** onset depression in the DSM as a separate category? It was likely included to confront and debunk the long-held myths that pregnancy offers women protection against depression and that treating depression during pregnancy should be avoided because it might put a fetus at risk.

Using a huge Danish population database, researchers showed that during the first three months **postpartum** there was an increased risk of first-time psychiatric contact and hospitalization among first-time mothers, relative to women one year **postpartum**. However, overall the rate of psychiatric contact during pregnancy and between three and twelve months **postpartum** was lower than for non-pregnant women. In a large US survey, pregnant and **postpartum** women were also found to have either a lower or not significantly different **prevalence** of psychiatric disorders relative to non-pregnant women, with one exception: **postpartum** women had a greater risk of major depression.

By some estimates, suicide accounts for 20% of **postpartum** deaths and startlingly, it is the **second most common cause of mortality among postpartum women.** One large literature review found the **prevalence** of **suicidal ideation** among pregnant women is as high as 33%. Unfortunately, there has not been comprehensive, high-quality research that has allowed us to fully understand the risks of suicide during pregnancy. **Postpartum** suicidal thoughts, attempts, and completed suicide are often preceded by suicidal behaviours before and during pregnancy. Women remain silent about their emotional distress and see suicide as their only option for many reasons, but I believe that chiefly their deaths are a result of **stigma**, fear of judgment, and lack of access to empathic, appropriate care.

Abundant research evidence clearly indicates that pregnancy does not protect women from depression, and that depression during pregnancy and in the year following childbirth must be taken very seriously, for the health and safety of both the mother and the child. Untreated depression may affect fetal development and heighten the risk of physical and mental illnesses in the child, including impairing brain development.

Mothers who have pregnancy-related depression are more likely to have reduced access to healthcare, poor nutrition, poor parenting practices, marital discord, poor self-care, and higher rates of smoking and substance abuse (illicit drugs and alcohol). Depression is also associated with more pregnancy complications, including pre-term birth, reduced likelihood of breastfeeding, and difficulties bonding with the newborn. Sadly, due to shame, **stigma**, and the myth that they should be insanely joyful and deeply bonded to their new baby within moments of the birth, up to one-half of new mothers with **postpartum** depression are not diagnosed.

The risk factors for pregnancy-related depression are, like for every mental illness, bio-psycho-social. Many studies have found that a previous history of **anxiety** or depression is the strongest risk factor for a new onset of depression during pregnancy and in the **postpartum** period. Nearly one-half of women who develop depression during pregnancy have a history of depression. In fact, if a woman has no history of mental illness, that suggests she is more likely to recover from a pregnancy-related depression. If nearly one-half of this group of women have previously been depressed, that means more than half haven't had a previous depression, and research indicates that it is common for a first episode of depression to occur during pregnancy.

Depression and **anxiety** commonly co-occur during pregnancy and the **postpartum** period. High **anxiety** during pregnancy is one of the strongest risk factors for depression; women who are highly anxious are three times more likely to suffer from depression during pregnancy.

Pregnancy-related depression can appear indistinguishable from depression that occurs at other times of life; however, co-occurring **anxiety disorders** are marginally more common. Generalized **anxiety**, obsessive-compulsive symptoms, **panic attacks**, and **psychotic** symptoms are slightly more prevalent in pregnancy-related depression, especially when it starts during the **postpartum** period, compared to depression occurring at other times during a woman's life. **Postpartum** depression might also be associated with the onset of **bipolar disorder.**

Women with a history of childhood sexual abuse are twice as likely to develop depression during pregnancy and the **postpartum** period, but childhood abuse of any kind (sexual, physical, or emotional) has been identified as a particularly strong predictor of pregnancy-related depression and **anxiety.** Other factors—such as the mother's age, particularly if she is still an adolescent; whether the pregnancy was intended and desired; and whether violence or abuse is present in her life currently—are also important risk factors for pregnancy-related depression.

Drug and alcohol abuse has, not unexpectedly, been associated with depression during pregnancy and in the **postpartum** period. Perhaps more surprising is the association between cigarette smoking before and during pregnancy and **anxiety** and depression when pregnant. The association appears to be even stronger for heavy smokers. It is unclear whether smoking increases the risk of depression or if depression and **anxiety** make unhealthy activities such as smoking cigarettes more likely. Fortunately, women who quit smoking during pregnancy might reduce their risk of depression in the peri- and **postpartum** period.

While a woman's risk of depression is virtually the same whether or not she is pregnant or **postpartum**, new fathers are nearly as likely to screen positive for depression as new mothers. Researchers reviewed studies conducted between the first trimester of pregnancy and one year **postpartum** and found a paternal depression rate of 10.4 percent, which was more than double the twelve-month **prevalence** for men in the general population (4.8 percent).

Risk factor	During pregnancy and peripartum	Postpartum
Biological:		
Age	Older age Younger age (especially adolescents)	Chronic medical illness History of a mental illness
Genetic/hormonal risk		Multiple births (e.g., twins, triplets)
Mental illness		Multiple children already at home
Medical illness		Preterm birth
Complicated pregnancy		Low birth weight infant IVF
Psychological:		
High level neuroticism personality trait	**History of mental illness or substance abuse**	**Depression/anxiety during pregnancy**
Negative coping style/ low self-esteem	**Anxiety during pregnancy**	**History of mental illness, especially depression**
	Substance abuse during pregnancy	History of substance abuse/smoking
Prior mental illness or substance abuse		Family history of a mental illness Neuroticism Style/quality of parenting during childhood
Social:		
Financial stressors	**Domestic violence**	**Domestic violence/previous abuse**
Current or past exposure to trauma, violence or stress	**Major stressful life events**	**Major stressful life events**
Lack of social support	**Low socioeconomic status/unemployment (self or partner)**	**Lack of social support/low intimate partner support/single mother**
Intimate relationship conflict	Lack of social support/low intimate partner support/single mother Pregnancy unintended/ unwanted	Low socioeconomic status

Bolded text indicates factors associated with the greatest risk. Adapted from Biaggi, A., et al. "Identifying the women at risk of antenatal anxiety and depression: a systematic review." *Journal of Affective Disorders* 191 (2016) 62–77; and Howard, L.M., et al. "Non-psychotic mental disorders in the perinatal period." *Lancet* 384 (2014): 1775–88.

Another study found that the **prevalence** of depressive symptoms among expectant fathers was 9.8 percent before delivery and 7.8 percent in the post-natal period.

Researchers have noted that the quality of the relationship with the mother and **anxiety** regarding the birth were significantly associated with a father's depression symptoms. Rates of depression are higher for mothers than for fathers, but a mother's depression appears to be the greatest risk factor for paternal depression. Other risks include a father's history of severe depression and the presence of symptoms of depression or **anxiety** before the pregnancy. As with all mental illnesses, there are clearly bio-psycho-social risk factors underlying paternal depression. Biologically, fathers-to-be might be at increased risk during their partner's pregnancy due to recognized changes in a man's testosterone, **cortisol**, and prolactin levels during the pregnancy.

Just as maternal depression can have long-term implications on a child's mental and physical health, there is also evidence that paternal depression can impact a child's behavioural, emotional, and social functioning, as well as heightening the child's risk for mental illnesses in the long term. Thus, the American Academy of Pediatrics now recommends that both mothers and fathers be screened for depression during and after pregnancy.

Does menopause heighten a woman's risk of depression?

As I wrote in chapter 2 (see page 35), women have a heightened risk of depression that has been largely attributed to **estrogen.** Women's depression risk increases significantly at **puberty**, mirroring the dramatic increase in **estrogen** that occurs at that time, and persists until **menopause.** Interestingly, despite the equally dramatic drop in **estrogen** that occurs at **menopause**, women's increased risk of depression persists into old age.

A 2016 review of high-quality research evidence found that women who experience early **menopause** were at greater risk for depression later in life. The early loss of **estrogen**, whether it happens naturally or due to the surgical removal of the ovaries, is a risk factor for depression and might be an important consideration when choosing a treatment. For instance, **estrogen**-replacement therapy might be beneficial for women whose depression was clearly provoked by the onset of **menopause**.

Is PMS a psychiatric disorder?

Many women experience mood changes in the days before their menstrual period begins, often referred to as **PMS** or **premenstrual syndrome**, which is not a psychiatric diagnosis. However, some women experience symptoms before their period begins that are so severe and distressing they are unable to function. The diagnosis of **premenstrual dysphoric disorder** (**PMDD**) was added to the **DSM-5** to identify women who experience severe and functionally impairing mood symptoms in the week before their menstrual period begins. PMDD symptoms usually lessen as bleeding starts and resolve mostly or completely as the period ends. Up to 5 percent of women experience a depressed mood, severe mood swings, irritability, anger, and **anxiety** during the premenstrual period. Additionally, PMDD may be associated with other common depression symptoms—such as changes in sleep and eating patterns, fatigue, difficulty concentrating, and **anhedonia**—and physical symptoms, such as pain, bloating, or breast tenderness.

I discuss the treatment of pregnancy-related depression in chapter 15.

Chapter summary

- Men and women may respond differently to antidepressants, which is likely due to differences in how their bodies absorb, distribute, metabolize, and eliminate medications.
- Women have twice the risk of developing depression compared to men, and that heightened risk is mostly related to the direct and indirect effects of **estrogen**.
- Pregnancy does not protect women from depression. Peri- and **postpartum** depression must be taken very seriously, for the health and safety of both the mother and the child.

Depression in women and men may differ in terms of lifetime risk, symptoms, and response to treatment, yet too often both doctors and patients fail to consider the power of estrogen and how it can impact both body and mind.

A real patient's story

ONE OF THE worst parts of having depression is the belief that no one cares. It is particularly hard to escape this feeling if you have reached out for help in the past and it didn't work.

I would say to someone with depression to reach out again. I guarantee you that there are people who care. They might not be able to cure you, but they can make your life much, much better. Finding the right person might not be easy, but they do exist and are easier to find than you think. What's more, as strange as it might seem, they want you to contact them. They want to help. They are waiting for you to call. When all seems lost, please do something for me: reach out one more time.

“Unless
someone like
you cares a whole
awful lot, nothing
is going to get
better. It’s not.”

DR. SEUSS
The Lorax

7

If I am depressed, where can I find help?

ONE OF THE greatest barriers to depression **recovery** is finding the right help. Whether you're looking for help for yourself or someone you care about, it's far more difficult than it should be to access appropriate psychiatric and psychological care. In this chapter, I discuss who to ask for help, what to expect from the professionals you're working with, and how you should prepare for your work with a professional to ensure it is truly beneficial.

If I am depressed, who can I ask for help?

Fortunately, many types of professionals are trained to treat patients struggling with a mental illness. When you need help managing depression, finding the professional that is right for you is an important first step.

Family doctors, also known as general or family practitioners (GP or FP), are often the first point of contact for someone wishing to access psychiatric services. Most are highly skilled, compassionate, and interested in assessing and caring for their patients who have a mental illness. In fact, due to the high **prevalence** of mental illnesses, a significant proportion of most family practices involves diagnosing and treating them. Some doctors take extra training and provide talk therapy as well as medication management. Other GPs are less interested or comfortable with psychiatric care, which is often evident soon after their patient breaches the topic.

Like family doctors, nurse practitioners (NPs) receive varying degrees of psychiatric training and have different levels of interest in psychiatry. However, I have found them to generally be highly motivated to build their psychiatric skills and care for mentally ill patients. NPs can prescribe, but some jurisdictions limit their prescribing of certain psychiatric medications. Some NPs also take a special interest in providing talk therapy.

Psychiatrists are doctors who, after medical school, complete residency training to become a specialist in the treatment of mental illnesses. During training, psychiatrists learn to prescribe medications as well as develop talk therapy skills. While most offer both to varying degrees, some psychiatrists might limit their practice to prescribing, while others focus entirely on talk therapy. In most jurisdictions, a referral from a GP or NP is required to access a psychiatrist. GPs and NPs generally refer to a psychiatrist only after they have tried to manage their patient's illness and the treatment has not been successful, or if their patient is severely ill and requires urgent, complex care.

Psychiatrists, GPs, and NPs are the only mental health professionals allowed to prescribe psychiatric medications. However, psychotherapy, also known as talk therapy, has a great deal of evidence supporting its use for the treatment of some mental illnesses. There are many practitioners who are trained to provide talk therapy, but they differ in terms of training, expertise, and scientific knowledge, which is an important consideration when choosing a therapist. There are also many different types of psychotherapy, which I describe in chapter 13.

Psychologists are therapists who have either a master of arts degree (MA) in psychology or a doctorate (PhD) degree, which means they have earned the honorific "doctor." It can help to know that if your therapist has a Dr. before their name, they likely are a psychiatrist (a medical doctor) or have a PhD level of training. PhD psychologists have completed a lengthier, more arduous training program than psychologists who have a master's degree, which means they should have the highest level of expertise in their field. PhD psychologists are psychotherapy experts and have the training and expertise to make a formal diagnosis.

I have worked with some incredibly talented, highly skilled psychologists over the years, forming strong relationships based on mutual respect. Some, but not all, patients require medication to treat their depression, and talk therapy isn't for everyone—it's important that mental health professionals recognize the value both forms of treatment may offer. If you find yourself sitting in front of a psychologist who doesn't believe in medication, or a psychiatrist who doesn't believe in the power of talk therapy, I'd respectfully suggest you run in the opposite direction.

A skilled psychologist is an incredible resource. When I am able to partner with a patient and their psychologist, I know the journey will be easier for everyone. I wouldn't want to take an unnecessary medication, so I don't want anyone else to take medication that is not required either. If it's possible to overcome a mental illness with psychological treatment alone, that is the best possible approach. However, for those who require medication, most will experience benefits from talk therapy as well.

There are other degrees that provide psychotherapy training, for instance an MA or a PhD in counselling or counselling psychology. Additionally, some social workers and nurses with advanced degrees have taken extra training in a specific type of talk therapy and offer counselling services.

Some members of the clergy offer spiritual support to those who gain strength from their faith, life coaches can help with planning and organization, and peer support workers can instill hope and provide encouragement, all of which may be an important source of additional social support for an individual recovering from depression. However, unless they have received specialized training and have a professional degree to back them up, I encourage you to use caution when engaging these sorts of services for the treatment of a serious mental illness. In fact, excellent faith leaders, professional coaches, and peer supporters will insist upon appropriate mental healthcare before they are comfortable providing services and will not overstate their abilities or what assistance they can offer.

It is important not to underestimate the potential of talk therapy to offer great benefits but also to cause great harm. Do your homework, and steer clear of individuals who are not members of their professional licensing body, for instance, a provincial or state **College of Psychologists** or **College of Physicians**, when seeking treatment for a serious mental illness.

If you live in an underserviced area, look for resources online. Make sure you use reputable websites; try the resources page on a local **mood disorders** society website for recommended providers, websites, books, or other services.

Keep in mind that websites that rate professionals are not always accurate. They tend to attract people on the extremes of the spectrum (they often either adore or despise the professional), so use those sites with caution. Likewise, asking family and friends if they know a good psychologist is sometimes a useful approach, but you and your mother or friend are different people and might not agree on what "good" means.

What if the professional I chose isn't a good fit for me?

When seeking a mental health professional,[4] it's important to keep in mind that not everyone will be a good fit for you. While

4 For the purposes of the discussion that follows, when I refer to a health professional, care provider, **clinician**, or practitioner, I recognize these terms are applicable to any number of professionals who provide treatment for patients with a mental illness.

unprofessional or disrespectful conduct is clearly a bad fit, sometimes fit is purely a style issue: if you're a more serious sort of person, you might not appreciate a therapist with a more lighthearted manner. Other times, the professional might have expressed a view that you felt was offensive, behaved in a manner that was off-putting, or put out the wrong vibe, and it's hard to put your finger on why you're not feeling comfortable.

Whatever the cause, working with a professional who isn't a good fit will not help you move forward and recover. If you've come across a bad fit, that doesn't mean the right person isn't out there, and you shouldn't feel that it's wrong to try someone else. **A professional should only be concerned that you get the help you need, not whether you like them.** However, unless the fit is glaringly bad, it's sometimes worth giving a potential **therapeutic relationship** another try, because first impressions may be clouded by **anxiety** or a bad day, on the part of the patient or the professional. I know I have personally started off on the wrong foot with a patient, yet with the next visit it is clearer to both of us that we will be able to work well together.

What should I expect from a therapeutic relationship?

The relationship between a professional from any field of medicine and a patient is referred to as a **therapeutic relationship.** This interaction is critically important and powerful, involving shared responsibilities, appropriate boundaries, and the development of trust, respect, and empathy.

Expectations regarding the likely benefits and potential harms of treatment, as well as an estimated timeline, should be addressed at the outset of a **therapeutic relationship** and reassessed at regular intervals. For instance, Jane might be seeing a psychologist for an initial assessment to treat her social **anxiety** and expect that she'll be ready to give a speech, necessary for her next promotion, the following week. Following a careful assessment of Jane's concerns, the psychologist should make clear that her expectation is unlikely to be met, but that progress should be expected after a certain number of sessions, along with a description of what progress might look like.

Likely because of a lack of familiarity with the complexity of psychiatric illnesses, some patients and their loved ones might have expectations regarding the speed and effectiveness of treatment that are not attainable. Much like many medical illnesses, the time it takes for psychiatric treatments, whether medications or talk therapy, to be effective is based on many factors, including: the type and severity of the illness, the rapidity of the individual's response to treatment, and their sensitivity to side effects.

The dental world can offer examples of individual responses to treatment. Consider braces: some lucky people need them for a year and their teeth are perfectly straight. Others require dental extractions, sometimes even jaw surgery, and then years of appliances and braces to attain that perfect smile. Psychiatric and psychological treatments are no different: every individual has their own needs and successful treatment might take weeks, months, or years.

Your first few visits with a therapist, when engaging in talk therapy, might have a more casual feel and might lead some to wonder, *What am I paying for? They're just chatting with me.* However, when working with a skilled therapist, that time is an opportunity for them to get to know you, assess how you are coping and functioning, and build rapport. The interaction should leave you feeling heard and understood and give you a better sense of the therapist's approach and the path ahead. However, if you've experienced months of chit-chat with no sense of a plan or symptom improvement, that is unlikely to be an effective **therapeutic relationship.**

There is an inherent power differential in any therapeutic relationship and that necessitates a strict adherence to professional boundaries. The power difference between a healthcare professional and their patient arises from different sources. A professional will know much more about the patient than the patient knows about the professional. Some will share their personal experience or provide a few details about themselves, such as whether they have children, but many will share very little about themselves because they wish to ensure that the interaction with their patient is centred entirely on the patient's needs. Personal disclosures are usually limited and are used to build rapport or a sense of understanding with the patient, for instance, "I have a teenager myself, so I know how challenging the teen years can be for any parent."

Another source of the power differential is related to the duties of a professional. In the course of treatment, they might be required to make decisions that could deeply impact the patient's life, for instance, whether they can work or travel, whether they will receive disability benefits, or whether they should be hospitalized. While decisions such as these are best made by seeking a patient's understanding and agreement, sometimes a very ill patient might not be able to participate in the decision-making process. It is therefore necessary for the professional to be able to act in the patient's best interests, without regard to their own personal needs.

Consequently, personal, especially sexual, relationships are never appropriate between two people engaged in a **therapeutic relationship**. If boundaries are not maintained, the professional's interest may supersede or replace the best interests of the patient, which can lead to exploitation and cause great harm.

While both members of the **therapeutic relationship** are responsible for maintaining appropriate boundaries, a patient struggling with a mental illness is likely vulnerable and distressed, thus the professional is ultimately responsible for ensuring a strict adherence to boundaries. Any boundary issues should be addressed immediately, in an empathic but direct manner. A couple of examples of boundary issues might include contacting the professional outside of appointment times for non-urgent matters or making comments or gestures that are irrelevant or inappropriate (e.g., sexual or excessively personal).

It bears repeating that there is no place for a "consensual sexual relationship" or sexual contact of any kind within a

therapeutic relationship. Much like a child is incapable of consenting to a sexual relationship, a patient is also considered unable to consent. Due to the power differential between professionals and their patients, governing bodies, such as **Colleges of Physicians or Psychologists**, have determined that sexual involvement is harmful to patients, even if the patient is an adult and capable of consent. Terminating a professional relationship to pursue an intimate relationship with a patient is also considered unethical.

Confidentiality is a key factor in the development of trust within a **therapeutic relationship.** The information shared by a patient must be kept in strict confidence and not disclosed to anyone unless there is explicit consent from the patient, if the patient is an imminent risk to themselves or others, or by a court order. However, physicians can communicate with a referring physician (for instance, a psychiatrist writing a clinical note to the referring family doctor). Additionally, in a hospital or community mental health team setting, **clinicians** from different specialities who are directly involved with a patient's care (e.g., doctors, nurses, social workers, occupational therapists) can communicate without specific consent from the patient. Those caregivers are within a circle of care, working as a team to help a patient recover. Some professionals, such as psychologists, have different rules regarding the sharing of patient information, and those rules should be understood at the beginning of a **therapeutic relationship.**

Respect is the cornerstone of any **therapeutic relationship** and it should be bidirectional. For instance, patients should arrive on time and the professional should adhere to their scheduled appointment times. While it's important to remember that sometimes when a patient is highly distressed or ill, scheduled appointments can run overtime, an ongoing pattern of extreme lateness on the side of a practitioner is discourteous and unprofessional. **Chronic** lateness on the part of a patient is likewise rude and is sometimes grounds for ending a **therapeutic relationship.**

Unfortunately, respect is sometimes missing within our medical system. Patients struggling with a severe mental illness are often highly vulnerable and they are not always treated with respect and dignity when they seek help. At times, their rights are removed unfairly, for the sake of expediency rather than for a real medical need or for safety. I have personally witnessed the derogatory, stigmatizing behaviour of a few of my colleagues, both fellow doctors and allied health professionals.

Treating patients in an inappropriate, disrespectful, or humiliating fashion is unacceptable and should be reported to a licensing body (e.g., the respective **Colleges of Physicians and Surgeons, Psychologists, Nurses,** or Social Workers) or the health authority. In reality, it is relatively rare for patients who have a mental illness to formally report abuse they suffered within the healthcare system. Those who are the most vulnerable are also the least likely to speak out, whether due to fear of retribution or loss of confidentiality, or because they are certain they will not be believed. It's important to note that family members and friends also have the right to send a letter of complaint to a professional body and may also choose to go to the media, if they're not satisfied by the response to their complaint.

How should I prepare for my first appointment to discuss my mental health?

Before your first visit with a new mental health professional, consider writing down your concerns in point form, so you don't forget anything that's important. If you're not sure you're able, consider asking someone to help you. You can also use your notes as a script, if you get emotional or feel overwhelmed, and it will allow you to get your experiences straight in case you're feeling under pressure to tell your story in a limited time. Have a list of previous times when you've had a similar problem and how you managed (e.g., medication, talk therapy, or no treatment).

If you're taking any medication, write down the name and dose or bring the medication with you. If you don't already know your family health history, ask a family member if anyone else has had a similar health concern.

Some people want to bring along a family member or friend, whether for support or, if required, to supply **collateral information. Collateral information** refers to information supplied by someone who knows you well, who can help a mental health professional to better understand your experiences or symptoms. This information is usually, but not always, provided by a family member or close friend.

Gathering **collateral information** is a challenging issue in psychiatry particularly, because sometimes a seriously ill patient will lose **insight**—they are so unwell that they don't realize how seriously ill they are. While this rarely happens in depression, it may, especially when the illness is very severe or when there are **psychotic** symptoms. Bipolar I disorder is also commonly associated with a loss of **insight**. In these situations, **collateral information** is invaluable. However, adults often don't want friends or family members to speak about them to a doctor or anyone else, especially if they don't believe they are ill.

As mentioned earlier, healthcare professionals are not legally allowed to share personal health information with anyone else, unless they have secured a patient's informed consent, the patient is at imminent risk, or by court order. Professionals can, however, receive information from a concerned family member or friend, without sharing any confidential information about their patient.

Collateral information is not just important for those who lack **insight**. Sometimes patients, for many reasons, understate their symptoms or don't recognize that their symptoms are as noticeable or severe as do the people who care about them. They might know they're ill but might not realize that their family is deeply concerned about their drinking or their irritability, for instance. A health professional should have this information, because it is essential for planning an approach to treatment.

Some professionals resist the presence of collateral sources, and sometimes that resistance is rational and necessary. For instance, if Mamta attends her appointments with her mother, and her mother does all the talking, or Mamta relies on her mother to speak for her without expressing herself, Mamta's mother might not be welcome to attend her appointments. Hopefully, in this situation, Mamta's doctor would take responsibility for creating an appropriate environment; however, this example does highlight a common challenge. It is important to respect a patient's requests in a **therapeutic relationship**, but if their request is standing in the way of progress, the issue must be thoughtfully considered and discussed.

More often than not, collateral sources are of value for the reasons mentioned above, as well as because the patient's friends and family might be more supportive of their treatment if they are able to meet with the professional and are helped to understand the decision-making process. Otherwise, they may undermine the **therapeutic relationship**, even unwittingly, by being critical of the treatment plan because they don't understand why decisions were made.

How does my doctor or psychologist know I am truly depressed?

> Eloise went to her family doctor because she was feeling hopeless. In fact, she had fleeting thoughts of suicide over the last few months, since she found her husband in bed with her best friend. Since the day she discovered their affair, she has had to start divorce proceedings, manage her own finances for the first time in her life, and cope with three young children who miss their father, all without the support of the two people she loved and trusted most. "I don't think I can go on living," she told her doctor. "I feel so lost. I'm devastated." Her doctor was not sure how to proceed, telling her, "I think anyone in your shoes would feel pretty terrible. Maybe this is something that has to run its course."

Medical illnesses, such as **hypertension** and high cholesterol, are often far easier to diagnose and treat than mental illnesses because doctors make the diagnosis and base their treatment choices on objective tests, such as blood pressure or cholesterol levels in the blood. In psychiatry, we have diagnostic guidelines such as the DSM-5 (see chapter 1), but the DSM-5 only provides lists of symptoms. Unfortunately, there are no evidence-based objective tests that can conclusively determine the presence or severity of a mental illness. There is no lab test, MRI scan, or electrical recording of the brain that can tell her doctor, "Eloise is depressed." They must rely on her subjective description of her symptoms, their own **clinical experience** talking to and treating depressed patients, and **clinical rating scales**, which can help to determine if an illness exists, its severity, and how to approach treatment.

Subjective experience of depression

It's important for Eloise's doctor to listen to and understand her subjective experience, but Eloise's account of her experience may also have some limitations as her doctor tries to gauge the severity of her symptoms. Eloise's current personal circumstances greatly impact how she experiences her symptoms. She's just lost her husband and best friend through a terrible betrayal that has left her alone and humiliated, and perhaps financially destitute. Who wouldn't feel depressed? But feeling depressed and unhappy isn't the same as having a DSM-5 diagnosis of major depression. To have a depression diagnosis, she must have a constellation of symptoms and resulting functional impairment.

Our subjective experience is, well, subjective. It's a reflection of everything that's happening to us at the time we're sharing an experience: anything from getting a divorce to stubbing a toe or finding a twenty-dollar bill on the sidewalk can impact what we feel, say, and do. Given that, Eloise's doctor must consider her subjective experience thoughtfully.

Do people struggling with a mental illness tend to embellish (overstate) or downplay (understate) the severity of their symptoms? Most people who aren't patients themselves say, "Overstate." Their impression is that people who are depressed tend to whine and focus only on themselves and how miserable they feel. Others believe that many people who claim to have a mental illness are lying to avoid their responsibilities. This view can reduce the likelihood that a patient will be willing to disclose their suffering, especially to colleagues, and represents a common stigmatizing experience, which I explore further in chapter 9. Importantly, research indicates that people who have a mental illness are just as likely to understate their symptoms as they are to embellish.

Often my patients tell me they're worried they might be overreacting, that their symptoms "aren't that bad," or that they should be able to "get over it." They're embarrassed by their illness and don't want anyone to know they're sick, including people very close to them. As a result, they might focus only on their physical symptoms and ignore their mental health, or they might attempt to ignore their illness entirely, resulting in its progression. Others are so fearful they won't be believed—and that, as a result, help will not be offered—that they overstate the severity of their symptoms. Some people lie about having a mental illness for secondary gain, for instance to obtain disability benefits or to avoid responsibility for criminal behaviour, but **malingering** or feigning illness is relatively rare outside these situations.

A professional's clinical experience

A professional's **clinical experience** is invaluable in helping to determine whether someone has less severe mood or **anxiety** symptoms associated with an emotional stressor or whether they have a diagnosis of major depression. Their **clinical experience** can help them to assess their patient's subjective experience; however, **clinical experience is also subjective.** Most of us want to see a health professional who has assessed and treated many patients with similar issues, yet professionals have the same challenges as other human beings and are fallible. We can focus on what we expect to see and exclude the unexpected, or make determinations before gathering all the necessary evidence, because of what we've seen before.

Measurement-based care

Because there are no blood tests or brain scans we can use to diagnose depression, we often rely on **clinical rating scales** to help to fill in some of the information gaps and more objectively assess the presence and severity of the illness. These extensively studied checklists do not replace a patient's words or a professional's **clinical experience**, but evidence clearly demonstrates that using a clinical scale, which is also referred to as measurement-based care, improves the likelihood of treatment success.

There are many validated clinical scales for depression. Validated means the scale has been used to assess large numbers of people and has been found to be sensitive (likely to correctly identify people who are ill) and specific (likely to correctly identify people who are not ill), reducing the risk of misdiagnosis. Additionally, some scales are patient administered, meaning they are completed by the patient, while others are **clinician** administered, which means the healthcare professional asks the questions and rates the response. These are not 100 percent objective measures, because the responses are open to a patient's or a professional's interpretation.

Depression rating scales are often designed to determine illness severity, and quantifying severity can help a **clinician** decide whether exercise, talk therapy, or medication might be the appropriate treatment to suggest to their patient. For instance, had Eloise's doctor suggested she complete a Patient Health Questionnaire (PHQ-9), one of the most user-friendly **clinical rating scales** for depression, he would have learned that she has a score of twenty, which suggests she has a severe depression and requires treatment immediately.

Furthermore, some depression scales can help determine how a patient is responding to therapy. For instance, if Eloise is prescribed a medication and three weeks later the PHQ-9 score has not improved, that medication was either not taken properly (or at all), needs to be increased, or isn't working and should be changed.

Finally, **clinical rating scales** can offer a sense of hope. Sometimes severely ill patients will respond very slowly to treatment or it might be difficult to find an effective treatment. Patients have said to me, after months of trying to find an effective treatment, "I am no better." Commonly, if we redo the PHQ-9, the questionnaire results will show there is a change. Certainly, if they still are not feeling well, we haven't reached the goal of **recovery**, but if the score went from twenty to twelve, it's reassuring to be able to say, "You're right that you're not all better, but we're moving in the right direction. Let's keep looking to find the right treatment for you."

Importantly, because clinical scales do not replace clinical judgment or experience, no one should rely on a PHQ-9 alone to make a depression diagnosis. Patients who are positively screened for depression using a PHQ-9 should then be offered a psychiatric assessment by a qualified professional.

A typical psychiatric assessment

In a typical psychiatric assessment, a health professional gathers relevant information to determine whether there is a diagnosis and its severity, and, based on that information, what the treatment plan should be moving forward. Some initial interviews are quite structured, which is most common in an initial psychiatric assessment. Other initial interviews, especially when the approach to treatment is talk therapy, might be more casual and have less of a "medical feel." A typical psychiatric interview includes the patient's subjective experience and uses the professional's **clinical experience** to answer the following questions.

Who are you? Your age, sexual orientation, marital status, whether you have children, current living situation (where and with whom), where you work or go to school (or, if you're retired, what your occupation was), and educational level. Some might want to mention their religious faith, cultural or ethnic background, or gender identity, if that feels important when answering this question.

What's going on right now? Current symptoms and how they are affecting your life, including their functional impact at home, work, school, and socially. Current life stressors, including work, school, financial, legal, health, or family issues. Current treatments, including talk therapy, psychiatric medications, and alternative treatments. If there is a current treatment, how is it helping and are there any side effects? What is your current support system and is it working for you?

Has this happened before? Previous psychiatric history, previous treatments, and the response to those treatments.

Any other important information. Current and past use of tobacco, alcohol, or illicit drugs and other addictive behaviours (e.g., gambling, gaming); a history of a serious traumatic event; information about childhood and school years. Family psychiatric history.

Are there any medical issues? Physical health (past and present, including past and current treatments); a history of head injury; menstrual cycle/**menopause** and current sexual health; family history of physical illness; level of physical activity; history of obesity.

In chapter 5, I discussed the mind-body connection and the fact that mental and physical illnesses commonly co-occur. As a result, a psychiatric assessment should include a discussion about physical health. Furthermore, physical illnesses can also be the cause of psychiatric symptoms. For instance, thyroid disorders (e.g., hypothyroidism), low iron (iron deficiency anemia), and obstructive sleep apnea can cause **chronic** exhaustion and mood changes. It is the standard of care for physicians to evaluate not just mental but also physical health when diagnosing a mental illness. This usually requires a lab workup and might include a screening test to determine the presence of illicit drugs, if drug abuse or dependence is an issue.

Treatment goals. What are your goals for treatment?

An example of a typical psychiatric history

Eloise is a forty-two-year-old woman from Shady Creek, where she lived, until recently, with her husband, Mac, and their three children, Doug (six), Glenda (two), and Maxi (six months). Eloise is a licensed auto-mechanic, and she and Mac own a paint and autobody shop, where she works forty to fifty hours per week. The children were cared for by Mac's mother on workdays; however Mac and Eloise recently separated, and his mother is no longer willing to provide childcare.

Eloise was referred by her family doctor with complaints of sadness and loss of interest in most activities over the last few months. She reported that her symptoms coincided with discovering her husband in bed with her best friend. Since the day she discovered their affair, she has had to start divorce proceedings, manage her own finances for the first time in her life, and cope with their three young children who miss their father, all without the support of the two people she loved and trusted most.

Eloise described herself as feeling "lost and devastated." She said she's never felt this way before. She's now having difficulty getting to sleep and staying asleep, she's lost twenty pounds, and her appetite is poor. She said she is feeling hopeless and worthless, and she described passive suicidal thoughts. She denied an active suicidal plan, stating, "I could never leave my children." She is also struggling with her memory and finds it difficult to follow conversations, which was never an issue in the past.

Initially, her family doctor recommended talk therapy, but Eloise didn't feel the psychologist was a good fit. She said she was unable to focus during sessions or follow through with homework. Now, her sadness and anxiety are so severe that she has taken time off work. She feels she might need medication and her family doctor wasn't sure it was necessary.

Eloise has a history of hypothyroidism and is prescribed Synthroid 0.05 mg daily. She takes no other medication. She has regular menstrual periods and had three normal pregnancies. All three of her children are healthy. She is a non-drinker and quit smoking seven years ago when she was pregnant. She smoked cannabis as a teen, but she has abstained from all drugs since she was in her early twenties.

Eloise's maternal grandmother had depression and was treated with medication, although she's not sure of the name. No one else in her family, that she's aware of, has had a mental illness.

She described her childhood as happy and peaceful, and she denied any childhood traumatic events. She has loving parents and they have been providing her with support and encouragement over the past several difficult months. She described her current relationship with Mac as acrimonious. She has a few close friends she tries to stay in touch with, but the loss of her best friend since childhood, along with her husband, has been a terrible blow.

Eloise is certain she is depressed. She wants to get better and feels she gave talk therapy an adequate trial but she's still not well. In fact, she says she is steadily feeling worse. She would like to learn more about other types of treatment for depression.

Chapter summary

- Help may take many forms, but a qualified professional is required to accurately diagnose and, depending on the severity, develop an appropriate treatment plan for managing depression.
- It's essential to have a good fit with your mental health professional.
- Strong boundaries help to create healthy and productive **therapeutic relationships**.
- Your subjective experience, your doctor's **clinical experience**, **clinical rating scales**, and a thorough interview are part of a complete psychiatric assessment.

The first line of depression defence is a family doctor, who can diagnose and provide treatment or, based on an individual's needs, make a referral for appropriate treatment. If you don't have a family doctor, reach out to the mental health services in your community. There are many listed at the end of the book in appendix 1.

A real patient's story

HOW CAN YOU help a friend or family member with depression? The single best thing a person can do is listen. If you think of depression as an abscess, a person can't "snap out" of an abscess. An abscess won't disappear by taking a vacation or counting blessings. Draining the abscess can be helpful for some people, by listening to your friend or loved one's experience. Some severely depressed people are very reluctant to talk about their situation for fear that they will be rejected, because they don't have the energy to start talking, or because they are convinced that no one cares.

Most importantly, to help someone you care about, stop talking. Just listen. The less you say, the better. The person might not answer immediately. They might not answer for many minutes. Perhaps they need to decide whether to trust you or gather enough energy to begin talking. Sit quietly and give your full attention to the person.

At some point, the person will likely stop talking for a while, perhaps to confirm that you are not judging or contradicting them. During this pause, sit quietly and continue to give the person your full attention. Use your body language to show your concern, to show that you are giving them your complete attention, and that you are listening. Empathic statements might be appropriate, such as "I had no idea you were going through this. This must be very difficult for you. I can't imagine how hard this must be for you." Reassure that person that everything they say to you will be kept confidential—and then be very sure to live up to your promise.

Never underestimate how powerful listening can be. The person might not show it, but they will feel better after speaking with you. They won't be cured, but they might be strong enough to make it through the rest of the day. Having someone listen to me was the first and most important step on my road to stability.

8

How do I talk about depression?

COMING TO TERMS with a diagnosis of depression can be a difficult journey, and the path is different for every individual. Some people are more open by nature, so if they're feeling consistently sad or down, or if they're concerned they might be depressed, they might quickly and candidly reach out to friends, loved ones, or their doctor. However, for many people the idea of talking to someone about their depression is daunting, even frightening. They might worry that they'll be judged or feel humiliated, or perhaps they'll be told they're overreacting or that they need to snap out of it. Once the diagnosis is confirmed, many will then need to address their illness with others, including their employer, which is, for many, another daunting task.

In this chapter, I consider the challenges of speaking to friends, family, doctors, insurers, and employers about depression or any mental illness. While everyone has their own unique circumstances, over my years of practice I have learned some approaches to these situations that might make them at least more tolerable and at best help to shore up support from those you might never have expected would understand and care.

How do I talk to my doctor about depression?

Desiree finally made an appointment with her family doctor, after putting it off for months. When the receptionist asked about the reason for the appointment, she said, "Back pain." However, as soon as her doctor closed the door and asked, "How are you doing?" Desiree began to cry. Her doctor became noticeably uncomfortable. When she said she was feeling "pretty blue" and she wasn't sleeping well, her doctor said, "We all have bad days sometimes." When she said she was feeling down almost every day for the last five or six months, he thumbed through her chart and said, "Let's get some lab work done and I'll see you when I get the results" and hurried off to see the next patient. Desiree left feeling disappointed in her doctor and in herself.

Most people struggling with depression will never have an opportunity to be assessed and treated by their doctor, either because they don't ask for help or they ask for help and the person they asked shuts them down. Deciding to speak up and ask for help is a critical first step in the process of recovering from depression. By reading this book, you'll see that depression is a real, serious illness, and help is available and worth asking for.

If you find yourself asking for help and feeling shut down, ignored, or dismissed, please ask someone else. Or, if there is no one else to ask, arm yourself with information, whether from this book or another reputable source, and ask again, this time more forcefully.

Ask your doctor for help by speaking directly. Outline your symptoms and their duration; for instance, "I have been feeling sad, down, disinterested, and crying a lot for the past few months." It's also okay to tell them, "I read about depression and I think that might be what I am experiencing." You can download and fill out a depression clinical rating scale, such as the PHQ-9, which I described on page 128. Bringing along a supportive friend or family member might help you to feel more comfortable and they can also provide **collateral information** to your doctor. Ask your doctor to refer you to a colleague or a psychiatrist if they're not willing to help. **It is your doctor's professional responsibility to provide you with appropriate care. If they are not comfortable providing that care, they must help you find someone who is.**

"Priceless pearls" for an excellent working relationship with your mental health professional

Whether you're just starting the treatment process and you have follow-up appointments with the person who is prescribing for you or providing talk therapy, the most important thing you can do is to be engaged and informed. My priceless pearls of wisdom for an excellent working relationship with your mental health professional include:

1. Before the first appointment, **write a point-form narrative of your symptoms and how they are impacting your life.** If you have **cognitive** symptoms that are making memory, motivation, and organization a challenge, consider asking a trusted friend or family member to **write your story down for you** as you dictate your experience. This can be valuable for your doctor, especially if it is in point-form, as well as for you when you're providing information to insurance companies or your HR department.
2. **Consider keeping notes between appointments.** A fifty-cent scribbler will do, so long as you keep it up-to-date and remember to take it along to your appointments. Recently it's become more common for people to use their phone to take notes.
    a. Before appointments, **think about how you're feeling,** both from a depression symptom perspective and, if you're taking medication, a treatment side effect perspective. Then write yourself a note in point form and bring it along. Better yet, use your mood tracker regularly (see appendix 2) and bring it along to your appointments.
    b. **If your therapist has given you homework, try your best to complete it.** They might ask you to complete specific tasks

("homework"), such as practicing CBT or keeping a mood tracker. In addition to doing your homework, note how it went. If you cannot complete your homework, write down why not, so your therapist will understand your treatment barriers and will be able to change the approach to improve your success.

c. During the appointment, **write down your doctor's suggestions.** If you aren't comfortable taking notes, **ask your doctor to write down their suggestions** in point form as they are speaking to you.

d. If you wish to **record the session**, for instance on your phone, please ask for permission, since recording without consent is offensive to many professionals and could lead to a break in your **therapeutic relationship.**

e. I often ask my patients, **"How do your friends/loved ones feel you're doing?"** If you don't know how people close to you feel you're doing, you should ask them.

f. **If you are prescribed medication,** know the names, the doses, what they do, and (if applicable) why you changed from one treatment to another.

g. Have your **pharmacy name, phone number, and fax number** accessible in your notebook or phone. It's a huge timesaver for your doctor.

3. If you don't wish to write down information about your medications, **bring them to your appointments with you** or take pictures of your bottles. Remember that your doctor will need to know *all* the medications you're taking, as well as any supplements, not just the psychiatric medications.

4. **Bring along a friend or family member**, if you feel that would be beneficial. **Collateral information** can be very helpful for your doctor (see page 124), but the accompanying person will also get a better sense of what the doctor is doing and why, increase their knowledge about the illness and treatment, and ask questions, all of which might encourage them to provide you greater support.

How do I talk to my family and friends about my depression?

Jenna Inski's uncle, I'll call him Bud Inski, was the family's resident expert on everyone else's life. When Jenna sold her house, he asked, "What price did you get?" and then, "I guess you waited to sell until the market was low, eh?" He had opinions on her boyfriends, carb versus protein diets, politics, and mental illness. When Jenna spoke of her treatment for depression, Bud Inski chimed in to remind the family that depression treatments are no better than taking a **placebo**, and he had never been depressed because of his daily mega-doses of vitamin C and echinacea. "How many of those pills are you taking anyway?" he asked her. When Jenna sheepishly admitted she was taking three medications since she was discharged from hospital, Bud Inski gasped. "That's way too much. It's those pills, not depression, that's gonna kill you!"

Patients often ask, "How do I talk to my family and friends about my depression?" and I now know that there are as many answers as there are families and friends. How to talk to family and friends depends mostly on whether they are usually supportive and understanding; if they aren't, perhaps they don't need to know anything about your depression. Importantly, it's up to every individual to decide if they wish to share, because like any personal medical issue, patients should feel completely in control of whether and how their private information is shared.

Learning to create clear, appropriate boundaries is an essential life skill, but if you've never been taught how to do so, it's a skill that's difficult to learn when you're depressed. Unless you have a very close and supportive family member or friend as a guide, a trusted professional might be helpful in developing a strategy for dealing with the unsupportive, the butt-in-skis (or in Jenna's case, Uncle Bud Inski), and the "Why not just try eye of newt? It worked for my best friend's second cousin" in your social circle.

Consider how inappropriate and rude it is for anyone to offer their opinion about the type and number of medications you are prescribed, when they have no knowledge or any way to evaluate medications or treatment combinations. Did Bud Inski's awareness of Jenna's three medications provide any profound **insight**? No. It just caused Jenna to doubt herself, her doctor, and her treatment.

If you have those sorts of people in your life, it is usually best to clearly and directly let them know that their input is not required. You don't have to be nasty, but your intention needs to be crystal clear. Saying, "Thank you for your thoughts, but I am working with a professional and I am going to follow their recommendations," should be all that is required. After that, there is no need to engage further on the topic of your depression. If you're asked further questions, it's fine to say, "I'd rather not talk about it" or "I'd rather not say."

If you've missed social events or another activity due to your depression, what should you say? If you're asked about your absence by someone who you're not particularly close to, don't feel the need to share your personal medical information. "I had a medical issue" is all that is required. Anyone who responds by asking, "What kind of medical issue?" is very rude, and the only answer I can think of, other than, "That's none of your business," is "explosive diarrhea." Usually people don't lean in after you drop that line and say, "Tell me more."

I wrote this book for those suffering from depression but equally for those who love someone who is depressed or just wants to learn more. Education builds understanding, so sharing this book or other reputable resources can be helpful in getting family members and friends "on side." Eventually, if they're not coming to understand that depression is real and serious and needs to be treated, it might be time to stop talking to them about it and find another means of support. This is often much easier said than done, but if you're committed and confident that you've chosen the right path to **recovery**, please don't let some misinformed, uneducated person—no matter how much they might care—derail your journey.

Someone I care about has been diagnosed with depression. How can I help?

If someone you care about has shared their depression diagnosis, the most important thing you can do is show compassion. Saying, "I'm sorry to hear that. I know depression is a really difficult illness to endure" immediately tells them that you understand depression is a real, serious illness and that you care.

Sometimes such a personal disclosure may lead even the closest friend or loved one to withdraw, perhaps because they're fearful they'll say the wrong thing, or because they have no idea what to say. However, ignoring someone's disclosure about their mental illness can make them feel much worse, because they might then feel they are a burden and become further isolated and hopeless. In my experience, **showing compassion and caring is never the wrong move.**

However, it is possible for well-meaning friends and family to make comments that are deeply hurtful, if they are sending the message that depression is the patient's fault. Comments like, "How can you be depressed when you have such a great life?" suggest the patient is somehow responsible for their illness. Likewise, offering unsolicited advice, especially if it has to do with the actual treatment of depression, can be harmful and even derail the **recovery** of a person struggling with depression.

Your friend or loved one might not want or need your help but will always benefit from your compassion and understanding. If they're already receiving professional care and they're working hard on their wellness, they might not want their relationship with you to become tangled up in their treatment. The normalcy of a supportive relationship might be all that is needed and is, indeed, a valuable gift.

Once someone you care about has shared their depression diagnosis, they might also share how they are managing their symptoms. If they're not seeking treatment or if they're expressing concerns about asking for help, it's a worthwhile time to share your belief that there is help available and ask if they'd like your assistance to find the help they need. Because depression is frequently associated with symptoms of poor motivation, low energy, and a sense of hopelessness, just making an appointment can feel overwhelming. Offering to make the appointment for them, driving them to an appointment, or reminding them about their appointment are thoughtful and often appreciated gestures. Depending on their circumstances, I know many of my patients have appreciated help with finding a psychologist or other mental health services, childcare support, assistance getting to appointments, financial support, and simply words of caring, hope, and encouragement from their close friends and loved ones.

Finally, if you're concerned that a friend or family member has suicidal thoughts or plans, do not avoid asking them about your concerns. You will not provoke suicidal thoughts in someone who does not have them already. However, you might prevent a suicide by opening the door for them to speak about their thoughts and letting them know there is help available.

I think someone I care about is depressed, but they have not been diagnosed. How can I help?

Only about one-third of people who have depression are ever diagnosed. This low percentage reflects many issues: an individual suffering from depression might fear judgment, they might worry they are overreacting or that they should be able to will themselves well, or they might not realize that their symptoms are related to depression. When you add on the lack of access to good medical care and the shame and fear rooted in **stigma** from families, communities, and within the medical profession, it's little wonder so few people seek help.

While your approach needs to be tailored specifically to the person you're concerned about, here are my suggestions for helping someone you care about to consider whether they are depressed.

1. **Do not make a diagnosis.** Even if you feel very certain, the person you care about might resent you saying, "I think you're depressed" and reject the idea immediately, closing down the discussion.
2. **Speak with compassion.** "I'm concerned about you."
3. **Speak about changes you have noticed**, not symptoms. "I've noticed you're sleeping much more than usual," or "You haven't been coming to our get-togethers over the past few months."
4. If they agree that they've been struggling, you can **suggest they talk to someone** (e.g., doctor, therapist, school counsellor, social worker, or spiritual advisor) to help them sort out what's going on.
5. If they're not willing to talk, **you might need to be more direct.** "The changes I've seen in you are really concerning me. Would you be willing to talk to your doctor, just to explore what might be going on?"
6. If they are willing to seek help, you can offer to **help to find a qualified professional, accompany them to an appointment, or help them to get to the appointment.**
7. Most importantly, let them know **you care and you're willing to help.**

What if my depressed friend or loved one is refusing help?

Unfortunately, it's usually impossible to force an adult, unless by a court order, to accept help if they don't want it, or if they don't believe they need help. In the context of a mental illness, **insight** refers to an individual's ability to recognize and accept that they are ill. **Psychotic** disorders in particular are associated with a loss of **insight.** As an example, you might recall that Phillip and Grace from chapter 1 both suffered from a **psychotic** depression and had lost **insight**, believing instead their illnesses were caused by outside forces—in Phillip's case, his mother's anger, and in Grace's case, the Russians.

In some jurisdictions, if an adult has lost **insight** due to a mental illness, they can be hospitalized against their will. A few jurisdictions also have laws that allow individuals who are so seriously mentally ill that they have lost **insight** to be treated without their consent.

However, a person's refusal to accept treatment might not be related to **psychosis** but due to fear, **stigma**, shame, lack of financial support (e.g., they can't take time away from work to be treated), or any number of other reasons. Ongoing substance abuse can be another factor, since they might not be willing to give up their addiction or they might believe that they'll be forced to abstain if they seek treatment for depression. Lack of access to resources or a poor previous experience with mental healthcare are other common reasons why patients refuse treatment.

As a friend, colleague, or loved one, you must realize that the only person you can control is you. You can offer to help, but you cannot make someone seek or accept help they do not want, even if it doesn't make any sense to you why they wouldn't want help, and the person is being terribly harmed by their untreated illness. Learning all you can about mental illness, making it known that you care and that you're willing to help, and trying to remain patient and nonjudgmental, which is difficult when we're frustrated, will help too.

When should I call 9-1-1?

If you are worried that your loved one or anyone else is at imminent risk of serious harm or death, call 9-1-1 immediately. The police are accustomed to managing situations that involve mental illness. Don't ignore your gut when it's telling you to call police. Explain the situation to the emergency operator and follow their instructions.

How do I speak to my employer or insurance provider about depression?

> Inoko, a thirty-four-year-old bus driver, didn't feel she was safe driving her route anymore. She'd driven through a couple of stop signs, once nearly running down an elderly woman pushing a child in a stroller. Her depression and anxiety symptoms were being treated, but they seemed to be getting worse. She wasn't sure whether she should speak to her boss, who was not a warm and fuzzy type, because she thought he might tell her colleagues she was "cracking up." She'd heard him make those comments about another co-worker who was on leave for depression. She also knew he was angry that the co-worker, as her boss put it, "went over my head" by speaking to HR rather than him about taking leave.

Many people continue to work, even when they're depressed. Depression makes getting out of bed difficult, let alone washing, dressing, eating, and getting to work on time. Throw a couple of kids and a partner on top of that load, and it might feel overwhelming, even impossible, to cope. Once at work, fatigue, low motivation, and **cognitive** symptoms can lead to underperformance, resulting in a greater sense of hopelessness, worthlessness, and uselessness. As I described in chapter 1, **"presenteeism"** occurs when, due to illness, your body is at work but your brain is not. When you can't perform your usual work in a timely, effective manner, it can lead to conflict with your boss and co-workers, making depression and **anxiety** symptoms worse. **Presenteeism** is believed to be much more expensive than absenteeism, costing society billions annually.

I am usually the one pushing my patient to take some time off work due to their illness. They are often fearful of work repercussions, loss of income, maintaining their privacy, and doubt that they're sick enough to need time off (or that others will believe they are sick enough). However, sometimes remaining at work can make patients more vulnerable to repercussions, if they're so ill that they aren't able to perform at work effectively.

Determining if it's necessary to take time away from work is a decision that must be made in concert with your doctor or therapist. When a patient is really worried about taking sick leave, I urge them to let me be the bad guy and blame me for insisting they take time off. Whenever possible, interacting with a company's human resources (HR) department is preferable, since their job is to deal with sick leave and they should be aware of the laws protecting a worker's privacy. Ultimately, a supervisor does not have the right to know your private medical information, and patients should carefully guard their confidentiality.

Additionally, I urge patients to allow me to provide information to their insurance company, rather than offering the information themselves, since dealing with insurers is provocative for pretty much everyone. Insurance companies are in the business of not spending their money—that's what makes them profitable. Case managers are paid not to spend any more of the insurance company's money than is absolutely necessary. Sometimes, they even receive financial bonuses based on their ability to get patients back to work. They follow basic guidelines and are not always concerned with an individual's unique issues that might be standing in the way of a rapid return to work. While it's preferable to interact with a case manager who sounds friendly and caring, it is very important to remember that they are not your friend and they will sometimes use what you say in a way you had not intended.

While some insurance companies are getting better at dealing with mental illness, overall, I'd say that most are a major source of **stress** and frustration for treating **clinicians** and their patients, requiring lengthy, excessively detailed reports and focusing on any minor improvement as a reason to end benefits. I urge my patients to have a friend or family member with them when interacting with insurers, to tape the conversation, and, most of all, not to overshare. Finally, it's wise to ask them to "Please contact my doctor," if they're asking questions that provoke **anxiety** or distress.

Sick leave is meant to allow patients the time needed to recover. This **recovery** time might include adjusting to new medications, having a course of ECT, or getting back on a normal sleep-wake cycle. Additionally, I usually encourage my patients to have some form of physical activity daily, even if it's just a brief walk to start, working their way up to a brisk walk for thirty minutes a day. Some fear being out and about while on sick leave, because they might be seen by colleagues. However, if your doctor is involved in your leave, they should include in any medical reports the importance that physical activity plays in your **recovery**. See chapter 13 for more on the mental health benefits of exercise.

The research is very clear: get back to work as soon as possible. The longer someone is off work, the less likely they are to ever return. I only need to consider how challenging I find it when I return to work after a few weeks' vacation. I can't barely recall how to turn on my computer! Then imagine someone who has had a serious depression, usually associated with impairing **cognitive** symptoms, and it's easy to understand why getting back to work as quickly as possible is so important.

After a sick leave, patients are often returning to a workplace where their colleagues are in the dark about why they've been off. In that case, a patient might be worried about how to answer their colleague's questions. If their colleagues know they've been off due to a mental illness, then a patient might be dealing with shame and embarrassment. Put all that on top of the worry and self-doubt because they haven't been at work for weeks or months, and it's clear that for some, returning to work can be a highly stressful experience.

Someone returning to work after a course of cancer chemotherapy might well expect they'll be met with a celebration and high-fives. Sadly, in all my years as a psychiatrist, I've never been told that my patient was greeted with a "welcome back" get-together, even when they shared the reason for their absence.

The best way to get back to work is slowly, following what is often called a *graduated return to work schedule*. Many insurers and HR departments are willing to consider this option, especially when it is clearly requested by the treating **clinician**. My experience tells me that rushing back to work too often results in depression **relapse** and another sick leave, sometimes a permanent one.

Finally, if someone asks, "Why were you off work?" and you don't wish to share, a simple "I had a medical issue" is accurate and should suffice. If they are rude enough to ask, "What kind of medical issue?" you have every right to respond, "That is none of your business," since (a) it isn't any of their business, and (b) it is incredibly rude to ask such a personal question. If you wished to share, you would have, and an adult should know better. If you're slightly more collegial than I might be, if faced with such a question, perhaps, "I'd rather not say, because it's a personal medical issue" will do.

How do I talk to other healthcare professionals about my mental illness and treatment?

One of my patients once told me she was fearful about an upcoming hip replacement surgery, which sadly was not about the surgery itself or its outcome. She was concerned about being shamed or humiliated by the hospital staff if she was asked about her psychiatric medications. She had recovered from a very severe depression and was very doing well. However, her wellness was maintained by exercise, social support, and several psychiatric medications. Her fear was well founded, because shaming happens frequently to my patients when they are seen by doctors and nurses who know nothing about their mental illness and the process of their **recovery**. She recently reminded me that at the time I had told her, "If they're mean, tell them I'll come over there and punch them in the nose." While I was not suggesting violence is ever the answer, I was making the point that she had *nothing* to be ashamed of, but those so-called healthcare professionals certainly should be ashamed of themselves.

It's important to realize that while psychiatry is a specialty that is completed after graduation from medical school, the **stigma** regarding mental illness is a major problem in all fields of medicine. The lack of knowledge regarding psychiatry, and the lack of respect for those who are suffering from a mental illness, is probably the greatest barrier to improved funding and adequate access to mental health services and treatments. The physician leaders and decision makers are rarely psychiatrists, and we as psychiatrists have historically failed to stand together and demand better for our patients. It is my sincerest hope that this will change, as we better understand the medical bases of serious mental illnesses and educate our colleagues, starting in medical school, especially regarding the scientific evidence demonstrating how mental health protects physical health. In short, early and effective treatment of mental illnesses saves lives *and* money.

When facing a healthcare professional who is making derogatory comments about your illness or treatment, you might not feel capable of standing up for yourself. If another physician raises concerns about your psychiatric treatment, you should report those concerns to your prescriber, who might choose to write to the culprit. Most importantly, please do not give someone like that the power to derail your progress and confidence. If concerns are raised, take them to your prescriber. They should be able to address those concerns and provide reassurance, and perhaps even a solid one-liner that you can use in the future and feel confident your doctor truly cares.

I am supporting a loved one who is depressed. How do I take care of myself?

Supporting a loved one who is severely depressed can be exhausting, highly stressful, and provoke mental and physical illness. I learned this most keenly when I worked for the Canadian Forces, treating patients who had severe post-traumatic **stress** disorder. I watched my patients' partners take over most of the household responsibilities, advocate for their loved one, and fear every day that their partner would never recover or that they would take their own life. Then, as their loved one slowly emerged from their debilitating illness, partner after partner descended into depression themselves.

If you love someone who is suffering or has suffered from depression, you will have watched them endure emotional, and sometimes physical, pain. I have learned through my experience as a psychiatrist that witnessing a loved one's struggle with mental illness can be an important and often unrecognized risk factor for depression. It's not only seeing a person you love in pain but also carrying the weight of the responsibilities that your loved one might be unable to manage due to their illness. Additionally, friends and family members often feel powerless to help, especially if the depression is very severe.

Intimate partners of depressed, anxious patients sometimes feel emotionally rejected and that their sexual desires are being ignored. Then they feel guilty, because they recognize it is the illness or the treatment that is responsible for the relationship challenges. Empathy, however, does have limits. When these pressures are unrelenting for months or even years, relationships can break down and families may be torn apart.

There are no easy answers for reducing the weight that caregivers carry. It's a burdensome job. However, these are my usual suggestions for limiting a caregiver's risk.

1. **Be involved in your loved one's care.** You will need to ask permission and discuss clear boundaries regarding what they view as acceptable input. More than any other comment, I have heard my patients complain about their partner asking, "Did you take your medication?" That's why it's best to discuss early on what you can say and do to be an active, involved, appreciated supporter.

   Why is a caregiver's involvement in treatment beneficial? Because information provides some sense of control over a situation that probably feels completely out of their control. If a loved one is suffering but you don't have any idea how they are being treated, by whom, or why they are taking a particular treatment, that could potentially provoke fear, helplessness, and frustration. Likewise, being left out of the process can cause a loved one to be less supportive of treatment, which might undermine **recovery.**

2. **Rather than complaining about a behaviour, try to be solution focused in your support of a depressed loved one.** As noted above, the question, "Did you take your medication?" seems to be incredibly annoying for just about everyone. However, it's also pretty annoying when your loved one is consistently missing their medication, especially when you have to deal with the repercussions. I suggest you try the same approach I use in my practice: I ask, "What can we do to make it easier for you to remember to take your medications?"; "What might help you to get up in the morning on time?"; or "How can I help you to get your lab work done for your next doctor's appointment?" If you get an "I don't know," you can follow up with "May I give you some suggestions that might help?"

3. **Make sure you have support outside of your relationship.** While your depressed loved one might not be socially active; you still need to see your friends and others who offer support. Likewise, exercise, faith, and other activities that provide pleasure, such as hobbies, must be maintained.

4. **Let your family doctor know what is happening in your life.** If you're fortunate enough to have a family doctor, share your burden with them. That will allow them to monitor your wellness and intervene before you're ill too.

5. **Don't be afraid to speak up if you fear for your loved one's safety.** Speaking up might save their life. Talk to them first, but if they do not have **insight**, call their doctor. Their doctor might not be able to tell you anything about them, but they can receive and act on your information or offer direction about how to handle the situation. If you or your loved one is at imminent risk, call 9-1-1 immediately.

Chapter summary

- Preparation can help to ensure you are heard and understood when you speak to a healthcare professional about depression.
- Just because someone is a friend or family member doesn't entitle them to know anything about your mental illness or how you are managing it. Strong boundaries make stronger relationships, especially if you have an Uncle Bud Inski.
- Taking care of yourself is crucial if you're trying to take care of someone else.

Seeking professional help for depression, surrounding yourself with supportive, understanding people, and keeping your distance from those who are unsupportive are all essential aspects of depression recovery.

A real patient's story

FOR FIVE YEARS I struggled with debilitating symptoms of depression, low thyroid, and **menopause**. I followed my doctors' treatment plan of antidepressant, **hormone**, and thyroid medications. I went to specialists and counsellors but couldn't think clearly enough to benefit. I felt like a dismal treatment failure.

The journey over five years to find a specialist who could help me find the right treatment was a long and painful process, fraught with misdiagnoses and **clinicians** with opinions and judgments but no answers. I was sent to a neuropsychiatrist for evaluation and it was only by chance—a favour one kind doctor was owed by another—that I finally came to be seen and treated by my present psychiatrist. She led me through the seventh ring of hell as she tried first one and then another medication and several combinations. She promised it would get better. That hell had an end because we found the right combination of medications to effectively treat the depression. That treatment helped to stabilize me and, in truth, saved my life.

The journey to wellness was a struggle, even with the right medication regimen. As my broken brain began healing, I could think again without huge effort. For the first time in five years, I could read again. I decided to set one physical goal I thought I could accomplish, even if I couldn't yet focus easily. I could swim in the lake I had loved when I was growing up, and I did. I swam and trained for the Across the Lake Swim, just one swim at a time. I remember it was the spring solstice. I went to the shores of the lake that day and I swam, not for long, but I went in the freezing cold water and felt more alive than I had for years.

9

What are the treatment options for depression?

BECAUSE I AM a psychiatrist, once a patient is in my office, the jig is up. They know they have a mental illness, they've usually already tried many treatments, and none of those treatments have worked adequately. Many have tried, with the help of their family doctor or a psychologist, to find an effective, tolerable treatment for some time, often for several years. From a medication perspective, what I do is often not that different from what their family doctor has tried, but as a specialist, I have more experience with making psychiatric diagnoses. I also have more time to see patients and perhaps a greater confidence in using some of the treatments at my disposal.

Medication treatments for mental illnesses are imperfect, but they are often necessary and can be lifesaving. Fortunately, psychotherapy (also known as talk therapy) with a qualified professional has a mountain of scientific evidence demonstrating it is a very effective treatment for many people struggling with depression. For some, talk therapy may be the only treatment that is required to recover. As well, everyday experiences and activities, like exercise, social interactions, meditation, a healthy diet, sleep, and faith, can provide an enormous benefit. Most importantly, understanding and having a sense of control over your mental illness, and a sense of hope that there is a path ahead, are powerful forces for **recovery** and sustained wellness.

In my **therapeutic relationship** with a patient, I am only the navigator. The patient is the captain of their own ship. My job is to chart the journey towards **recovery**, by knowing the appropriate treatment options and sharing that information with my patient, so they can make a decision that is informed. This means they know what the treatment is supposed to offer and the potential side effects, and why one treatment is being suggested over another. Then the ship's captain (my patient) takes the helm and says either "Full steam ahead!" or "Man overboard!"

I am a strong advocate for **evidence-based treatments**, but frankly I can get behind just about anything else, so long as it is safe and doesn't involve a pseudo-professional dishonestly lining their pockets by taking advantage of vulnerable individuals. However, if you truly need a prescription medication, nothing else will do. Some other treatment options may be helpful **augmentation** strategies for severe mental illness, but they cannot carry the weight alone. One lovely patient once said to me, "I tried so hard, but I finally had to accept that I couldn't yoga my way out of my depression."

In this chapter, I describe some of the common challenges and questions I hear every day from my patients who are considering taking an antidepressant. I often hear the same questions from patients who have been prescribed antidepressants for a long time, because it's hard to stick with long-term treatment without ongoing support and encouragement.

What are some of the challenges that patients face when starting a medication to treat depression?

Ideally, GPs and NPs, and especially psychiatrists, should possess the knowledge and expertise necessary to treat serious mental illnesses with medication. These are essential tools of our trade, yet prescribing is not always well taught or well executed, which can cause harm to patients and to society.

Psychiatric medications are now commonly regarded, even among educated adults, as dangerous, unnecessary, intolerable, or ineffective. Anti-medication and anti-psychiatry zealots, egged on by irresponsible media reports, have powerfully perpetuated the **stigma** and burden of mental illness, adding to the weight of hopelessness and shame that mentally ill patients already carry.

The too-frequent headline "Psychiatric drugs are no more effective than **placebo**" is utterly false for most patients, but sadly, this belief has permeated our society. In all areas of medicine, media reports often highlight snippets of negative research, without considering the larger body of evidence and **clinical experience** demonstrating the benefits of a treatment, which I believe can and does cause tremendous harm. Fear of medication is endemic, most especially for drugs used to treat mental illnesses, because they impact how you think and feel. Patients fear psychiatric medications might alter their personality, make them feel like a zombie, or impair their ability to think clearly and function normally. However, the right medication should improve or resolve symptoms, including **cognitive** symptoms associated with mental illness, and help patients to regain their optimal functioning.

The trouble is there is no recipe for prescribing psychiatric medications. Every individual is unique, so with the guidance of their doctor, patients must find the treatment that's right for them. If a drug makes them feel worse, it's not the right drug, but that doesn't mean there are no other options. The right treatment must be found and sometimes that takes time, effort, and creativity. Feeling like a zombie is never an acceptable outcome.

Inappropriate prescribing, inadequate resources to monitor treatment, delayed treatment, failure to manage side effects, and symptoms of anxiety add to the risk of developing negative perceptions about psychiatric medications. In the wrong hands, any medication can cause harm, but when prescribed appropriately,

psychiatric medications are compassionate, effective, and sometimes lifesaving.

When depression doesn't get better with the usual treatments prescribed by a GP or NP, a patient might be referred to a psychiatrist. If there isn't a psychiatrist to refer to, or the wait is months or even years, the patient may remain untreated or continue to take ineffective or intolerable treatment, reinforcing their belief that medications don't work or that they cause more harm than good.

I encourage my new patients to start the search for the right treatment by providing them with education and by trying to instill a sense of hope. I say, "I want you to love your drugs," because with the right treatment there is hope for a full and sustained **recovery**. For my work to be a success, my patients shouldn't feel medicated. Ultimately, they should feel and function like they did before they got ill. The journey begins when my patient is armed with a plan, information, and a sense of optimism.

Unfortunately, sometimes within hours of our meeting, that optimism is shattered. Whether by a pharmacist making an ill-advised comment; a confidante voicing an indignant, uninformed opinion; or Dr. Google; my patient's lingering fears are reignited. Comments like, "You don't need that drug. I have a homeopath/shaman/vitamin B complex that worked wonders for my friend" can powerfully undermine an anxious, ill patient's resolve, causing their new **insight** and game plan to be forgotten.

A serious mental illness that is not appropriately and fully treated can result in prolonged suffering, further functional decline, the destruction of important relationships, unemployment, **cognitive impairment**, more **refractory** illness, and a heightened risk of suicide. These are clearly not trivial issues. The suffering associated with an untreated or even an under-treated illness is real and frankly heartbreaking in such a rich, truly privileged society. Yet, it is the reality for so many.

While I truly hope my patients will ultimately love their medication, not everyone does, and the search for their best treatment must continue. Sometimes the journey requires that they muster seemingly infinite patience, which is so difficult when you feel miserable. I ask them to never, never, never give up, and I won't either.

Once the right treatment is found, then the challenge changes. I now have to ask them to take the treatment every day, unfailingly. Patients I have known for many years, who trust me and tell me they feel far better with treatment than without, have commonly shared that they face a daily internal struggle when deciding to take their medication. I will admit to feeling truly bewildered by this struggle, likely because I have such faith in the scientific evidence regarding the power of wellness and the risks of **relapse.** However, some people despise the fact that they need to take medication. I feel their struggle is rooted in self-**stigma.** That's my own term for what I see as a patient's enduring belief that they should be able to get better without treatment, that they're well enough to be able to stop treatment, or perhaps they forget how ill they were or how terrible it was to be severely depressed.

Selling in a tough market

After twenty years as a psychiatrist, I have learned that my job is essentially sales. Unfortunately, I'm selling something that no one really wants to buy, so I've been selling in a tough market all these years.

No one asks to be mentally ill or wants a mental illness, so helping my patients to accept their diagnosis is often my first "sales" challenge. I tell patients that their depression is a real, serious, potentially progressive, medical illness. It can become an inflammatory illness and cause a real brain injury. There is no shame in having a mental illness. It happened because of a combination of genetics, psychological make-up, and their environment. With treatment, it's possible, in fact likely, to live a normal, healthy, happy life.

Then I must "sell" the treatment. If selling treatments were like selling cars, I could say I have a number of models that patients can choose from. They could consider the medication model: drugs that they've only ever heard were dangerous and no better than **placebo**. I have another possible model:

ECT, where I electrocute their brain, but it works wonders. They can choose model number three: talk therapy, where they share their deepest, most private thoughts and feelings with someone they don't know, or perhaps even a *group* of people they don't know if they choose the group therapy model. Talk about a hard sell! But if I'm unable to engage my patient to find the most effective, safe, tolerable treatment, I know they are vulnerable to more pain and suffering, so I keep on pitching.

Finally comes the "after-market sales": please don't stop your treatment! Put yourself first when it comes to self-care: get a good night's sleep, wake up at the same time every day, and eat a healthy diet. Keep going with that daily exercise. Don't drink too much. Please don't smoke pot. Create and maintain appropriate boundaries with friends, family, and at work or school, and, most especially, with Uncle Bud Inski.

While it's still a buyer's market, I believe there are some positive market indicators: young people seem more open and accepting of mental illness, major corporations are confidently partnering with organizations to destigmatize mental illness, and leaders in sports and celebrities are publicly (and bravely) disclosing their personal struggles with mental illness. Until the time when anyone can tell their friends, family, colleagues, or surgeon that they have a mental illness, I'll keep on selling my wares.

How do Health Canada and the American Food and Drug Administration (FDA) evaluate and approve medications for depression?

Melissa went to see her psychiatrist because she wasn't sleeping well. After discussing Melissa's symptoms, her psychiatrist thought Melissa's sleep disturbance was probably related to her ongoing anxiety and depression, so she recommended an antidepressant medication that would help mood and anxiety, and because it was also sedating, it would likely improve her sleep. When Melissa went to pick up the prescription, her pharmacist asked her why she was taking the medication. She replied, "For my sleep," to which the pharmacist said, "That drug isn't indicated for sleep problems. It's an antidepressant." Melissa was very upset, believing her doctor had made a mistake by prescribing the wrong medication, when she just wanted a treatment for her sleep.

When a drug company develops a new treatment for depression, it must secure approval from a government **regulatory agency** that assesses and monitors the safety and efficacy of medications. **Health Canada** is the Canadian **regulatory agency**; in the United States, it's the **Food and Drug Administration (FDA)**; and in Europe, the regulator is called the **European Medicines Agency (EMA)**. To demonstrate a drug's safety and effectiveness, drug companies conduct clinical trials, which are studies evaluating the medication in large numbers of subjects suffering from depression, often in comparison with a **placebo.** An antidepressant is given a **Health Canada**, FDA, or EMA **indication** for the treatment of depression, because the evidence the drug company presented satisfied the requirements of the **regulatory agency.**

Regulatory agencies are not always aligned regarding drug **indications.** Canada may lag behind the United States because drug companies often apply to **Health Canada** to get a drug approved for sale months or even years after they apply to the FDA. The reason for this delay is often a matter of money: the market in the United States is ten times larger and therefore far more profitable than the market in Canada. Additionally, regulatory agencies might differ in their evaluation of the research provided by the drug company.

Every **regulatory agency** develops its own **product monograph**, which contains all the critical information regarding the medication, including its **indications**, dose, possible side effects, and **mechanism of action**. The Canadian and US **product monographs** are similar but may differ regarding official **indications.**

When determining if a drug should receive an official **indication**, regulators evaluate the research evidence they receive from the drug company seeking approval. A drug might be very effective for depression and **anxiety**, but if the company is only seeking approval for depression, even if they have research evidence demonstrating it works well for **anxiety**, it will only receive a depression **indication.**

In the past, drug companies would work to secure as many **indications** as possible, because that allowed them to market the drug for a broader range of disorders. However, over the last few decades, the cost of bringing a drug to market, including drug discovery, clinical trials, and the regulatory application process, has skyrocketed to more than $1 billion. Consequently, most new antidepressants are approved for depression only, even though they might be an effective treatment for another disorder, such as **anxiety.**

Understanding official **indications** is important, because Melissa's experience is very common. If your doctor recommends an antidepressant medication for **anxiety**, pain, or sleep, and you mention that to your pharmacist, they might tell you, "It's not indicated for that disorder." Make sure to speak to your prescriber if you're concerned. They should let you know if they're prescribing a medication "off-label," which means they are prescribing it for a reason that is different from the official **indication.** Generally speaking, if your doctor is prescribing you a treatment off-label, that implies that they have experience using the medication in that circumstance, their colleagues are also using the treatment in a similar manner, likely there are scientific reports or smaller studies demonstrating a potential benefit when the drug is used off-label, and that they believe the treatment is both effective and safe.

Prescribing treatments off-label is an extremely common practice in psychiatry. A medication indicated for one disorder may be found to be useful for treating another disorder, by conducting clinical trials and by patient experience that occurred after the drug was approved. If the drug is no longer covered by patent protection, no drug company is going to apply to a regulator for another official **indication.** Likewise, even if a drug still had patent protection and the research evidence was available, some companies will not seek another official **indication**, following a careful cost-benefit analysis.

What dose will I need?

When **Health Canada** or the FDA gives an official **indication** for a medication, they also approve an official **product monograph**, which includes the recommended dose range. The dose range is based on the research provided by the drug company, including dose finding studies, which are used to establish the safety and efficacy of different doses.

Once a new medication is approved and available for sale, the drug company will usually offer education to prescribers that is based on the **product monograph**. However, I also rely heavily on the experiences of my colleagues. I want to know how they are using a drug in their practice to optimize their patient's benefits and minimize side effects. Most experienced prescribers will tell you it takes time to determine how to use a new medication most effectively in their practice. Keep in mind that all research studies are artificial situations. Patients in the real world often have more complicated illnesses, with overlapping medical and psychiatric symptoms and disorders. Prescribing a medication in the real world isn't a one-size-fits-all affair. It requires a thoughtful, nuanced approach, and that requires time and experience. It's called a medical *practice*, after all.

As a general rule, I tend to initiate new medications, including antidepressants, at a very low dose, often lower than what is recommended in the **product monograph**, to ensure my patients tolerate the medication well. It can be common to experience some minor side effects when a drug is initiated, but these usually resolve within a few weeks, at most, and may be fully manageable using my antidepressant Golden Rules (see page 217). If there are side effects, I only increase the dose when they have resolved. Starting low and increasing slowly has only one drawback: it might take a little longer to see the full benefits of a treatment. However, no drug will work if it's not taken, so I feel it's better that the treatment is well tolerated, since that increases the likelihood it will be taken. Increasing a patient's dose of a particular medication to achieve the desired effects is called **titration**.

With each dose increase, there should be symptom improvement and tolerability. If the dose is increased and there are side effects that are intolerable or don't resolve, or there is no additional symptom improvement, the last dose is the optimized dose. Once we know the optimized dose, the discussion turns to whether the medication is doing its job fully or whether it needs to be changed or augmented.

While I always strive to keep doses as low as possible, I sometimes prescribe medications at higher doses than recommended by the **product monograph.** This prescribing reflects my **clinical experience**, because after treating many patients with a medication, I know that some will truly benefit from higher doses and tolerate those doses well. Treating at doses above the range found in a **product monograph** is a common practice in psychiatry, particularly for some antidepressant medications. Additionally, I always prefer to squeeze everything I can out of one medication before adding another or having to switch to something else, which takes time (when people want to feel better *now*) and might lead to more side effects.

Because dose optimization, particularly when it involves doses above the recommendations in the **product monograph**, is a practice associated with **clinical experience**, it can sometimes lead to confusion. Some colleagues or allied professionals, such as pharmacists, may be unaware or uncomfortable with common psychiatric doses of certain medications. Your doctor should let you know if they are prescribing a higher than usual dose of a medication and they should give you their rationale. However, if you're told by another healthcare professional that your medication dose is way too high or outside the normal range, be sure to check with the person who prescribed the medication. It could be a mistake, but it could also reflect their experience with your illness and that drug.

As an example, the **Health Canada product monograph** for the antidepressant medication venlafaxine XR recommends a maximum dose of 225 mg. However, it is common practice to prescribe doses of 300–450 mg for patients with depression and **anxiety**, so long as the medication is more effective and well tolerated at those doses.

How long should it take for my antidepressant to work?

If you ask mental health professionals how long it takes for an antidepressant to work, the most common response you will hear is "four to six weeks." However, most antidepressants should start working more quickly; some benefit should be apparent within two weeks. At two weeks, it's unlikely there will be a complete **recovery**, but research suggests that symptoms should be about 20 percent better, which translates to a minor but noticeable change. Patients sometimes tell me, "I'm a little less tearful" or "I'm a little less on edge." Using **depression rating scales** at this stage of treatment can be very valuable (see page 128): it's much easier to calculate a percentage improvement from a score on a rating scale than from a subjective experience.

If no benefit at all has occurred within two weeks, the dose should be increased. If after another two weeks, there is little or no improvement in symptoms, the medication is very unlikely to be beneficial and another treatment should be tried.

How can I monitor my progress in between doctor's visits?

There are many ways that you can keep track of your treatment progress, including whether you're experiencing symptom improvement and whether you're tolerating the treatment well. Good mood trackers also monitor many other aspects of depression **recovery**, including exercise, **anxiety**, drug or alcohol use, sleep time, and mood changes associated with a menstrual cycle. Often, it's difficult to remember how you've been doing, especially if you're not seeing your doctor very often. Using a mood tracker for even four to six weeks can be very useful in determining whether your treatment is on the right track.

One of the easiest ways to monitor your progress is by using a paper mood tracker, such as the one found in appendix 2. Keep a pencil and a copy of this chart on your bedside table, so you remember to fill it in every night. It can be invaluable for both you and your doctor, so long as you remember to bring it to your appointments; consider keeping an updated picture of it on your phone. Remember to fill it out even when you feel well.

For those who have evolved beyond the paper and pencil approach to the world, there are many apps that can help you to keep track of your progress. Some offer great tools, including medication and appointment reminders, as well as daily suggestions regarding improving self-care. One of my favorites is MoodFx, developed by my colleague Dr. Raymond Lam at the University of British Columbia.

Once I feel better, how long should I continue the medication?

In chapter 4, I described **neurogenesis** (growing new **neurons**), which is an essential aspect of recovering from depression. Once the right treatment is found, the depression symptoms have resolved, and the brain has recovered, with healthy new **neurons** functioning normally in the brain, is the job of the antidepressant done? Maybe, but likely not. It really depends on the severity of the depression, whether every symptom has resolved, and the number of previous episodes of depression.

Those who have a first depressive episode and experience full symptom resolution without **residual symptoms** should continue the medication, at the dose that got them well, for nine to twelve months from the time they are well and then slowly **taper** the medication over several weeks.

About 50 percent of those who recover from a first episode of depression will eventually get depressed again. Once there have been two episodes of depression, research suggests that those patients should continue treatment for at least two years from the time they are perfectly well. Approximately 80 percent of those who have had two episodes of depression will have another

recurrence if they stop treatment, and once you've had three episodes of depression, you're pretty much guaranteed to have another depression if treatment is discontinued.

Because of the near certainty of **recurrence** once there have been three or more depression episodes, and the fact that with each **recurrence** the illness often becomes more difficult to manage, treatment should continue indefinitely. This is why it is so important to find a depression treatment that is not just effective but also well tolerated, because no one wants to continue taking a medication that causes really bothersome side effects.

As a reminder, sometimes the first depression is very severe, and the brain changes associated with the episode look indistinguishable from what you might expect from a third episode of depression. Earlier and more severe structural and functional brain changes are more likely when a first depression is difficult to treat, if it is associated with **psychotic** symptoms or a serious suicide attempt, if there is ongoing substance abuse, or when the depression is associated with another psychiatric diagnosis, such as an **anxiety disorder**. Patients who have had a very difficult to treat or life-threatening depression should be treated as if they have had three depressions, and they should seriously consider staying on their treatment, at the dose that got them well, indefinitely.

Will the medication used to treat my depression harm my physical health?

This question is very common, and I am happy to report that it is one I can usually answer confidently with a firm "no." As you might recall from chapter 5, mental illnesses may provoke physical illnesses, and the reverse is also true. Additionally, some psychiatric medications can cause side effects like movement disorders, weight gain, and metabolic disorders (e.g., **diabetes**, high cholesterol), especially the older **atypical antipsychotics**. Additionally, lithium has rarely been associated with kidney damage. However, research has clearly demonstrated that good mental health protects physical health. For more on the side effects of antidepressants, see chapter 11.

Your doctor should inform you if the medication you are prescribed has been associated with serious side effects, including significant movement disorders, weight gain, **diabetes**, high cholesterol, or kidney damage. If you're taking lithium, your doctor should recommend regular lab screening to ensure your kidneys continue to function normally. It is important to raise concerns about side effects with your doctor and to ask about any long-term potential consequences related to taking your prescribed medication. There is always a risk-benefit calculation you and your doctor must work through to ensure you're making the best treatment choice possible. Getting your information from reliable sources increases the likelihood you'll make an informed choice and the best choice for your future well-being.

Are antidepressants addictive?

Addictions are serious **chronic** brain illnesses associated with an inability to abstain from a substance or behaviour, impaired behavioural control, and craving. Many individuals suffering from an addiction lack **insight** regarding the severity and impact of their **dysfunctional** behaviour is having on their life and the lives of others. Too often, addictions ultimately result in physical and mental illnesses, impaired functioning, and damaged relationships. An addiction to a drug or alcohol may wax and wane, but over time, especially without effective treatment, addiction tends to progress and cause significant disability and premature death.

Drug dependence refers to physical dependence, whereby the body adapts to the drug, requiring more of it to achieve an effect (tolerance) and provokes physical or mental symptoms if drug use is abruptly stopped (withdrawal). Physical dependence can happen with the **chronic** use of many medications, even when they are taken as prescribed. Physical dependence is not the same as addiction, although it often accompanies an addiction.

Whether antidepressant tolerance (the need to increase the dose to maintain the same benefits) actually exists is hotly debated. The research is mixed and emotions run high regarding this topic, but my interpretation of the data and my **clinical experience** has led me to believe that what is sometimes referred to as tolerance is not tolerance at all. Almost without exception, my patients who are prescribed an antidepressant and have been very well for an extended period get ill again for these reasons: they've stopped their treatment or reduced the dose; they've been switched to a less effective generic alternative (often without their knowledge or consent); they have the wrong diagnosis (most often bipolar); they've experienced a serious life stressor; or they have an undiagnosed or untreated co-morbid condition (especially **anxiety** or an addiction). Finally, severe and **chronic** mental illnesses, such as depression and **bipolar disorder**, do progress if not fully treated (see **residual symptoms** on page 224).

Antidepressants are not associated with addiction, dependence, drug-craving, or drug-seeking behaviour. They do not cause individuals to feel stoned or euphoric in the manner seen with cannabis, cocaine, or heroin. They can provoke mania and hypomania in patients who have untreated **bipolar disorder**, but this is not the same as provoking a drug-induced euphoria associated with an illicit drug. While very unpleasant **discontinuation symptoms** may occur (see page 212), particularly with some of the older antidepressants, these are usually mild and short-lived, resolving within a few days to two weeks. If severe, there are strategies that can help to overcome these symptoms.

I can't afford my psychiatric medication. Do I have any options?

Each province and territory in Canada has its own pharmacare program, and the coverage of psychiatric medications can vary greatly between provinces. Some provinces have programs that cover the cost of some psychiatric medications for those who have a lower income. Be sure to ask your prescriber what options are available to you where you live.

Most drug companies that are currently marketing a depression treatment offer medication samples, which doctors can provide to their patients. Furthermore, many of those companies also have generous assistance programs that will provide their drug to patients who are unable to afford it and do not have a drug plan through their work. Doctors can reach out to a pharmaceutical company to find an application for patient assistance. Most forms are available online.

I am not a believer in the benevolence of generic (non-brand) companies and their saintly role in saving Canadians money. These companies exist entirely for profit. They don't conduct novel drug research and development, unlike innovative pharmaceutical companies that invest heavily in new drug development. To bring a drug to market, generic companies use the drug developer's research and test their product on a small number of healthy volunteers. That's it!

Generics are often priced just below the price of the branded product despite costing far less, usually pennies a pill. Pharmacies make far more profit and special bonuses by dispensing generics, which is why they rarely, if ever, ask customers if they want a branded product when a generic is available. Many chain pharmacies mandate automatic generic substitutions.

My greatest concern, however, is that while generic drugs are supposed to contain exactly the same amount of drug and produce the same effect as the branded product, I know that this is not always the case. The most problematic products are the generics that attempt to copy branded products that have a special delivery system, like extended release (e.g., drugs with SR, XR, or XL in their name). However, over the last several years, many generic companies have moved their production to countries where there is little or no quality control, further compromising drug quality and safety. In my opinion, regulators are not adequately ensuring the safety and efficacy of the generic drugs supplied to consumers, and I know there have been devastating consequences.

There are programs available in some provinces and US states that pay the difference between the branded and generic product. In Canada, the innoviCares program pays the difference (or most of it) between many generic and branded drugs for consumers. Given the countless occasions when my patients have been unwittingly moved from a branded to a generic drug, or between generic drugs, and that has precipitated a serious **recurrence** of their illness, whenever possible I try to ensure my patients are able to access a branded product.

Chapter summary

- Antidepressants are one possible treatment for depression. A thoughtful and careful assessment will help to determine what is best for each individual, whether it is a medication, talk therapy, exercise, or another form of treatment.
- Antidepressants are effective treatments for depression, but every antidepressant does not work for every person.
- **Health Canada** and the FDA are federal agencies that approve medications, based on their safety and whether they are proven to be effective.
- The dose and length of a medication treatment is dependent on the response to the treatment, illness severity, and the number of previous depression episodes.

Depression treatment must be personalized to meet each individual's needs. There are many options available, and while there is no single perfect treatment, there is one that is best for you.

A real patient's story

RECOVERY FROM DEPRESSION, in my experience, requires patience, perseverance, flexibility in thinking, and faith in your doctor and the medications they may prescribe.

I recommend that you:

- Ask for help and keep asking for help until you get some.
- Find a doctor you like and trust.
- Be willing to try different medications.
- Stay on the medications, even if there are negative side effects, but talk to your doctor about your concerns.
- Move your body every day, if you can.
- Surround yourself with people who support you.
- Find activities that can distract you or even buoy you up when you are feeling really down.
- Forgive yourself for your shortcomings.

10

What are antidepressants and how do they work?

THERE ARE MANY different types of medications used to treat severe depression. The term "antidepressant" is vague and doesn't accurately describe the breadth of potential benefits these treatments can provide. Likewise, the term says nothing about how these treatments actually work, which is known as the **mechanism of action.**

When depressed, a patient might be prescribed one of a number of different types of antidepressants, **antipsychotics**, **anticonvulsants**, or stimulant medications—or a combination of two or more of these medications. In the pages that follow, I provide an overview of the different medication treatments currently available for depression, including their **mechanism of action** and why you and your doctor might choose one over another. Notably, I only include medications that have reputable research evidence for their safety and effectiveness. If you don't find a treatment listed here, that's because the scientific evidence is non-existent, shoddy, or clearly demonstrates it is not safe or effective. Then you might find it in the myths section in chapter 14.

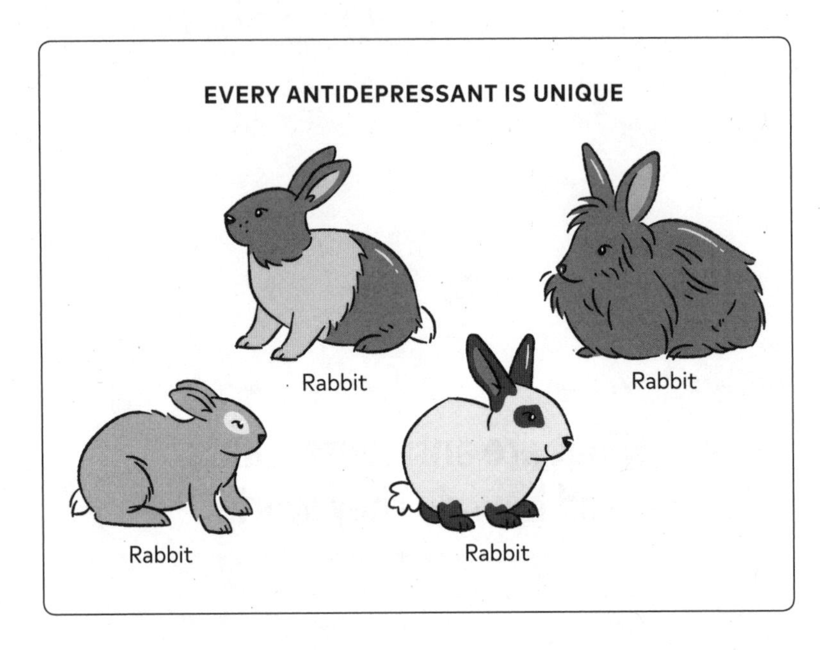

There are several large classes of antidepressants—for instance, SSRIs (selective **serotonin** reuptake inhibitors), SNRIs (**serotonin-norepinephrine** reuptake inhibitors), and TCAs (tricyclic antidepressants)—but even within these classes, each medication is unique, despite having a similar effect on the brain. One SSRI might work well for a particular patient while another SSRI might not. Similarly, if three people are taking the same medication, one might have no side effects, another might have diarrhea, while the third complains of constipation. Each antidepressant is a distinct chemical entity, which interacts with a unique individual's brain. The resulting overall benefits, as well as the side effects, are also likely to be different for every individual. This unique response is referred to as **inter-individual variability**, which tends to be extremely common for psychiatric medications.

Do antidepressants work?

Antidepressant treatments have been available for more than sixty years, and over that time they have advanced, becoming easier to take, with fewer intolerable side effects and a lower risk of death if taken in overdose. However, as a group, antidepressants are not getting more effective. When large populations are studied, antidepressants are clearly effective, which means they outperform a **placebo** in clinical trials. Additionally, some antidepressants manage specific symptoms, such as **insomnia** or pain, better than others. However, on an individual level, there is **inter-individual variability** regarding whether a specific patient will respond to a specific antidepressant.

It's important to know that a **placebo** is not the same as no treatment. In fact, a **placebo** can have a powerful impact on a patient's symptoms. In a clinical trial, subjects aren't handed a pill, either the drug or a **placebo**, and told, "Take this," and then sent on their way. They are met by the research team, treated respectfully, given a diagnosis, offered a treatment (which may or may not be a **placebo**), and then they are seen regularly to assess how they're doing by the same kind people who welcomed them into the study.

The **placebo** effect has been known for centuries and is well documented in many areas of medicine, but especially for the management of pain. Interestingly, the **placebo** effect is increasing in US clinical trials particularly, which has been hypothesized to be associated with longer, larger, and more expensive clinical trials, which might enhance subjects' expectations of a treatment's effectiveness. Additionally, the way research is conducted in the United States, which is now a highly lucrative industry staffed by specialized research assistants, whose primary job is to support their study subjects, might also be fuelling the enhancement of the **placebo** effect.

Canadian researchers reviewed eighty-four clinical trials, published between 1990 and 2013, studying new medications for the treatment of **chronic** neuropathic pain. They found that the study medications had similar analgesic effects over the twenty-three-year period, but **placebo** responses rose. Medications were superior to **placebo** by 27 percent in 1996, but by 2013, the difference between **placebo** and study drug dropped to just 9 percent. Interestingly, the massive change in the **placebo** response was entirely driven by the thirty-five studies that were conducted in the United States. The remainder of the studies were conducted in Asia and Europe and did not show the same powerful **placebo** effect. It's not that the treatments are getting less effective, but that **placebos** are becoming more effective.

Unfortunately, this increase in the **placebo** effect is proving to be a serious barrier to new and promising treatments getting to market. Over the past ten years, more than 90 percent of potential drugs for the treatment of neuropathic and cancer pain have failed at advanced phases of clinical trials.

As you read in chapter 5, depression hurts. Many depressed patients suffer from painful physical symptoms, and patients suffering from **chronic** pain are at greater risk for depression. Importantly, **placebos**, psychiatric medications, and analgesic medications work in similar brain areas, which might mean that the growing **placebo** responses can mask a drug's therapeutic benefit.

Antidepressant trials are highly restrictive. In fact, the entry criteria for those trials has become so narrow that up to 90 percent of patients in clinical practice wouldn't be acceptable subjects for a research study. Clinical trials are conducted on "pristine" patients, meaning people who have no other medical or psychiatric issues other than the one that is being studied. In reality, most people are far more complicated and may have multiple issues, whether medical (e.g., obesity, **diabetes**) or psychiatric (e.g., depression and **anxiety** or ADHD). For this reason, the findings in clinical trials do not always align very well with the **clinical experience** of those practicing medicine in the community.

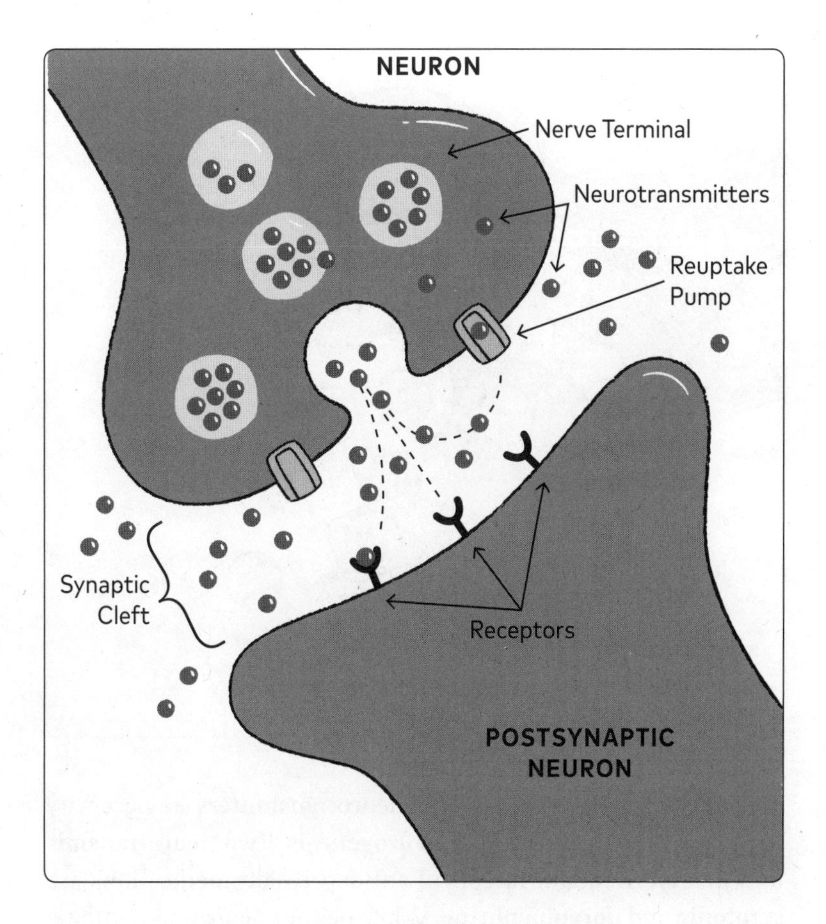

How do antidepressants work?

There are several distinct classes of antidepressants, and those classes differ based on how they do their job—the **mechanism of action.** For instance, some are reuptake inhibitors, others act directly to alter the sensitivity of receptors, while others inhibit a specific enzyme. Regardless of a medication's specific **mechanism of action**, all antidepressants have one key effect: they increase certain **neurotransmitters.**

As I discussed in chapter 4, antidepressants grow brain cells (**neurons**) through a process called **neurogenesis.** However, growing new **neurons** is a complicated business, requiring many steps

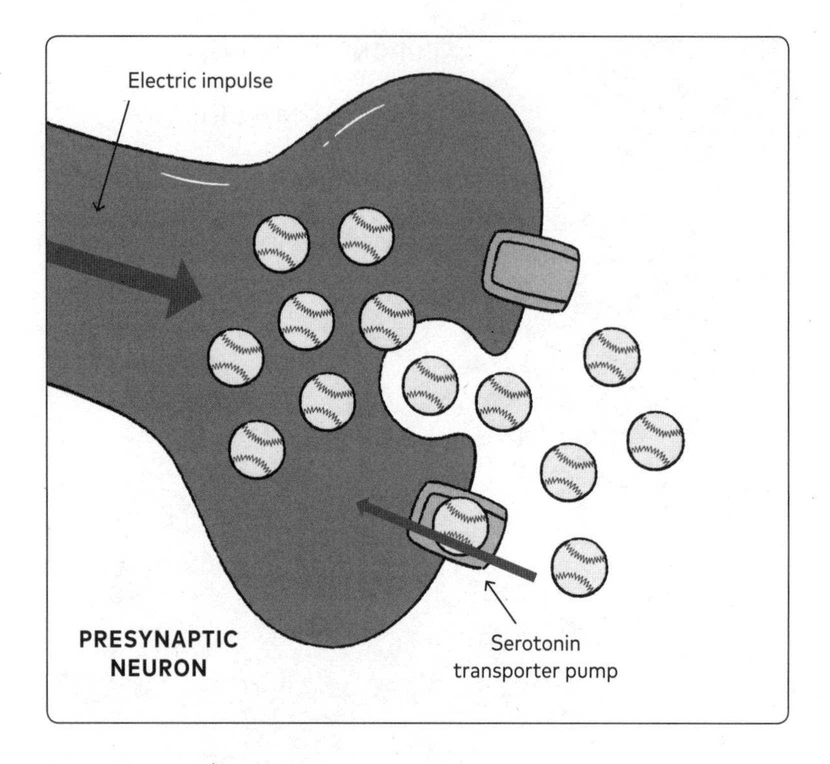

over weeks or months. A variety of **neurotransmitters** are necessary participants in the process of **neurogenesis**. Two **neurotransmitters** that are frequent targets of antidepressant medications are **serotonin** and **norepinephrine**. While neither **neurotransmitter** is the cause or the cure for depression alone, both may play a critical role in the **recovery** from depression.

You might want to look back at chapter 2 to remind yourself that **neurons** use electricity and **neurotransmitters**, such as **serotonin** and **norepinephrine**, to send messages around the brain. Using **serotonin** as an example, when an electrical message reaches the end of a **serotonin neuron** (called the **nerve terminal**), it provokes the release of **serotonin**, which moves across the synaptic cleft (the gap between **neurons**) and attaches to the **serotonin** receptors on adjacent **neurons**. In a non-depressed brain, there is a normal amount of **serotonin** being released from a **nerve terminal** and

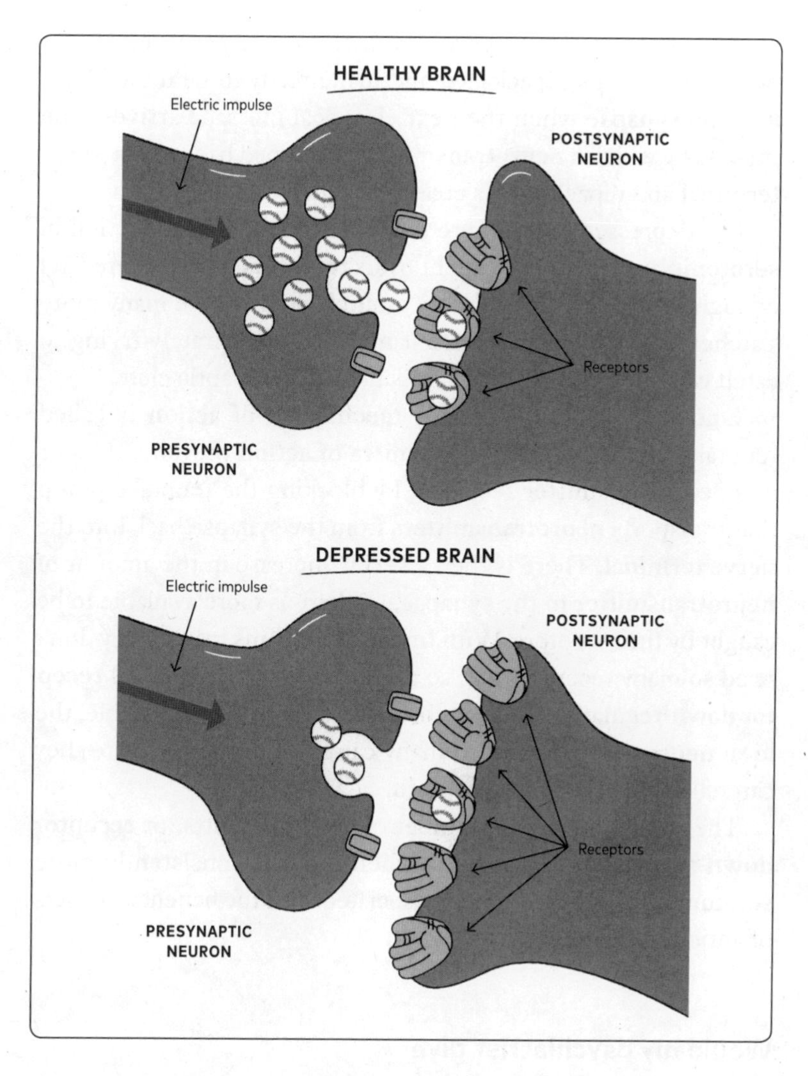

there is a predictable number of **serotonin** receptors on the adjacent **neurons.**

If you think of **serotonin** as being like a baseball, the receptors are catcher's mitts. The **nerve terminal** throws the **serotonin** balls into the **synapse**, and receptors on adjacent **neurons** catch them, pass on their message to the **neuron**, and then pass the **serotonin** ball back into the **synapse**. The **serotonin** is then recycled by being pumped back into the **nerve terminal**, via the **serotonin transporter**, where it's repackaged and made ready to be tossed back into the **synapse** when the next electrical message arrives. The process by which a **neurotransmitter** is pumped back into a **nerve terminal** and repackaged is creatively called reuptake.

In a depressed brain, there is a well-documented reduction in **serotonin** available to be caught by its receptors. When there isn't enough **serotonin**, its receptors multiply so there are many more "catcher's mitts" on the adjacent **neurons**, desperately trying to catch what little **serotonin** is available in the synaptic cleft.

One type of antidepressant **mechanism of action** is called reuptake inhibition. This **mechanism of action** prevents the normal **neurotransmitter** recycling by blocking the reuptake pump that transports **neurotransmitters** from the **synapse** back into the **nerve terminal.** There is then a steady increase in the amount of **neurotransmitter** in the **synapse**, so there is more available to be caught by the receptors. With time, the **neurons** realize they don't need so many receptors and so make fewer, which is called **receptor down-regulation.** When more **serotonin** balls are available, the local **neurons** don't need so many catcher's mitts to ensure they can reliably catch some **serotonin.**

The reduction in the number of catcher's mitts, or **receptor down-regulation**, that occurs when there is consistently more **serotonin** available is strongly associated with the beneficial effects of antidepressants.

Would my psychiatrist give that drug to someone she loves?

I adhere to this Golden Rule in my relationships with patients: "Whatever is hurtful to you, do not do to any other person."

Whether I'm prescribing for a patient for the first time or the fifth time, they're understandably concerned that the treatment we decide on will work quickly so they'll feel better soon and want to know if they'll have side effects. I try to reassure them, whether it's to let them know all the reasons I'm hopeful it might be the right treatment choice, or how other people have found it to be helpful, as well as letting them know that if it's not the right medication for them, we have many other options we can try.

Often the words that seem to be the most reassuring for my patients are the ones that come from my heart. I tell them I would not suggest something I wouldn't take myself or give to someone I love. When I am treating my patients, I always try to think about how I would like my child or another loved one to be treated. I think, *Would I want my kid to take this medication?* For that reason, I have included a section called "Would I take it?" in the charts that follow. While we have many antidepressant choices, from my **clinical experience** (and some clinical research), I know that some are better tolerated, and maybe even more effective, than others.

I see many patients who are very ill, often after they've bravely and patiently endured many trials of medications. Usually they've come to me because previous treatments have not been helpful, or they've caused intolerable side effects. That is often the time when we must look to medications that aren't at the top of my list. Sometimes the only treatment that works is one that is not my first, second, or even my third choice. However, if a treatment works and the side effects are not severe, many people prefer to live with that, rather than living with unrelenting depression.

If you are already taking an antidepressant that is not listed as a good first choice on a chart below, please don't stop taking it, especially if it's working and you're tolerating it well. For you, that antidepressant might be the best choice and highlights the fact that every antidepressant is unique, just like every brain is unique. If you wish to reconsider if it is the best medication for you, please speak to your prescriber before changing the dose or stopping the treatment.

What are selective serotonin reuptake inhibitors (SSRIs)?

The name of the antidepressant class called selective **serotonin** reuptake inhibitors perhaps now makes sense to you, because it literally means that the drug selectively blocks the reuptake of only **serotonin**, leading to a sustained increase of **serotonin** in the synaptic cleft. The longer the reuptake is blocked, the more **serotonin** accumulates, which can interact with the nearby **serotonin** receptors. When there is a sustained increase of **serotonin** for at least several weeks, it causes down-regulation of **serotonin** receptors, which sets into motion various brain changes that can lead to the improvement of depression and **anxiety** symptoms.

There are six SSRIs available in North America. They all have the same **mechanism of action** and they have similar side effects, but each SSRI is chemically distinct. All SSRIs have a **Health Canada** and FDA **indication** for depression. Many also have **indications** for other disorders (see the following table). However, as I discussed on page 161, the lack of an official **indication** doesn't necessarily mean the drug is not helpful for a disorder.

SSRIs have a **class effect**, which means that, as a group, they are useful for the treatment of a particular disorder, in this case, depression and **anxiety disorders.** You'll notice that the older agents, especially sertraline and paroxetine, have many **indications,** but doctors often prescribe all SSRIs for **anxiety disorders**, even without an official **indication.** The **class effect** doesn't apply to all disorders, thus only fluoxetine seems to be particularly beneficial for the eating disorder bulimia nervosa.

The **class effect** extends to medication side effects as well, although, again, every SSRI is chemically distinct, and each medication may have its own unique side effects. As noted previously, there is also a great deal of **inter-individual variability** regarding the likelihood of having a particular side effect. When I describe usual medication side effects associated with each antidepressant class or a specific medication, it's important to remember that they usually occur in a small percentage of patients, and many are transient and resolve quickly. I describe usual antidepressant side effects in depth, and highlight which medications are more or less likely to cause them, in chapter 11.

Generic name	Brand name	Health Canada indications						
		Depression	Generalized anxiety disorder	Social anxiety disorder	Obsessive-compulsive disorder	Panic disorder	Post-traumatic stress disorder	Other
Citalopram	Celexa	X						
Escitalopram	Cipralex (Canada) Lexapro (USA)	X	X		X			
Fluoxetine	Prozac	X			X			Bulimia nervosa
Fluvoxamine	Luvox	X			X			
Paroxetine	Paxil	X	X	X	X	X	X	
Sertraline	Zoloft	X			X	X		

SSRIs as a class

- ***The up side:*** SSRIs are generally safe and effective for depression and anxiety. There is a very low risk associated with overdose.
- ***The down side:*** Some patients will experience weight gain, sexual side effects, sleep disturbance, and **discontinuation symptoms**.

Citalopram

- ***The down side:*** Citalopram has the greatest risk of causing heart-rhythm problems compared to other SSRIs.
- ***Would I take it?:*** Other SSRI options are better.

Escitalopram

- ***The up side:*** Escitalopram is usually very effective and well tolerated. It has the FDA **indication** for the treatment of depression in children.
- ***The down side:*** Excessive sweating is not uncommon.
- ***Would I take it?:*** A good first choice SSRI.

Fluoxetine

- ***The up side:*** Missing a dose is less of a concern because fluoxetine leaves the body very slowly. It has the FDA **indication** for the treatment of depression in children.
- ***The down side:*** Slower onset of antidepressant effect.
- ***Would I take it?:*** Not my first choice SSRI except for bulimia nervosa.

Fluvoxamine

- ***The up side:*** Fluvoxamine is usually reserved for the treatment of OCD.
- ***The down side:*** Fluvoxamine has a greater risk of drug interactions than some other SSRIs.
- ***Would I take it?:*** Other options are better, but it is useful for OCD.

Paroxetine

- ***The up side:*** Paroxetine has many official **Health Canada** and FDA **indications**.
- ***The down side:*** Paroxetine has the greatest risk of weight gain, sexual side effects, and **discontinuation symptoms** compared to other SSRIs. It is not recommended for children or pregnant women.
- ***Would I take it?:*** Other SSRI options are better.

Sertraline

- ***The up side:*** Sertraline is generally very effective and well tolerated. It is often a first choice for pregnant or breastfeeding women.
- ***Would I take it?:*** A good first choice SSRI.

What are serotonin norepinephrine reuptake inhibitors (SNRIs)?

The **mechanism of action** of SNRIs is to block the reuptake of both **serotonin** and **norepinephrine**, which leads to a sustained increase of both **neurotransmitters** in the synaptic cleft. The longer the reuptake is blocked, the more **serotonin** and **norepinephrine** accumulates in the cleft that can interact with nearby receptors, which eventually causes **receptor down-regulation**, resulting in various brain changes that will alleviate depression and **anxiety** symptoms.

There are four SNRIs available in North America. They all exert their effect in the same way and may have similar side effects, but each SNRI is chemically distinct.

All SNRIs block the **serotonin transporter** and increase **serotonin** in a clinically meaningful way at low doses. However, for most SNRIs, the dose must be much higher to increase **norepinephrine** to a level where depression symptoms are improved. For example, **Health Canada**'s maximum recommended dose of venlafaxine XR is 225 mg; however, the **norepinephrine** effect only starts to be evident at that dose. Consequently, psychiatrists commonly prescribe much higher doses of venlafaxine XR. Below 225 mg, venlafaxine XR is acting only as an SSRI, while at or above that dose, patients will experience the benefit of increasing both **serotonin** and **norepinephrine.**

The usual recommended dose of duloxetine is 60 to 120 mg, but it only becomes a true SNRI, with a meaningful **norepinephrine** effect, at 120 mg. Likewise, desvenlafaxine becomes an SNRI at 100 mg and might be more effective for some patients at higher doses. The only SNRI with therapeutically beneficial **norepinephrine** effects at lower doses is levomilnacipran.

SNRIs also have some unique **class effects**, because not only are they beneficial for the treatment of depression and **anxiety**, they are also effective treatments for some pain disorders. For instance, the SNRI duloxetine has several pain **indications**, including diabetic neuropathic pain, migraine, fibromyalgia, osteoarthritis of the knee, and lower back pain.

Another **class effect** of SNRIs is their risk of provoking an increase in blood pressure and heart rate. Many studies have demonstrated that SNRIs very rarely cause a clinically significant increase in blood pressure, also called **hypertension.** In my practice, I have occasionally found increased blood pressure readings with the addition of an SNRI in patients who already have **hypertension**, but it is very unusual to provoke **hypertension** in people who don't already have higher readings. As a class, regulators suggest that SNRIs should be avoided in patients who have uncontrolled **hypertension**, a recent major cardiac event (e.g., heart attack), a history of stroke, severe congestive heart failure, or an uncontrolled abnormal heart rhythm.

Generic name	Brand name	Health Canada indications				
		Depression	Generalized anxiety disorder	Social anxiety disorder	Panic disorder	Other
Desvenlafaxine	Pristiq	X				
Duloxetine	Cymbalta	X	X			Pain
Levomilnacipran	Fetzima	X				
Venlafaxine XR	Effexor XR	X	X	X	X	

SNRIs as a class

- *The up side:* Generally, SNRIs are safe and effective for depression and anxiety. Most are helpful for the treatment of pain at higher doses.
- *The down side:* Some patients will experience weight gain, sexual side effects, sleep disturbance, excessive sweating, and **discontinuation symptoms**. Increased blood pressure is another possible side effect, although this is rarely clinically significant.

Desvenlafaxine

- *The up side:* Desvenlafaxine is usually well tolerated and it tends to have a lower risk of sexual side effects, weight gain, sleep disturbance, and **discontinuation syndrome** than some other SNRIs. It has also been helpful for hot flashes in perimenopausal women.
- *Would I take it?:* A good first choice SNRI.

Duloxetine

- *The up side:* Along with its benefits for depression and anxiety, duloxetine is often very helpful for painful physical symptoms, including fibromyalgia, migraines, joint pain, and diabetic neuropathic pain.
- *The down side:* Some patients experience excessive sweating, which is especially bothersome in the summer months.
- *Would I take it?:* A good first choice SNRI.

Levomilnacipran

- ***The up side:*** Levomilnacipran tends to have a lower risk of sexual side effects, weight gain, and **discontinuation syndrome** than some other SNRIs. It is also helpful for improving motivation and energy, even at lower doses.
- ***Would I take it?:*** A good first choice SNRI.

Venlafaxine XR

- ***The up side:*** Venlafaxine XR has many **Health Canada** official **indications**.
- ***The down side:*** It has the greatest risk of weight gain, sexual side effects, excessive sweating, and **discontinuation symptoms** compared to other SNRIs. It is frequently under-dosed. It should be avoided in pregnant women due to the risk of **discontinuation symptoms** in newborns.
- ***Would I take it?:*** Other SNRI options are better tolerated and easier to dose.

Why might your doctor suggest an SNRI instead of an SSRI?

Because **norepinephrine** offers some significant benefits for some patients, SNRIs are sometimes preferred over SSRIs. Back in chapter 4, you learned about the "flee, freeze, or fight" response, which allows our brain and body to react rapidly to protect us in a threatening situation. Because this response requires a burst of **norepinephrine**, some people mistakenly think that **norepinephrine** causes **anxiety**. A burst of **norepinephrine**, in response to a scary situation, provokes fear, which we need to react quickly and appropriately to a threat. However, bathing receptors in **norepinephrine** over three or more weeks has a potent anti-**anxiety** effect. If you have difficult to treat **anxiety**, your doctor might suggest you try an SNRI.

If you have **chronic** pain, your doctor might suggest an SNRI, especially at higher doses, to ensure you benefit from the **norepinephrine** effect. Increasing **norepinephrine** in the spinal cord and **neurons** leaving the brain and moving out into the body (called descending pathways), especially over several weeks, can be enormously beneficial for many kinds of pain.

What are multimodal antidepressants?

There are some new kids on the block in the antidepressant community, which are medications that have somewhat unique mechanisms of action. Vilazodone and vortioxetine are called multimodal antidepressants because they are both SSRIs, but they also have an additional activity that causes changes in specific **serotonin** receptors.

Vilazodone is the last antidepressant to enter the Canadian market, and its claim to fame seems to be related to tolerability (e.g., lower risk of weight gain and sexual **dysfunction** compared to other SSRIs), while maintaining the **class effect** of improving depression and **anxiety** symptoms.

Vortioxetine has an additional benefit compared to other antidepressants: **cognitive** improvement. Recall from chapter 1 that depression is commonly associated with **cognitive** symptoms, including difficulty with memory, concentration, organizing, and planning, as well as slowed thinking. Vortioxetine has a great deal of research evidence demonstrating its benefit in improving **cognitive** symptoms associated with depression. In fact, even if vortioxetine doesn't improve depression symptoms, some patients still notice they're able to think more clearly and thus function better.

Generic name	Brand name	Health Canada indications	
		Depression	Other
Vilazodone	Viibryd	X	
Vortioxetine	Trintellix	X	Cognitive improvement

Multimodal antidepressants as a class

- *The up side:* Multimodal antidepressants are generally effective for depression and anxiety.

Vilazodone

- *The up side:* For many, vilazodone has a much lower risk of sexual side effects and a lower risk of weight gain compared to other SSRIs and SNRIs.
- *The down side:* Vilazodone must be taken with food to be adequately absorbed and some patients will experience nausea and/or diarrhea, especially when initiating the medication. However, this side effect tends to be short-lived and usually resolves within a few weeks.
- *Would I take it?:* A good first choice antidepressant.

Vortioxetine

- *The up side:* Vortioxetine had strong evidence for improving depression-related **cognitive** symptoms. For some patients, there is a lower risk of sexual side effects and weight gain compared to other SSRIs and SNRIs.
- *The down side:* Nausea and vomiting may be significant but usually resolves. Starting at the lowest possible dose, taking with food, and increasing slowly all help to reduce the risk.
- *Would I take it?:* A good first choice antidepressant.

Novel antidepressants

There are a couple of oddball antidepressants called **novel antidepressants:** they're in classes by themselves when it comes to their mechanisms of action. That's a good thing in my books, because if an SSRI or SNRI isn't an option for a patient, due to side effects or because they're not effective, it's good to have other treatments to try that are completely different. Additionally, these medications, because they have unique mechanisms of action, may be used in combination with an SSRI or SNRI.

Bupropion XL is a **norepinephrine** and **dopamine** reuptake inhibitor (NDRI), but most of its benefit is derived from increasing

norepinephrine. Dopamine is another **neurotransmitter** that is implicated in depression, but it also plays a critical role in promoting motivation, pleasure seeking (e.g., love, lust, and joie de vivre), reward seeking (**dopamine** plays a major role in addiction), attention, learning, and fluidity of movement.

Bupropion XL is a very well-tolerated antidepressant for most patients, because it doesn't cause sexual side effects or weight gain, which are among the most frustrating side effects that patients face. Bupropion XL is not just helpful for depression symptoms but has also been demonstrated to effectively treat seasonal patterns of depression. For some patients with **seasonal depression**, bupropion XL is only required in the fall and winter months and may be discontinued during the spring and summer, when there are longer days and more sunlight.

Bupropion XL can be useful for managing mild to moderate **anxiety** symptoms or **generalized anxiety disorder**, especially if it's helping to reduce depression symptoms. However, it is usually not very useful for treating severe **anxiety** or **anxiety disorders**, such as **panic disorder**, PTSD, OCD, or **social anxiety disorder**. In these situations, **serotonin** is almost always required, if the symptoms are severe enough that medication is deemed necessary.

The seizure risk associated with bupropion XL is frequently mentioned, but the research evidence does not support those concerns, especially at usual doses. The concern arose from a poorly conducted study that included patients with electrolyte abnormalities related to an eating disorder. The evidence suggests that using the long-acting bupropion (this is why I specify bupropion XL) at usual doses (300–450 mg) is safe, even for a patient who also has a seizure disorder. This is good news for those who want to take this antidepressant, because of its superior tolerability.

Mirtazapine is a noradrenergic and specific serotonergic antidepressant (NaSSA). Usually, when there is enough **serotonin** and **norepinephrine** in the synaptic cleft to interact with the adjacent receptors, the release of **neurotransmitters** from the **nerve terminal** stops. NaSSAs work by blocking the message that tells the

neuron to stop releasing **neurotransmitters**, so more and more are released. This is a positive thing in a depressed brain, because the level of **serotonin** and **norepinephrine** is too low.

Mirtazapine does not usually cause sexual side effects, which is a major problem for many antidepressants. Additionally, it has an anti-nausea effect, so it's a good choice for patients who are very sensitive to nausea when prescribed other antidepressants. Mirtazapine can also help to improve sleep, although when it is initiated many complain that it is much too sedating. This side effect usually resolves after a few weeks and thereafter patients continue to get a better sleep. However, those first few weeks can be a serious challenge.

Weight gain is only a good thing if depression has resulted in a loss of appetite and serious weight loss. However, mirtazapine routinely causes excessive weight gain; for many patients, that is a serious problem that often results in treatment discontinuation. Mirtazapine should be avoided in patients who are already struggling with their weight or who would find any weight gain to be unacceptable. For more on the side effects of antidepressants, see chapter 11.

Trazodone is a **serotonin** antagonist and reuptake inhibitor (SARI). It is rarely used as an antidepressant, because high doses are required to have a robust antidepressant effect. At those doses, trazodone is generally not as well tolerated as other antidepressants. It is primarily used in Canada, at the very low end of the dose range, as a treatment for **insomnia** (see page 209).

Generic name	**Brand name**	**Health Canada indications**	
		Depression	Other
Bupropion XL	Wellbutrin XL	X*	
Mirtazapine	Remeron	X	
Trazodone	Desyrel	X	Insomnia

* including prevention of seasonal depression episodes

Bupropion XL

- *The up side:* Bupropion XL has the lowest risk of any antidepressant for sexual side effects and weight gain. It is also a useful treatment for **seasonal depression**.
- *The down side:* Bupropion XL is not generally helpful for **anxiety disorders**, such as **panic disorder**, OCD, PTSD, or social **anxiety disorder**. However, mild or generalized anxiety might benefit from bupropion XL.
- *Would I take it?:* A good first choice antidepressant.

Mirtazapine

- *The up side:* Mirtazapine has a very low risk of sexual side effects as well as a low risk of nausea. It might be useful for patients who are highly sensitive to antidepressant-related nausea. Mirtazapine is a good choice for patients who have **insomnia** and significant weight loss due to depression-related loss of appetite.
- *The down side:* Mirtazapine is amongst the worst antidepressants for causing weight gain. It is also commonly excessively sedating when initiated, which may take several weeks to resolve.
- *Would I take it?:* Other options are often better tolerated. Mirtazapine is most useful when weight gain and significant sedation are desirable.

Trazodone

- *The up side:* Trazodone is helpful at lower doses for improving sleep but at higher doses, its side effects may make it intolerable.
- *The down side:* Higher doses of trazodone are required to provide an antidepressant benefit, but the side effects at higher doses limit its use.
- *Would I take it?:* Trazodone is not recommended as an antidepressant because other choices are likely more effective and tolerable. However, it is often very helpful as a treatment for **insomnia**.

Tricyclic and tetracyclic antidepressants (TCAs)

Among the oldest antidepressants, TCAs are named for their chemical structure—either three circles (tricyclic) or four circles (tetracyclic). The TCAs have a similar **mechanism of action** to

SSRIs and SNRIs, which is to block reuptake of **serotonin** and/or **norepinephrine.** However, they have largely been replaced by SSRIs, SNRIs, and newer, **novel antidepressants**, because the TCAs tend to be less well tolerated and, as a class, they have a greater risk of lethality in overdose.

TCAs are very effective antidepressants and offer some added benefits, especially related to neuropathic pain relief, prevention of migraines, and improved sleep. Aside from amitriptyline, which also has the **indication** for OCD, TCAs are only indicated for the treatment of depression but they have been used off-label for decades for a variety of disorders.

Generic name	Brand name	Health Canada indications	
		Depression	Other
Amitriptyline	Elavil	X	OCD
Clomipramine	Anafranil	X	
Desipramine	Norpramin	X	
Imipramine	Tofranil/ Surmontil	X	
Nortriptyline	Aventyl	X	
Trazodone	Desyrel	X	Insomnia

TCAs as a class

- ***The up side:*** TCAs are generally effective for depression.
- ***The down side:*** TCAs as class tend to have more bothersome side effects (e.g., dry mouth, blurred vision, constipation, urinary hesitancy (hard to pee), weight gain, sexual side effects). As a class, they are associated with a higher risk of lethality in overdose compared to most newer antidepressants.
- ***Would I take it?:*** Not if a newer antidepressant worked as well, since they tend to be better tolerated.

Amitriptyline

- ***The up side:*** An effective treatment for neuropathic pain and very severe/ **psychotic** depression.

Clomipramine

- *The up side:* Often used for the treatment of **obsessive-compulsive disorder**.

Desipramine

- *The up side:* An effective treatment for very severe/**psychotic** depression.

Nortriptyline

- *The up side:* An effective treatment for neuropathic pain.

Monoamine oxidase inhibitors (MAOIs)

Monoamine oxidase inhibitors (**MAOIs**) are an interesting group of older antidepressants that have a unique **mechanism of action. Monoamine oxidase** (**MAO**) is an enzyme involved in the breakdown and removal (also called **metabolism**) of **neurotransmitters**, such as **serotonin, norepinephrine**, and **dopamine**. When the action of MAO is blocked (or inhibited), it results in an increase in these **neurotransmitters** in the **nerve terminal** and in the bloodstream. There are two types of MAOIs: A and B type. Inhibiting the A type appears to be necessary for its antidepressant effect.

Tranylcypromine and phenelzine are non-selective MAOIs, which means they block both the A and B type of MAO enzyme, rather than just the A type required to treat depression. They are also irreversible, which means they permanently block the MAO enzyme. The only way to overcome their effect is to stop the drug and wait for more MAO to be produced, which takes up to four weeks, depending on which MAOI is prescribed. Tranylcypromine, for instance, rapidly produces an antidepressant effect, and it takes about a week for new MAO enzymes to be produced once the drug is withdrawn. Phenelzine tends to work more slowly and leaves the system more slowly as well.

Irreversible MAOIs are reserved for the most ill patients, including those with **psychotic** depression, because this type of antidepressant is associated with some serious risks (see page 198).

MAOIs may also be very helpful for **atypical** depression and some **anxiety disorders**, such as **panic disorder** and social **anxiety disorder.** I have found them most helpful for patients who have **treatment-resistant depression (TRD)** (to read more about TRD, see chapter 12), which means several other types of antidepressants or other treatments have not been helpful for their depression symptoms.

Certain drugs and foods contain a precursor of **norepinephrine**, called **tyramine**, which must be broken down by MAO. When taking a MAOI, **tyramine** from foods or drugs will not be broken down and that leads to an accumulation of **norepinephrine**, which can result in extremely high blood pressure, called a **hypertensive crisis.**

A **hypertensive crisis** is potentially deadly and may be associated with a constellation of other symptoms, including headache, heart racing, palpitations, slowed heart rate, chest pain, sore or stiff neck, nausea, vomiting, sweating (sometimes with fever and sometimes with cold, clammy skin), dilated pupils, and light sensitivity.

Due to the risk of serious side effects, irreversible MAOIs should not be taken in combination with other medications that can cause an increase in **norepinephrine**, **dopamine**, or **serotonin.** Consequently, they are not prescribed together with other antidepressants. Many other medications, including some **over-the-counter treatments**, should also be avoided, which is why it's important to speak to your doctor or pharmacist before taking any other medications if you're prescribed an MAOI.

It's also necessary to allow time for the MAOI to be cleared out of the body before starting another antidepressant, and for another antidepressant to be completely cleared from the body before starting an MAOI. This might mean that a patient will have to be antidepressant-free for up to four weeks to safely make the switch, depending on the medication in question. For someone who is very ill, that length of time may be intolerable.

Tyramine occurs naturally in some foods or may be produced when bacteria breaks down the protein in fermented, aged, or spoiled food. Consequently, fermented food and drink, like beer, wine, aged cheeses, and cured meat, must be avoided when taking an MAOI, because they contain **tyramine** which can provoke increased blood pressure (see below).

Foods that are high risk in combination with MAOIS

- All matured or aged cheeses. Cheeses made from pasteurized milk are less likely to contain high levels of **tyramine**, so cottage cheese, cream cheese, ricotta, and processed cheese are considered MAOI-safe. All non-cheese dairy products can be consumed providing they are fresh, including milk, yogurt, and ice cream.
- All aged, cured, or fermented meat, fish, or poultry. Any meat, fish, or poultry that was bought fresh, stored correctly, and eaten fresh and has not undergone aging, curing, or fermenting is considered safe.
- All fermented soybean products (e.g., soy sauce, miso, fermented tofu or tempeh) and fava or broad bean pods.
- Sauerkraut.
- Banana peel (but not the pulp). If you're eating banana peels on a regular basis, perhaps there are some other issues that need to be discussed?
- Concentrated yeast extracts (e.g., Marmite or Vegemite spread). Apologies to Aussies and Brits!
- All tap/draught beers; unpasteurized beer (e.g., canned or bottled draught beer); Belgian, Korean, European, and African beers; and homemade beer and wine. Some bottled beers, including non-alcoholic beer, may also pose a risk. Patients are generally advised to minimize or avoid use of all alcoholic beverages. One drink per day of domestic bottled or canned beer, red or white wine, fortified wines, and spirits (e.g. rum, vodka, gin) is generally considered to be safe.

Many of the foods listed above are deliberately aged as part of their production and must be avoided. Other foods may also naturally age over time, even if they are refrigerated, so it is very important to buy and eat only fresh foods or those that have been properly frozen when prescribed an MAOI. Avoid eating foods if you are unsure of their freshness and be very cautious of new foods, even if they have been refrigerated. When there is any doubt, either avoid the food or eat only a small amount.

Tyramine levels may vary between food brands or even between different batches of the same brand. This means that you can accidentally eat a prohibited food on one occasion and have no reaction, but another time that same food might cause a serious hypertensive reaction.

Over the last many years, new research has suggested that the concerns regarding the dangers of using MAOIs are overstated and have unfortunately limited the use of these very effective and generally well-tolerated treatments. Importantly, the need for dietary restrictions appear to have been developed based on poor evidence and many researchers believe they are vastly overstated, which is good news for depressed banana peel eaters everywhere!

Medication regulatory agencies (e.g., **Health Canada**, FDA) recommend that MAOIs, as a class, should be avoided in patients who have uncontrolled blood pressure, a recent major cardiac event (e.g., heart attack), a history of stroke, severe congestive heart failure, or an uncontrolled abnormal heart rhythm.

While I tend to offer MAOIs only to those who have TRD, they are extremely effective medications, so patients are often willing to give an MAOI a try because their depression is causing them anguish. If the drug works and is well tolerated, most patients incorporate the MAOI into their lives seamlessly.

If you are prescribed a MAOI, consider wearing a medical alert bracelet or carry a notice in your wallet to let first responders know, in case you're in an accident and require resuscitation. Drugs that are sometimes used in this situation can provoke a **hypertensive crisis** when combined with a MAOI.

The other MAOI: The reversible inhibitor of monoamine oxidase type A (RIMA)

Moclobemide, the newest MAOI, is also known as a RIMA, which stands for reversible inhibitor of MAO-A: it preferentially inhibits only MAO-A. This effect lasts twenty-four hours at most and is reversible. That means that if there is too much **tyramine** around, the MAO enzyme will be able to function and break it down, preventing a **hypertensive crisis.** However, at higher than usual doses (above 900 mg per day), moclobemide can block both MAO types A and B irreversibly, so most doctors suggest that their patients prescribed higher doses follow the careful food and drug safety measures that those prescribed irreversible MAOIs are asked to follow.

Generic name	Brand name	Health Canada indication
		Depression
Moclobemide	Manerix	X
Phenelzine	Nardil	X
Tranylcypromine	Parnate	X

MAOIs as a class

- *The up side:* MAOIs are generally very effective for depression and anxiety and are usually well tolerated.
- *The down side:* The irreversible MAOIs have a risk of drug and food interactions that may result in a **hypertensive crisis**. Due to this risk, patients must follow dietary restrictions and exercise special care when taking other prescription and **over-the-counter medications**.
- *Would I take it?:* Not if I found a newer antidepressant that worked as well, since they tend to be better tolerated and the MAOI food and drug restrictions are a bother.

Moclobemide

- *The up side:* Low risk of weight gain and sexual **dysfunction**, and not excessively sedating.

- ***The down side:*** At higher doses, patients should follow the same dietary and drug interactions as are required for irreversible MAOIs.
- ***Would I take it?:*** Yes, this is a well-tolerated treatment, especially if lower doses are effective.

Phenelzine

- ***The up side:*** Phenelzine is a very effective treatment for severe depression and anxiety, including **panic disorder** and social **anxiety disorder**.
- ***The down side:*** Phenelzine has a risk of drug and food interactions that requires dietary restrictions and care with prescription and **over-the-counter medications**. It may also be excessively sedating and cause weight gain.

Tranylcypromine

- ***The up side:*** Tranylcypromine is a very effective treatment for severe depression and anxiety, including **panic disorder** and social **anxiety disorder**. It has a lower risk of weight gain than phenelzine.
- ***The down side:*** Tranylcypromine has a risk of drug and food interactions that requires dietary restrictions and care with prescription and **over-the-counter medications**. It may also be excessively sedating.

Investigational depression treatments

Ketamine

Currently available antidepressants work primarily through their effect on the **neurotransmitters serotonin, norepinephrine,** and (to a lesser extent) **dopamine.** But research indicates that there are other important **neurotransmitters** involved in the development and maintenance of depression. **Glutamate** is the most abundant excitatory **neurotransmitter** in the brain and plays a critical role in many normal brain functions, including **neurogenesis, neuroplasticity,** and **cognitive** functions, such as learning and memory. It is critical that the amount of **glutamate** in various brain regions is kept at an optimal level for normal brain functioning, because excessive **glutamate** can damage or kill **neurons. Glutamate** has been implicated as a cause of depression, **bipolar disorders,**

anxiety disorders, **schizophrenia**, substance abuse, and other serious neurodegenerative disorders, such as Alzheimer's disease and amyotrophic lateral sclerosis (ALS).

Like the other **neurotransmitters** involved in depression, **glutamate** is released from the terminal end of a **neuron**, binds to receptors on adjacent **neurons**, and is then transported back into the **nerve terminal** from the synaptic cleft by reuptake pumps, where it is repackaged and prepared to be released again when needed (see chapter 10). There are several different types and subtypes of **glutamate** receptors, so drugs can bind to different receptor subtypes and impact **glutamate** function in different ways, depending on the specific drug and receptor involved. Thus, one drug that impacts **glutamate** receptors could potentially have several very different, and even opposite, effects.

As I described in chapter 4, **chronic stress** can cause the brain support cells, called **glial cells**, to stop functioning properly. One of their critical roles is to ensure that the amount of **glutamate** is tightly controlled. It is likely that the nerve cell injury and death associated with **chronic** depression is mediated, at least in part, by the accumulation of **glutamate** in sensitive brain areas that results from the failure of **glial cells** to suck up excessive **glutamate**.

Ketamine is a drug that has typically been used for anesthesia, pain management, and sedation for adults and children in a hospital setting. It seems to have unique effects in different brain regions, and it interacts with a number of **glutamate** receptors, including the NMDA and AMPA receptors. Ketamine is referred to as a high-affinity NMDA **receptor antagonist**, which means it attaches itself very effectively to the NMDA receptor and blocks its effects. However, there are likely multiple effects of the drug that explain its therapeutic benefits in depression. For instance, ketamine is also thought to substantially increase the amount of **brain-derived neurotrophic factor** (**BDNF**), which is an essential requirement of effective antidepressant treatment (see page 77). It also improves how effectively **neurons** communicate and promotes the growth of new connections between **neurons**, called **synaptogenesis**.

Although ketamine has been used in medicine for more than fifty years, its use in psychiatry is relatively recent, and represents an exciting advancement because at low doses it very rapidly produces an antidepressant effect, even for patients who have **treatment-resistant depression** (**TRD**). (To read more about TRD, see chapter 12.) Research suggests it may significantly reduce the risk of suicide in patients with severe depression. Its use for the treatment of depression is not approved by **Health Canada** or the FDA. Ketamine is administered via an intravenous infusion over about forty minutes, and a robust antidepressant effect can be experienced within four hours of receiving the treatment and may last up to two weeks. The benefits may be extended for weeks, months, and even years when treatments are given every two to seven days. Those who don't have an initial robust response might experience a benefit after several treatments or with the use of slightly higher doses.

Intravenous ketamine, when used as an antidepressant, has generally been very well tolerated. Some patients experience perceptual disturbances or dissociation, but these side effects, if present, usually peak within an hour of treatment and are almost always fully resolved within a few hours. Likewise, increased heart rate and blood pressure is possible but also tends to be mild, short-lived, and rarely results in treatment discontinuation. The most common side effects are drowsiness, dizziness, nausea, feeling strange or unreal, poor coordination, and blurred vision. However, a review of studies that included 234 patients found no difference in discontinuation rates for those treated with ketamine and those treated with traditional antidepressant medications.

Ketamine has been misused and abused, and it must be used with caution in individuals at risk for substance abuse. As a street drug, ketamine produces a variety of effects including hallucinogenic-like effects and dissociation, which might include a sensation of floating or of being separated from your body. The drug effects are very short-lived, usually between one to two hours.

Despite the exciting research and benefits for the most ill patients with depression, the availability of ketamine intravenous infusions is still very limited in Canada. Some provinces have research centres where the treatment is available for patients with TRD. There are also some for-profit clinics offering ketamine infusions. Most programs follow a ketamine infusion protocol, where patients are initially given treatments every few days for several weeks and the ultimate dose and frequency of treatments are determined by the patient's experience.

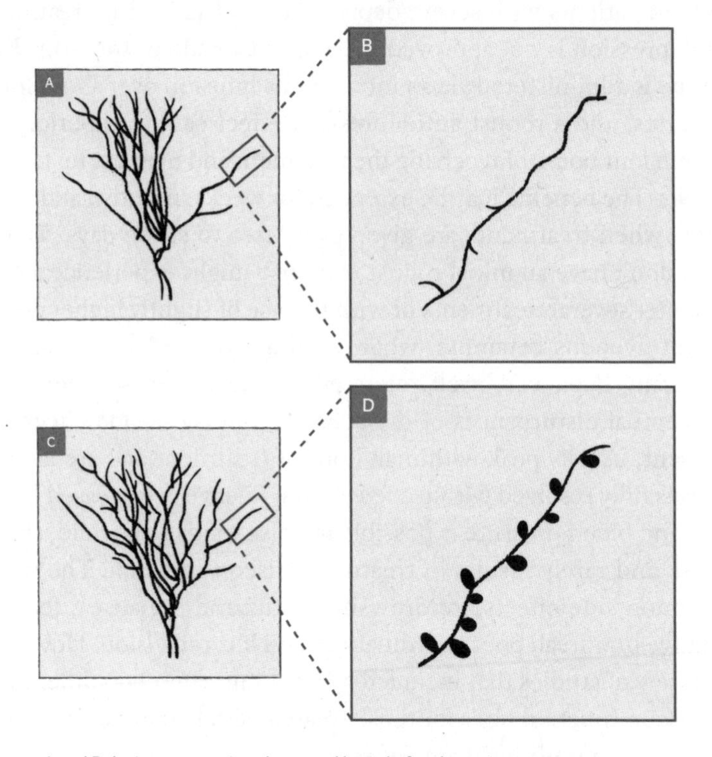

Images A and B depict a neuron in a depressed brain before ketamine treatment.

Image A shows a neuron from a depressed brain with a reduced number of dendrites (projections that interact with other neurons).

B is a close-up of a dendrite from the depressed brain showing atrophy. It has fewer, less dense branches so it is less able to pass on messages to adjacent neurons.

C and D are depicting a neuron in a depressed brain twenty-four hours after ketamine treatment.

C shows more numerous and dense dendrites and D is a close-up of a dendrite that has already started to recover and become more able to pass on messages to adjacent neurons.

Esketamine

Ketamine is made of a mixture of two enantiomers, which are mirror images of each other, called S-ketamine and R-ketamine. Esketamine contains just the *S*-enantiomer, which has a much higher affinity for the NMDA receptor than ketamine (the R+S mixture). While ketamine is administered through an intravenous infusion, esketamine is dispensed as a self-administered nasal spray.

While intranasal esketamine has similar antidepressant benefits as compared to ketamine, its ease of use and early robust research data led the FDA to consider it a depression treatment breakthrough. In March 2019, the FDA-approved esketamine (Spravato®) nasal spray, to be used in conjunction with an oral antidepressant, for the treatment of depression in adults who have TRD. This represents the first new antidepressant **mechanism of action** in thirty years.

To date, there have been three short-term trials and two long-term trials assessing the safety and effectiveness of esketamine for TRD, and two studies are underway assessing the drug's benefits for patients at imminent risk for suicide. In the TRD trials, patients were maintained on an antidepressant medication along with the esketamine. Like ketamine, the robust therapeutic benefits of esketamine are rapidly apparent, usually within days, and continue to improve over six to eight weeks. The studies found that standard doses of 56 to 84 mg produced robust antidepressant effects. The drug is given twice a week for a month and then every week to two weeks once the antidepressant effect has been established. Elderly patients should be initiated at a dose of 28 mg, but they will ultimately likely require the standard dose of 56 to 84 mg.

Esketamine will be administered in a clinic where patients are monitored for up to two hours after treatment. The side effects of esketamine are similar to those of ketamine; they are also short-lived and almost always resolve within a few hours of treatment. The monitoring post-treatment is required because, like with a ketamine infusion, some patients will experience perceptual disturbances and increased blood pressure. For nearly all patients, these effects peak within forty minutes and resolve completely within ninety minutes. Patients must not drive after receiving esketamine until, as the drug developer will recommend, they have had a restful night's sleep.

Esketamine is a major breakthrough for the treatment of the most severely ill depressed patients. It is now available in the United States, and it should be available for use in Canada in 2019.

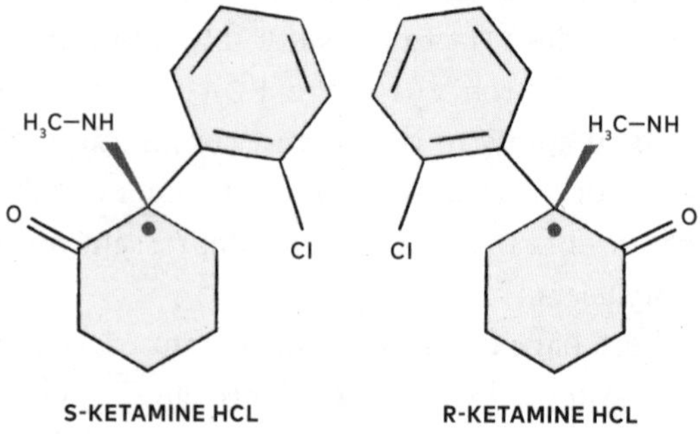

S-KETAMINE HCL

R-KETAMINE HCL

Chapter summary

- Each antidepressant is unique. The right medication for an individual is one that fully manages the depression symptoms and doesn't cause intolerable side effects.
- If one medication doesn't work or isn't well tolerated, it's likely another will.
- What doesn't work for one person might be the very best treatment for someone else.

The key to finding the right medication for depression is communication. It's important to listen carefully to your prescriber and ask questions if you have concerns. Make sure to report symptom changes and side effects. When both team members are fully and honestly engaged, recovery is not just possible but likely.

A real patient's story

"I JUST NEED TO sleep," I cried to anyone who'd listen. While it was true—I did need to sleep—I also needed more than that: I needed professional help.

A cancer scare a few months earlier had resulted in a total hysterectomy, which plunged me into instant **menopause**. Whether it was the sudden loss of **hormones**, the difficult **recovery**, a return to work too soon, or the fear of cancer itself (fortunately, I had endometriosis, not cancer) in the weeks that followed, I'd become increasingly anxious about everything. Throw in bladder issues and broken sleep, and it was a breeding ground for depression and **anxiety** to take hold. But instead of letting people know that I was struggling, I did the opposite and assured everyone that I was doing *great!*

I was far from great. In the past, whenever I'd faced a difficult challenge or experienced a devastating loss, I'd push down my emotions and pretend that everything was fine. I believed that to do otherwise would make me seem ungrateful, whiny, or—worse of all—weak. For years, this mindset worked for me.

Until it didn't.

I arrived at the emergency room of our local hospital with debilitating **insomnia** and **anxiety** so severe I could barely walk, my mind as broken as my body.

I wish I could say I got the help I needed, but I didn't. Lucky for me, my husband refused to give up until he found a doctor who did provide the help and medication I required. This allowed me to not only sleep but calm down enough so that I could start putting the pieces of my fractured life back together again.

As I write this, it's been a little over four months since the day I crash-landed in the emergency room, scared and fearing for my life. Without the caring attention of the medical professional who intervened, I honestly don't know what would have happened. Happily, what I've since learned is that while depression and **anxiety** is a terrifying experience to go through, there is always room for hope because help is out there. I'm still not well, but thankfully I'm having more good days than bad. While I'd love nothing more than to be better now, I've learned to appreciate the progress I've made and have accepted that true healing takes time.

A friend who has gone through something similar before recently told me that I'll never be the same again. My heart sank, imagining the worst. He then assured me that what he meant was that I would be a stronger and better person because of this. He told me that while his breakdown was the hardest thing he's ever been through, it taught him a lot about himself and that he learned to value what really matters in life.

There have already been unexpected gifts that have come from this. I'm more open with people, less guarded and judgmental, more willing to ask for help. I've developed closer, more genuine relationships with my family and friends. Some have also generously shared with me their own journeys with depression and **anxiety**. Knowing so many others have walked this path before—and continue to walk this path—humbles me and gives me hope. And I now know that no one is ever truly alone, as long as they can summon the courage to reach out.

11

What are the common side effects of antidepressants?

ANTIDEPRESSANTS EXERT their beneficial effects by increasing **neurotransmitters** in the brain, but those same neurotransmitters may also provoke side effects. Most side effects resolve after the first few weeks of treatment, while others may lead you and your doctor to try another medication. In the pages that follow, when I state that a treatment is tolerable or well tolerated, that means it is not provoking unpleasant side effects.

There is a great deal of inter-individual variability in how people tolerate antidepressant medications: most people have little or no problem with side effects, while others have a far greater challenge finding a medication that is tolerable for them. If one medication has side effects that you find intolerable, ask to try another option.

Some of the more common antidepressant side effects include:

Nausea

While nausea is most often due to an increase in **serotonin**, it can be provoked by many causes, including **anxiety** (see functional gastrointestinal disorder (FGID) on page 89). Nausea is nearly always transient and is often mitigated by following my Golden Rules (see page 217). If antidepressant-associated nausea is severe or persistent, another medication should be tried.

Lowest risk: mirtazapine, bupropion XL, MAOIs.
Major culprits: vortioxetine, any SSRI or SNRI.

Headache

Headaches can be caused by so many different factors, including medical causes and **anxiety**, that it's almost impossible to suggest a single likely source. However, antidepressant-related headaches are nearly always transient and often mitigated by following my Golden Rules. There is a beneficial **class effect** for appropriately dosed SNRIs, which may help to reduce pain, including a reduction in headaches and migraines. If headaches are severe or persistent and their onset coincided with the initiation of an antidepressant, another medication should be tried.

Lowest risk: SNRIs (especially duloxetine and levomilnacipran).
Major culprits: Any other antidepressant.

Drowsiness

There are some antidepressants that are more likely to cause drowsiness, which can be very useful if you're not sleeping well. However, if the drowsiness persists, even after your mood improves, that may be a serious barrier to improved functioning. You might also be drowsy because you're depressed and not sleeping well, or because you have a medical issue, such as low iron (anemia), low thyroid (hypothyroidism), or sleep apnea. These disorders should be ruled out as part of an initial assessment, which should include lab tests. If antidepressant-associated drowsiness is severe or persistent, another medication should be tried.

Lowest risk: bupropion XL.
Major culprits: mirtazapine, quetiapine, TCAs.

Restlessness/agitation

Any antidepressant can cause these side effects, especially those that increase **norepinephrine**, but such symptoms can also be related to depression and severe **anxiety**. Restlessness and agitation is nearly always transient and often mitigated by following my Golden Rules. When initiating an antidepressant, "start low and go slow" is particularly helpful. If antidepressant-associated restlessness or agitation is severe or persistent, another medication should be tried.

Lowest risk: mirtazapine.
Major culprits: bupropion XL, SNRIs.

Dry mouth

Dry mouth can be caused by so many different factors, including **anxiety**, but increasing **norepinephrine** seems to be a major provocation. Dry mouth may be transient, but if persistent can result in major dental problems, including cavities, gingivitis, and bad breath. Using an over-the-counter dry mouth treatment may not be particularly helpful, although chewing sugarless gum may offer some relief. If dry mouth is severe or persistent, another antidepressant should be tried.

Major culprits: bupropion XL, SNRIs, TCAs.

Insomnia

Insomnia is a common symptom of depression but can also be provoked by certain antidepressants, especially related to **serotonin.** If you believe your antidepressant is making you sleep poorly, first try to switch the timing. That means if you're taking it at night, try taking it in the morning, and if you're currently taking it in the morning, try taking it at night. If **insomnia** is severe or persistent and the onset coincided with the initiation of an antidepressant, another medication should be considered.

Lowest risk: mirtazapine, quetiapine, trazodone, newer antidepressants (desvenlafaxine, levomilnacipran, vilazodone, vortioxetine), TCAs.
Major culprits: SSRIs, bupropion XL.

Constipation/diarrhea

Bowel symptoms may be associated with depression and **anxiety**, but some individuals can be sensitive to increases in **serotonin** and **norepinephrine**, resulting in altered bowel motility. Additionally, as you read in chapter 5, depression has been associated with irritable bowel syndrome, which is commonly associated with alternating constipation and diarrhea.

The most effective treatments for constipation are exercise (even a little bit of walking), lots of water, and increased dietary or supplemental fibre (now available in tablet form taken with lots of water). The short-term use of a laxative or a stool softener may help, but if constipation is severe or persistent, another antidepressant should be considered.

Loperamide is an extremely effective **over-the-counter treatment** for diarrhea, but if diarrhea is severe or persistent, another antidepressant should be considered.

Potential culprits: Any of them.

Sexual dysfunction

Sexual **dysfunction** can take many forms: loss of sexual interest or desire, anorgasmia (slow to reach orgasm or inability to orgasm); for women, vaginal dryness or pain during intercourse; and for men, an inability to obtain or sustain an erection.

A loss of sexual interest or functioning is a common symptom of depression but can also be a problematic side effect associated with antidepressant treatments, mostly related to increasing **serotonin.** It's important to tell your doctor about what your sexual desire/functioning was like before the depression started; otherwise, a drug might be blamed for a pre-existing issue. While depression might be the initial cause, as the depression resolves so should the sexual problems. Unfortunately, the antidepressant treatment might then prolong or worsen the problem.

There is a great deal of **inter-individual variability** related to how a medication impacts sexual functioning. Two people taking the same medication may have very different experiences. For some people, antidepressant-related sexual **dysfunction** may be transient, but more often it persists, so it's important to discuss sexual issues with your doctor because it's a major reason why people discontinue treatment. Several possible options might help to reduce this extremely frustrating side effect. Because sexual **dysfunction** tends to be dose-dependent, lowering the antidepressant dose might help, so long as a lower dose doesn't result in worsening depression or **anxiety** symptoms. Alternatively, switching to a lower-risk antidepressant might help, so long as it also manages the depression. Another option is to combine an antidepressant that has a lower risk of sexual side effects with a lower dose of the antidepressant that is causing the sexual side effects. If the sexual **dysfunction** is severe or persistent, another antidepressant should be considered.

If you've tried other antidepressants and sexual problems persist, men have the option of using treatments such as sildenafil (Viagra®), tadalafil (Cialis®), or vardenafil (Levitra®) which improve the quality and longevity of an erection, and don't interfere with the effectiveness of the antidepressant. Interestingly, I have prescribed these drugs often, and many men report that their sexual desire has improved, simply by having an erection they can count on. Unfortunately, these treatments don't work for women, and currently there are no effective treatments available to manage a woman's medication-related sexual **dysfunction.**

Flibanserin (Addyi®) is a medication developed for women with low sexual drive, known officially as hypoactive sexual desire disorder (HSDD). According to the **product monograph**, flibanserin is intended for women who have not gone through **menopause**, who have not had problems with low sexual desire in the past, are troubled by their low sexual drive, and who have low sexual desire no matter the type of sexual activity, the situation, or the sexual partner. The drug's **product monograph** also states that flibanserin should be used only if low sexual desire is not due to a medical or mental health problem, problems in the relationship, or medicine or other drug use, and it should not be used to improve sexual performance. Frustratingly, the **product monograph** warns that women who drink alcohol should not take flibanserin—so much for a nice glass of wine with a delicious meal before getting busy with your partner!

It's important to consider whether a woman's change in sexual desire or functioning is related to **perimenopause** or **menopause.** A reduction in **estrogen** can affect sexual desire as well as cause vaginal changes that result in discomfort during intercourse. **Estrogen** replacement, sometimes by using **estrogen** locally (e.g., intra-vaginal creams or a slow-release **estrogen** ring), can provide enormous benefit.

It's also important to discuss antidepressant-induced sexual side effects with your partner, since they might feel your lack of interest or difficulty with sexual functioning reflects your feelings for them, rather than being due to the medication. Importantly, there is ample evidence demonstrating that partners who have their sexual needs met are more engaged and supportive, so your sexual functioning is a very important factor to consider and discuss with your mate.

Lowest risk: mirtazapine, bupropion XL, newer antidepressants (desvenlafaxine, levomilnacipran, vilazodone, vortioxetine), MAOIs.

Major culprits: SSRIs, SNRIs.

Discontinuation symptoms

Because there may be a constellation of unpleasant symptoms that result from the discontinuation of an antidepressant, the experience is often referred to as **discontinuation syndrome.** While any antidepressant can cause **discontinuation symptoms,** this sometimes highly distressing side effect occurs much more often with some of the older antidepressants, such as the SSRI paroxetine and the SNRI venlafaxine XR. Those two medications can sometimes provoke **discontinuation symptoms** after a patient has missed only one dose or by taking a dose a little later than usual. For other medications, discontinuation side effects might take a few days to become apparent. Mercifully, this problem is less commonly associated with newer antidepressant medications.

Discontinuation symptoms are non-specific and may include flu-like symptoms (nausea, vomiting, diarrhea, body aches, headaches, dizziness, sweating), restlessness, jitteriness, sleep disturbance, **anxiety**, depressed mood, electric shock–like feelings that project into extremities and into the face and jaw, and just about any other awful feeling you can think of. From that list, it's probably apparent that having those symptoms can be very confusing: one might wonder, *Am I getting depressed again?*

There is a great deal of **inter-individual variability** related to **discontinuation symptoms.** Two people discontinuing the same medication may have very different experiences; one might have no problems, while the other might have very unpleasant symptoms.

The best way to avoid **discontinuation symptoms** is to lower the antidepressant dose slowly, over a few weeks, if possible. If one antidepressant isn't working well and another is going to be tried, the new medication should be initiated before the old treatment is stopped, which should eliminate the risk of **discontinuation symptoms.** Because **discontinuation symptoms** are so unpleasant, I try my best to avoid prescribing antidepressants that have the potential to provoke a severe reaction. There are many other effective antidepressants that have a far lower risk.

Importantly, **discontinuation symptoms** are distinctly different from the classic withdrawal syndrome associated with alcohol or illicit drugs. Antidepressants are not associated with dependence or drug-seeking behaviour; they do not cause individuals to feel stoned or euphoric in the manner one would expect from cocaine or heroin; and I've never, ever had a patient tell me they craved their antidepressant during discontinuation. While **discontinuation symptoms** are sometimes very unpleasant, they are almost always mild and short-lived, usually resolving within a few days to two weeks.

Lowest risk: bupropion XL, mirtazapine, newer antidepressants (desvenlafaxine, levomilnacipran, vilazodone, vortioxetine), MAOIs.

Major culprits: some SSRIs (especially paroxetine), some SNRIs (especially venlafaxine XR).

Weight gain

Weight gain is another extremely frustrating side effect that may affect some people taking a particular medication, but not others. Some of the older medications are more likely to cause weight gain, while the newer antidepressants tend to have a comparatively lower risk. As discussed in chapter 5, just having a depression diagnosis is associated with an increased risk of obesity and other metabolic disorders, such as **diabetes.** Using a depression treatment that provokes weight gain should be avoided whenever possible. If weight gain is significant and the onset coincided with the initiation of an antidepressant, another medication should be considered.

There is a great deal of **inter-individual variability** related to how a medication impacts weight. Two people taking the same medication may have very different experiences. It's important to discuss weight concerns with your doctor because it's a major reason why people discontinue treatment. In situations where multiple treatments have not been effective, and the only effective depression treatment is provoking weight gain, it's important to discuss the issue with your doctor. There are many possible treatments that can help with weight control.

Lowest risk: bupropion XL, newer antidepressants (desvenlafaxine, levomilnacipran, vilazodone, vortioxetine), moclobemide.

Major culprits: mirtazapine, quetiapine, some SSRIs (especially paroxetine), some SNRIs.

Emotional flatness or inability to feel

Shouka was prescribed an SSRI for depression, which was started at a very low dose and slowly increased until her symptoms fully resolved. She no longer felt sad; she had a renewed interest in cooking, which she had always loved to do; and she was able to keep her home clean and complete her tasks at work. However, she also noticed she could no longer cry or feel what she described as "a normal range of emotions." She told her doctor, "My daughter graduated from law school last week. I'm very proud of her, but I just don't feel as excited and joyful as I think I normally would. I feel dull, like I can't feel really happy or really sad. I'm glad I don't feel depressed anymore, but I'd like to be able to experience normal feelings of joy and sadness."

Shouka's experience is not uncommon for patients who are prescribed an SSRI or an SNRI at a very low dose. In fact, about 30 percent of patients report that while an antidepressant improved their mood and **anxiety** symptoms, they have lost the ability to feel intense emotions. This flatness is caused by increasing **serotonin** in the **prefrontal cortex (PFC)**, the brain area behind the forehead. For the 30 percent of patients who have extra-sensitive **serotonin** receptors in the PFC, increasing **serotonin** causes a reduction in two other **neurotransmitters**, **norepinephrine** and **dopamine**, and that leaves them feeling emotionally flat, apathetic, or unmotivated.

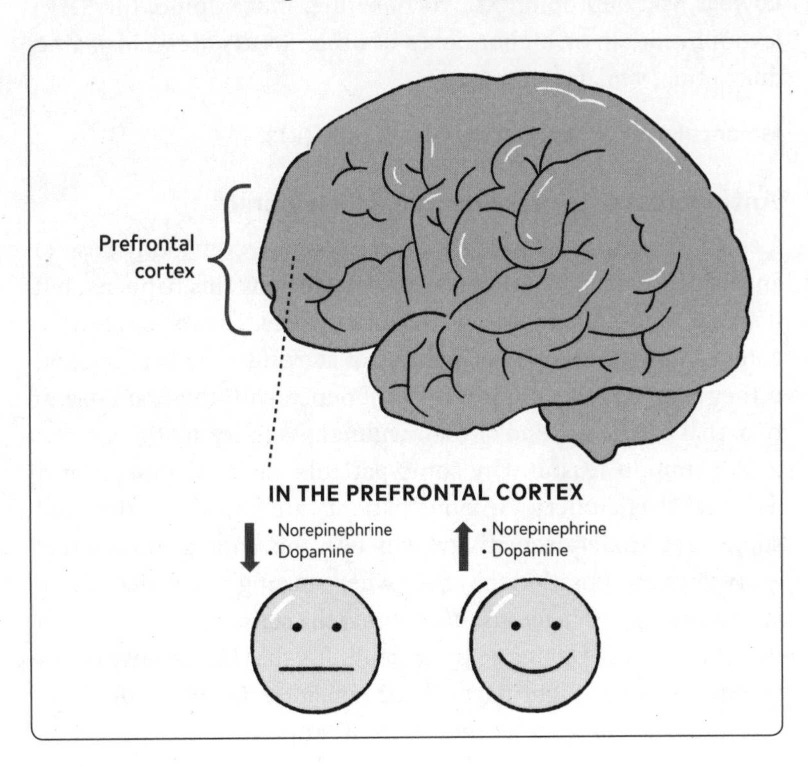

Sometimes, a prescriber might be concerned that their patient's inability to feel intense emotions means their depression is under-treated, so they increase the SSRI dose, which will only make the problem worse. However, if the cause is an SNRI, that is probably because the dose is too low (so it is increasing only **serotonin** and not **norepinephrine**) and increasing the dose might help. Lowering the antidepressant dose, in the hopes of lessening the side effect, often leads to a return of the depression or **anxiety** symptoms.

If the inability to feel is medication-induced, it can be resolved by several different strategies: switch to one of the low-risk antidepressants or a higher dose of an SNRI (or if already prescribed an SNRI, increase the dose), or your prescriber might choose to add another medication that boosts **norepinephrine** and **dopamine** in the PFC.

Lowest risk: bupropion XL, vortioxetine, mirtazapine, the SNRI levomilnacipran or higher doses of other SNRIs (desvenlafaxine, duloxetine, venlafaxine XR).

Major culprits: SSRIs and low doses of SNRIs.

"Antidepressants make me feel much worse"

A small percentage of patients cannot tolerate even a tiny dose of an antidepressant. There are a few reasons why this happens, but it's sometimes difficult to sort out exactly why. The issue is further confused by a patient's normal fear of starting a medication, and if they then have an unpleasant experience with the first dose or two, that can be the end of their willingness to try anything else.

A common reason why some patients can't tolerate an antidepressant is **anxiety**. Anxious patients are already fearful, and some have **anxiety** sensitivity, which in this context means that every physical sensation they have when starting a new medication is interpreted as dangerous. It's not that the sensation is not real, or that the patient is trying to be difficult. It's that the **anxiety** is real and makes what might normally be considered a mild side effect feel far worse, and sometimes even life-threatening. This feeling can sometimes be mitigated by education, the short-term use of an anti-**anxiety** treatment (see **benzodiazepines** on page 235), or by starting the antidepressant at a very low dose and increasing the dose very slowly.

Another common reason why patients might not be able to tolerate an antidepressant medication is because they actually have **bipolar depression**, not unipolar depression (see page 19). For some patients with **bipolar disorder**, an antidepressant can make them feel very uncomfortable, physically and mentally; in the worst case, an antidepressant can flip a bipolar patient from depression or a normal mood into mania or hypomania.

Lowest risk: bupropion XL, MAOIs, **atypical antipsychotics.**

Major culprits: SSRIs, SNRIs, and all antidepressants that impact **serotonin.**

My antidepressant Golden Rules

These are my important tips to ensure you have *minimal or no side effects* from an antidepressant:

1. **Start low and go slow.** Ask your doctor to start your antidepressant medication at the lowest possible dose and increase slowly. If you're in the over sixty-five-years-old set, start lower and go slower. However, remember that starting lower and increasing more slowly might mean it takes a little longer for the medication to have a therapeutic benefit. Thus, you must follow rule #2.
2. **Try your best to be patient.** It's really difficult to wait any longer than *right this minute* to feel better, but by initiating treatments slowly, you're more likely to tolerate them well and less likely to end up on a higher dose than necessary.
3. **Take with food.** With few exceptions, psychiatric medications can be taken with food, which reduces the risk of nausea. The largest meal is most often the best choice. Some medications

should always be taken with food, or they will not be adequately absorbed. If your doctor or pharmacist asks you to take a medication with food, be sure to do so, at least until you've asked them if it's okay to make a change.

4. Taking medication at the **suppertime meal** often allows you to sleep through any early side effects. There are a few medications that are best dosed in the morning, because they can impact sleep, but the majority can be taken in the evening.
5. If you're concerned the medication you are taking later in the day is **negatively impacting your sleep**, try switching it to breakfast (still with food to reduce nausea). Likewise, if you're taking a medication in the morning and you're concerned it's negatively impacting your sleep, change it to the evening.
6. **Do not increase the dose until any side effects have resolved.**
7. **Don't listen to non-professionals regarding medication.** Non-professionals include some websites. You can ask your pharmacist for advice, but if that advice doesn't align with what you were told by the person who prescribed your medication, contact them before taking any drastic steps, like stopping the medication.
8. Remember that **nearly all side effects resolve within a few weeks.** Keep your health professional updated on the side effects, and hang in there.
9. If one treatment isn't tolerated or doesn't work, **there are many others to choose from.** Don't give up. If you've tried a few antidepressants and they're ineffective or intolerable, you and your doctor need to consider whether your diagnosis is correct. One of the most commonly missed diagnoses is **bipolar disorder.**
10. **Take your antidepressant every day.** If you forget it one day, take it as soon as you remember. To avoid forgetting, **set your phone with a reminder** and *do not turn off the reminder until you take it*! If you're not in a place where you can take it right away, click the "remind me later" option. Once you turn the reminder off, if you're anything like 99 percent of the population, the reminder is forgotten.

11. If you keep forgetting if you've taken your medication, **use a plastic dosette** or ask your pharmacy to **blister-pack** your medications. Missing a dose can provoke discontinuation side effects for some medications, and they're not enjoyable. More importantly, missing doses makes your medication less effective and can result in a failure to recover or depression **relapse.**
12. **Keep a dose in your purse and/or desk at work**, stored safely (ask your pharmacy for another labelled bottle), if you're prone to forgetting. While not ideal, it's better to be able to take it immediately when you remember.
13. Once you find a treatment that you tolerate well and it's helping, it's essential to treat every symptom. To read more about **residual symptoms of depression**, see page 224.
14. **Anxiety can provoke physical symptoms**, and patients may believe those symptoms are caused by their medication. Remember that anxiety is often more difficult to treat than depression and commonly requires higher doses of an antidepressant to fully manage. For more information about the connection between anxiety and depression, see chapter 5.

Chapter summary

- There is a great deal of **inter-individual variability** regarding side effects, so medications must be chosen based on each individual's experience.
- Most side effects are transient (short-lived), resolving within a week or two.
- It is important to follow my antidepressant Golden Rules, because no drug will work if it's not taken.

Any treatment can cause unwanted effects, including psychotherapy and exercise (unless you've never rolled your ankle taking a brisk walk). By taking the time to find the depression treatment that's best for you, you'll protect both your mental and physical health.

A real patient's story

SINCE ADOLESCENCE, I have suffered from periods of totally debilitating depression—for different lengths of time—that had a considerable impact on me, plus my family and friends. I would withdraw and sink into a void of anguish and have a sense of meaninglessness. I wanted to protect the people around me from what I couldn't protect myself from. I couldn't be the mother, partner, daughter, sister, or friend I wanted to be in that condition. I knew I needed help but wasn't sure where to turn—I didn't even know if there was help to be had and whether I had the energy to find it. I was exhausted.

I am grateful that I was given a referral to a psychiatrist. Though it took some time to get in to see her, I knew right away that the doctor could offer me some hope. She listened carefully, asked pointed questions, and immediately recognized my many symptoms in the context of my past.

It took some time to achieve a life balance with the ability to interact meaningfully with family, friends, and colleagues again and to recover some of the memory loss that had resulted from years of untreated disease. However, the doctor's pharmaceutical approach has allowed me to feel stable and grounded again.

To anyone experiencing the pain of depression, I can unequivocally say there is hope. But you do have to acknowledge that you (most likely) have a **chronic** condition that will require lifetime adherence to the treatment plan. On one occasion not long ago, I stopped taking my medication and landed right back in the pit I started in.

I implore anyone with similar symptoms to see a psychiatric professional who understands the neurology of depression and related diseases. When I hear of people like me—who think there is no light at the end of the tunnel or, even worse, are considering suicide—it breaks my heart. I know, from experience, that there is a path to wellness they could take. I continue to touch base with my psychiatrist regularly, but with her guidance I have learned how to manage my mental health and lead a meaningful life while accepting that I have a **chronic** illness. I am eternally grateful to her for what she has offered me: a road to **recovery**, to a life of wellness and stability.

12

What is treatment-resistant depression?

FOR ABOUT 50 percent of patients treated for depression, the first antidepressant prescribed doesn't work adequately, and for some, the second one doesn't work adequately either. In fact, for patients with a moderately severe or severe depression who are taking a single antidepressant, only about one-half will experience improved symptoms and only about one-third will experience **remission** of all of their symptoms.

When depression symptoms don't improve following an adequate trial (e.g., an optimized dose for four to six weeks) of at least two different antidepressants, the diagnosis is changed to **treatment-resistant depression (TRD)**. Up to 30 percent of depressed patients will ultimately be diagnosed with TRD. Most patients referred to a psychiatric practice due to depression have TRD and have tried many treatments, resulting in frustration and a sense that they might never recover.

It bears repeating: hang in there! There is always a path ahead, although I know it can sometimes be a very frustrating journey. You will find a treatment that works. Please don't give up the search.

Why is it necessary to treat every symptom?

Cosette, thirty-four, was treated for depression for the last few months and reported to her doctor that she was no longer depressed. She was interested in reading again and she had just contacted her book club, hoping to get back to her "normal routine." However, Cosette was worried about her inability to focus when reading, telling her doctor, "I have tried to start a novel, but my mind seems to wander almost immediately, and I can't get past the first few pages. I also worry about my memory. Do you think it's possible I have Alzheimer's disease?" She had also emailed her tennis partner but worried she might not have the energy to play, telling her doctor, "I'm still not sleeping well, and I feel really tired every day."

Residual symptoms are those that remain after the core depression symptoms (such as a depressed mood and **anhedonia**) have resolved. A patient might meet the criteria for **remission** on a **depression rating scale** but continue to experience **residual symptoms**, which are bothersome and sometimes very distressing. The most common **residual symptoms** include fatigue, **insomnia**, and **cognitive** symptoms.

Research clearly demonstrates that failing to treat depression fully, by not addressing **residual symptoms**, is a powerful predictor of depression **relapse.** In fact, some high-quality, long-term research concluded that the presence of **residual symptoms** is the most powerful predictor of **relapse**, even greater than the number of previous episodes of depression.

So why don't doctors treat every symptom? Sometimes it's because they're not comfortable with optimizing the dose, switching antidepressants, or combining treatments. However, often it's their patient who's refusing to be appropriately treated. "I think I'm already on a high enough dose," or "I read on the internet that drug X can cause Y terrible side effect," or "My mother/husband/ grocer told me I shouldn't need any medication, and you're asking me to take more?" I often hear those kinds of comments when I attempt to explain why treating every symptom is beneficial in the long run. Unfortunately, patients often don't have the support from family and friends, or they rely on Dr. Google or their grocer when they're making their treatment decisions.

What is pharmacogenomics?

There is an important new tool that prescribers can use to help find the right medication for a patient who is not tolerating or not responding to usual depression treatments. **Pharmacogenomics** combines the study of how drugs work (pharmacology) and how **genes** function (genomics) to understand how a patient's **genes** can affect their response to medications.

In chapter 6, I described the **cytochrome P450 enzymes (CYP)** that are necessary for drug **metabolism**. Recall that while most people's CYP system works in a pretty standard manner, some of us have CYP enzymes that are much more active than usual (called rapid or extensive metabolizers), while others might have enzymes that function more slowly or less effectively than usual. Many, but not all, psychiatric medications are metabolized by CYP enzymes.

You might also recall that when regulators give a drug an official **indication** (see chapter 9), they include a usual dose range in the **product monograph**. This dose range is based on research provided by the drug company and tends to reflect what works for most people in the population. However, we know drug doses are not "one dose fits all." That's due to a number of factors, but one important reason is that some people metabolize drugs at different rates.

Until recently, we didn't have easy access to information regarding how a patient metabolizes medications, or specifically whether they have CYP enzymes that work rapidly or extensively, or whether they have sluggish, ineffective enzymes. Knowing this information can help to predict who will benefit from a drug, who will not respond, and who is more likely to experience side effects.

If you are prescribed a medication that is metabolized by a CYP enzyme, and your enzyme works faster and more vigorously than usual, regular doses of that medication might be too low to be effective. Likewise, if you have a sluggish, ineffective CYP enzyme, a drug that is metabolized by that enzyme is more likely to accumulate and might be intolerable or provoke more serious side effects.

Additionally, some medications can impact how effectively a specific CYP enzyme will do its job. For instance, if you are prescribed the antidepressant duloxetine, which is metabolized by CYP1A2, and you are also taking a medication that inhibits (blocks the activity of) CYP1A2 (e.g., the antidepressant fluvoxamine), the level of duloxetine in your blood will increase significantly. If your doctor prescribed these two medications together, lower doses of duloxetine might be necessary and better tolerated. Just to add to any confusion you might already have, while duloxetine is *metabolized* by CYP1A2, it also *inhibits* the activity of the CYP2D6 enzyme. Thus, if you are taking duloxetine and your doctor adds a medication that requires CYP2D6 to be metabolized (e.g., aripiprazole or brexpiprazole) you would likely require a lower dose of the new medication being added, but the duloxetine dose would not need to be changed.

Certain foods and smoking cigarettes can also affect how CYP enzymes function. Smoking induces CYP1A2 enzyme activity, which means it causes the enzyme to work much more effectively. As a result, smoking can reduce the amount of duloxetine in the blood by 30 percent. By quitting smoking, the blood level of duloxetine would increase. One food that powerfully impacts the activity of a CYP enzyme is grapefruit, which inhibits (reduces the activity) of CYP3A4 and has been responsible for severe side effects associated with drugs that are metabolized by that enzyme. The effect of having a glass of grapefruit juice can last for twenty-four hours.

The CYP enzymes that most commonly impact psychiatric medications are CYP3A4, CYP1A2, CYP2D6, and CYP2C19. The following table includes psychiatric medications that are metabolized by these CYP enzymes; however, the list does not include every medication. No medication decisions should be made before discussing them with your prescriber. Not all CYP drug interactions are clinically relevant, which means they might be possible but they are unlikely to cause a problem for the patient.

Finally, **pharmacogenomics** testing can be expensive and is not usually covered by provincial health plans. As such, in Canada, it is usually reserved for patients who have not been able to find an effective, tolerable psychiatric treatment.

CYP3A4	CYP1A2	CYP2D6	CYP2C19
Antidepressants that affect the activity of a CYP enzyme			
	Imipramine	Fluoxetine	Citalopram
	Fluvoxamine	Paroxetine	Amitriptyline
		Duloxetine	Clomipramine
		Venlafaxine	Imipramine
		All TCAs	
		Fluvoxamine	
CYP3A4	**CYP1A2**	**CYP2D6**	**CYP2C19**
Antipsychotics that affect the activity of a CYP enzyme			
Aripiprazole	Clozapine	Aripiprazole	
Brexpiprazole		Brexpiprazole	
Haloperidol	Haloperidol	Haloperidol	
Quetiapine	Olanzapine	Perphenazine	
Ziprasidone		Risperidone	
CYP3A4	**CYP1A2**	**CYP2D6**	**CYP2C19**
Others psychiatric medications that affect the activity of a CYP enzyme			
Buspirone		Atomoxetine	Diazepam

Why have I been prescribed two antidepressants?

When there hasn't been improvement in depression symptoms after an initial trial of an antidepressant, most experts recommend trying another antidepressant, perhaps from another class, as the next step. For instance, if a trial of an SSRI is unsuccessful, most prescribers would consider switching to an SNRI or a multimodal antidepressant next. It's important to ensure that whichever antidepressant is tried, it be given at the optimal dose. However, after two or more trials of different antidepressants have not produced a benefit, or there's been just a partial benefit from an antidepressant, despite optimizing the dose, most experts suggest employing a combination of two treatments.

Combining two antidepressants is a common practice, but to make a difference, the antidepressants should have distinct mechanisms of action. For instance, combining an SSRI or SNRI with a NaSSA (mirtazapine) or an SSRI with an NDRI (bupropion XL) makes good sense because these drugs work differently. Combining two SSRIs or an SSRI with an SNRI is not usually done, because this rarely adds much benefit.

Combining two antidepressants with distinct mechanisms of action might also allow the doses to remain lower than when using either drug alone. Additionally, the second antidepressant might help to mitigate a side effect caused by the first antidepressant. For instance, the rationale behind prescribing mirtazapine or bupropion XL along with an SSRI or SNRI might be to mitigate sexual side effects. Unfortunately, this approach doesn't always work, and there may be unintended side effects, such as weight gain from the mirtazapine.

While combining two antidepressants is a common strategy when managing TRD, the scientific evidence supporting this approach is not strong. Employing an **atypical antipsychotic** (see below) in combination with an antidepressant has much higher quality evidence but is more likely to provoke side effects. For this reason, antidepressant combinations might be attempted first. However, if a patient is very ill, the most rapid and likely the most effective approach is to follow the science.

What other medications are commonly prescribed for TRD?

Atypical antipsychotics

There are several types of medications that may be prescribed in combination with an antidepressant for patients with TRD. One type is called **atypical antipsychotics (AAPs)**, a name that sometimes provokes fear and avoidance among patients suffering from depression. The name is truly a misnomer. While they are very effective treatments for **psychotic** symptoms, many AAPs are at least as effective for the treatment of depression. Several also have official **Health Canada** and FDA **indications** for depression, either alone or in combination with an antidepressant.

There are two different classes of antipsychotic medications. The older group are alternately called conventional, typical, or first-generation **antipsychotics.** These drugs were modern-day miracles, resulting in the reawakening of patients suffering from severe **psychotic** disorders, such as **schizophrenia.** Prior to the use of chlorpromazine, the first antipsychotic, these patients were often institutionalized for long periods (sometimes for their entire adult life), and psychiatrists routinely used extreme measures, including lobotomy, to manage their **psychotic** or manic symptoms.

The main **mechanism of action** of the older **antipsychotics** is to act as **dopamine receptor antagonists**, which means they block the effects of the **neurotransmitter dopamine**. When **dopamine** is present at relatively higher levels than normal in the most ancient, reptilian part of the brain, called the limbic region, it can cause **psychotic** symptoms. Older **antipsychotics** block the **dopamine** receptors in that brain region, providing an antipsychotic effect.

However, while the first **antipsychotics** provided incredible benefits for many patients, they also came with some serious, sometimes irreversible, side effects. For instance, by blocking **dopamine** in other brain areas, **conventional antipsychotics** can provoke movement disorders, including tremors and stiffness, severe restlessness (called **akathisia**), and a serious, sometimes irreversible movement disorder called **tardive dyskinesia (TD)**.

Schizophrenia is associated with **psychotic** symptoms but also with what are known as negative symptoms, such as apathy, a flattened **affect** (very little or no emotional expression), lack of motivation, difficulty with getting started with activities, and other **cognitive** symptoms. These symptoms are caused by a lower than normal level of **dopamine** in the **prefrontal cortex (PFC)** and are commonly experienced by many people diagnosed with **schizophrenia.** Unfortunately, older, **conventional antipsychotics** also cause a reduction in **dopamine** in the PFC. This means that a treatment used to manage **psychotic** symptoms associated with **schizophrenia** can cause a significant worsening of negative symptoms. Clearly, feeling chronically apathetic and not being able to motivate yourself, get started on activities, and express emotions would have a serious impact on the day-to-day functioning of a patient suffering from **schizophrenia.**

The **conventional antipsychotics** also affect other **neurotransmitters** and their receptors, which provide little or no benefit but may provoke unpleasant side effects, including sedation, blurred vision, and constipation.

Eventually, newer, better tolerated antipsychotic medications were developed, that are referred to as second-generation or **atypical.** These drugs also block **dopamine** in the limbic area of the brain, which provides an antipsychotic effect. However, they also impact other **neurotransmitters** and their receptors, especially **serotonin,** and that is what makes these drugs so different from their predecessors and useful for the treatment of other disorders, including depression. AAPs are less likely to worsen negative symptoms of **schizophrenia,** because they are designed to prevent the lowering of **dopamine** in the PFC, which causes worsening negative symptoms with **conventional antipsychotics.**

The first group of AAPs included the medications olanzapine, risperidone, clozapine, and quetiapine, which were better tolerated than the conventional drugs in some respects, particularly because they have a lower risk of movement disorders, including **tardive dyskinesia.** However, they have other serious side effects, including significant weight gain and, for some, an increased risk of type II **diabetes** and high cholesterol. As discussed in chapter 5, having a serious mental illness is associated with an increased risk of obesity and **diabetes,** even before medication is involved. These medications further heighten that risk.

Fortunately, a new group of AAPs has been developed that are far less likely to cause weight gain, and their risk of **diabetes** and high cholesterol is similar to **placebo.** The risk of movement disorders with these newer AAPs is also lower than the rates seen with **conventional antipsychotics.**

Most importantly, when AAPs are prescribed at lower doses, they can be very effective depression treatments for patients who haven't fully responded to an antidepressant alone.

There is an international society developed for the sole purpose of properly naming psychiatric medications, the ECNP's Neuroscience-Based Nomenclature Task Force. Instead of calling these **atypical antipsychotics**, it describes them by their **mechanism of action.** Unfortunately, the uptake of this new naming system has been very slow, and the term antipsychotic, laden with negative connotations, remains the common terminology. Regulatory agencies like **Health Canada** and the FDA still use the term antipsychotic, despite giving these drugs official **indications** for depression.

If you or someone you love is prescribed an antipsychotic for depression, please know that there is a mountain of evidence underlying that choice. In fact, the AAPs have more research evidence than any other class of medications for use in managing TRD. These drugs do come with some risks and side effects, so the decision to use them should only follow a thoughtful discussion with your prescriber.

Generic name	Brand name	Health Canada indication
Aripiprazole	Abilify	Indicated for depression when combined with an antidepressant
Brexpiprazole	Rexulti	Indicated for depression when combined with an antidepressant
Lurasidone	Latuda	Indicated for bipolar depression
Olanzapine	Zyprexa	Not indicated for depression in Canada
Quetiapine XR	Seroquel XR	Indicated as a mono-therapy or when combined with an antidepressant
Risperidone	Risperdol	Not indicated for depression in Canada

Atypical antipsychotics (AAPs) as a class

- ***The up side:*** AAPs are usually very effective treatments for TRD. Most work to improve both depression and anxiety symptoms. Lower doses are usually required when treating depression compared to the doses required to manage a **psychotic** disorder.

- *The down side:* Taking a medication that is called an "antipsychotic" for depression might cause patients to fear they will be judged. Some AAPs pose a serious risk of weight gain, increased blood sugar levels, and increased cholesterol. The risk of movement disorders, including **tardive dyskinesia**, is an important consideration.

Aripiprazole

- *The up side:* Aripiprazole is usually a very effective, tolerable treatment for TRD. It is not usually sedating and has a lower risk of weight gain than some AAPs. Its impact on cholesterol and blood sugar is similar to **placebo**. It has a **Health Canada** and FDA **indication** for the treatment of depression when used in combination with an antidepressant.
- *The down side:* Aripiprazole has a moderate risk of weight gain.
- *Would I take it?:* A good first choice as an add-on to an antidepressant.

Brexpiprazole

- *The up side:* Brexpiprazole is usually a very effective, tolerable treatment for TRD. It is not usually sedating and has a lower risk of weight gain than some AAPs. Its impact on cholesterol and blood sugar is similar to **placebo**. Brexpiprazole also poses a lower risk of severe restlessness (**akathisia**) than some other AAPs, such as aripiprazole. It has the **Health Canada** and FDA **indication** for the treatment of depression when used in combination with an antidepressant.
- *The down side:* Brexpiprazole poses a moderate risk of weight gain.
- *Would I take it?:* A good first choice as an add-on to an antidepressant.

Lurasidone

- *The up side:* Lurasidone has some evidence supporting its use for in TRD, but it is not indicated for unipolar depression by the FDA or **Health Canada**. It poses a lower risk of weight gain compared to other AAPs.
- *The down side:* Lurasidone may be excessively sedating (but it might also help sleep). It must be taken with food (350 calories) to be adequately absorbed.
- *Would I take it?:* A good second-line choice as an add-on to an antidepressant.

Olanzapine

- *The up side:* Olanzapine has evidence supporting its use for TRD when taken in combination with the antidepressant fluoxetine.
- *The down side:* Olanzapine poses a high risk of weight gain, **diabetes**, increased

cholesterol, and excessive sedation.

- ***Would I take it?:*** Avoid if possible. Other AAPs are better tolerated and likely more effective.

Quetiapine/Quetiapine XR

- ***The up side:*** Quetiapine is usually a very effective treatment for TRD and anxiety. It is also helpful if sedation is required. Quetiapine has evidence for its use as a monotherapy for depression, but it is often used in combination with an antidepressant.
- ***The down side:*** Quetiapine poses a moderate to high risk of weight gain and **diabetes**. While sedation might initially be a desirable side effect, in the long term it might be excessive and cause functional impairment.
- ***Would I take it?:*** Very effective, but due to weight gain and excessive sedation, I reserve it as a second-line treatment and prescribe it most often in combination with an antidepressant.

Risperidone

- ***The up side:*** Risperidone has evidence supporting its use for TRD.
- ***The down side:*** Risperidone poses a high risk of weight gain, **diabetes**, increased cholesterol, and excessive sedation. It may also cause unwanted breast growth in men and lactation. Risperidone has a higher risk of restlessness and movement side effects compared with other AAPs.
- ***Would I take it?:*** Avoid if possible. Other AAPs are better tolerated and likely more effective.

Lithium

Lithium is a well-known treatment for **bipolar disorder** but has also been used as an add-on medication for TRD. The evidence for its use is not as robust as that for **atypical antipsychotics**, but some patients find it helpful. Much of the research evaluating lithium for TRD involved its use in combination with the older antidepressants, such as TCAs. Lithium requires regular blood monitoring because it can cause kidney damage when used over the long term and can be highly toxic in overdose. Additionally, the use of lithium has been associated with an annoying tremor, acne, weight gain, and frequent urination. If lithium is going to be a useful **augmentation** strategy, its effects are usually apparent within two weeks.

Thyroid

Much like the limited evidence for the use of lithium for TRD, thyroid **hormone**, specifically triiodothyronine (T3), has been used for many years but has limited evidence. Some patients find it helpful, and it has few side effects. Like lithium, if T3 is going to be a useful add-on to an antidepressant, its effects are usually apparent within two weeks.

Stimulant medications

These medications are used most commonly for the treatment of **attention deficit hyperactivity disorder** (ADHD) and include two different drug classes: methylphenidate and dexamphetamine. While there is limited evidence that stimulant medications treat the core symptoms of depression, they can be very helpful for improving motivation and reducing fatigue and apathy. Stimulant medications have a great deal of research evidence supporting their safety because they are commonly prescribed for children and they are usually very well tolerated. However, they may increase heart rate and blood pressure, so they should be used with caution in individuals who already have high blood pressure or an unstable heart condition.

What medications are commonly prescribed or depression associated with anxiety?

You have likely noticed that **anxiety** has figured prominently in this book. That's because it is commonly associated with depression, it's a miserable experience, and it gets in the way of effectively managing depression. All antidepressants may improve **anxiety** symptoms as well as depression. However, the antidepressants that impact **serotonin** are the most effective at managing **anxiety** and **anxiety disorders**, although **norepinephrine** can also be very helpful. Likewise, most **atypical antipsychotics** can help to manage **anxiety** symptoms.

Because **anxiety** makes depression more difficult to treat, often requires higher antidepressant doses to manage, and heightens patients' sensitivity to medication side effects, I sometimes prescribe another type of medication to help to manage **anxiety** in the short term.

Benzodiazepines

Benzodiazepines are among the most misunderstood and unfairly vilified medications in psychiatry, which is truly unfortunate for so many suffering patients who are not offered these compassionate medications. If you have been prescribed a psychiatric medication that ends in "-pam," such as lorazepam, clonazepam, or diazepam, you have been prescribed a **benzodiazepine.**

Benzodiazepines are used for many purposes: anti-**anxiety**, muscle relaxant, the treatment of alcohol withdrawal, sedation, **anticonvulsant**, and mood stabilizer. They are also used to treat restless legs syndrome and **acute** agitation and may be employed intravenously for anesthesia. They rapidly and very effectively manage **acute anxiety**, arguably better than any other treatment. They are also inexpensive and extremely well tolerated by most patients. They carry a low risk of lethality in overdose, unless they are used at high doses in combination with an opioid pain medication or alcohol.

I think of **benzodiazepines** as a bandage: they manage the **anxiety** while the antidepressant treatment fixes the **anxiety** and depression more permanently, and then the **benzodiazepine** "bandage" can be removed. Used correctly, **benzodiazepines** should rapidly reduce **anxiety** and improve a patient's ability to cope and function. Too low a dose will do nothing, and too high a dose will make the patient sleepy and feel dopey. It can take a few days to find the optimum dose, but the rapid relief from **anxiety** can be lifesaving. Recall that **anxiety** heightens suicide risk, so I don't make that comment lightly.

Unfortunately, **benzodiazepines** have sometimes been prescribed inappropriately, which has resulted in a backlash against these valuable medications, leading some **clinicians** to refuse to prescribe them. However, the issues with **benzodiazepines**, when used to treat **anxiety**, are almost always related to poor prescribing practices (the doctor), not due to patients misusing them. In fact, it is most common in my practice that patients stop their **benzodiazepine** before I ask them to, because they're no longer required. While that is my **clinical experience**, long-term research evidence backs this up, demonstrating that most patients stop their **benzodiazepine** quickly and most patients do not use excessive doses.

Sometimes my patients express fear that they will become addicted to a **benzodiazepine.** However, when used appropriately, lorazepam and clonazepam (which are the ones I prescribe for **anxiety**) have a low risk of abuse or addiction. Again, the misuse and abuse of **benzodiazepines** is most often related to poor prescribing practices. If **benzodiazepines** are the only treatment used to manage depression and **anxiety**, they will not resolve the underlying illness and, as a result, over time some patients will need higher doses to relieve their **anxiety.**

The most common situation I encounter when **benzodiazepines** are used inappropriately is when a patient has **bipolar disorder**, but they have instead been diagnosed with unipolar depression and **anxiety.** These patients commonly have severe **anxiety** and antidepressants have not been effective or tolerable. The **benzodiazepine** initially helped the **anxiety**, but because their **bipolar disorder** has not been appropriately treated, they use more and more **benzodiazepine** to gain some benefit. When I meet them, they are taking a high dose of a **benzodiazepine** and tell me, "It used to work, but now it's doing nothing." It's easy to blame the patient for misusing the medication, but they are trying to find some relief with a medication that they tolerate and that gave them some benefit in the past. I believe this situation demonstrates the failure of the prescriber, not the failure of the suffering patient.

When prescribed appropriately and monitored carefully, many psychiatrists believe in the value of **benzodiazepines.** They are preferred for patients who are at low risk for substance abuse, so they are not using them in combination with opioids or alcohol.

However, **benzodiazepines** are highly effective when employed to help patients to overcome alcohol abuse and effectively prevent the life-threatening withdrawal symptoms associated with **chronic** alcohol dependence.

When comparing the efficacy of **benzodiazepines** and antidepressants for adults with **generalized anxiety disorder**, a large 2018 review found that **benzodiazepines** are more effective than SSRIs or SNRIs. Likewise, international treatment guidelines for **anxiety** recognize that **benzodiazepines** are extremely effective, have a low side-effect burden, are a low risk in overdose, and are very inexpensive, but that they must be prescribed and used appropriately.

Research indicates that prescribing a **benzodiazepine** as an add-on treatment when initiating an antidepressant can be very helpful, likely because **anxiety** can lead to early antidepressant discontinuation. Patients co-prescribed a **benzodiazepine** in the short term tend to stay on the antidepressant treatment because they tolerate the early side effects far better and their symptoms stabilize more rapidly. To read more about the frequent co-occurrence of **anxiety** and depression, see chapter 5.

While most patients tolerate **benzodiazepines** very well, they may cause daytime sleepiness and fatigue, especially if they are dosed too high. They may also slow reaction time and have **cognitive** impacts, so they must be used with great caution when driving or doing other tasks that are safety sensitive. Extra caution must be used when prescribing **benzodiazepines** for elderly patients, due to their effects on **cognition**, reaction time, and balance. However, older patients may experience terrible **anxiety** in association with depression, and they have the highest rate of completed suicide, so aggressively managing **anxiety** symptoms is appropriate and compassionate, and **benzodiazepines**, even at very low doses, can be lifesaving in this role. Short-term use, meaning for periods of one to three months, is preferred.

Specific benzodiazepines for anxiety

Clonazepam (Rivotril® in Canada; Klonopin® in the USA)

- *The up side:* Compared to other **benzodiazepines**, clonazepam has a relatively gradual onset of anti-anxiety benefit, and its effects gradually **taper** off as well. It may be taken two or three times daily, at low dose, and slowly tapered over several weeks as other treatments (e.g., an antidepressant) begin to manage the depression and anxiety symptoms.
- *The down side:* Clonazepam is usually reserved for short-term use. Its **cognitive** side effects and the risk of falls can be a concern, especially with older patients. When **benzodiazepines are prescribed or used inappropriately**, they can be habit forming and **they should never be used in combination with alcohol or opioids.**
- *Would I take it?:* Yes.

Lorazepam (Ativan®)

- *The up side:* Lorazepam has a more rapid onset of effect than clonazepam, especially if the sublingual form is used. It may be taken two or three times daily, at low dose, and slowly tapered over several weeks as other treatments begin to manage the depression and anxiety symptoms. It is often useful for alcohol withdrawal and to provide rapid sedation and manage agitation for patients with **bipolar disorder** or **acute psychosis**. For **acute** agitation, lorazepam is sometimes given by intramuscular (IM) injection. The sublingual form may be employed for the treatment of **acute** anxiety, including **panic attacks**. Lorazepam can also be invaluable, now and again, for those who have life-limiting phobias (e.g., if you're terrified of flying or unable to visit the dentist due to anxiety).
- *The down side:* Lorazepam is usually reserved for short-term use. Its **cognitive** side effects and the risk of falls can be a concern, especially with older patients. When **benzodiazepines are prescribed or used inappropriately,** they can be habit forming and **they should never be used in combination with alcohol or opioids.**
- *Would I take it?:* Yes.

Alprazolam (Xanax®)

- *The up side:* Alprazolam has a very rapid onset of effect.
- *The down side:* Because of its very rapid onset of effect, this is a difficult drug to discontinue and has a higher risk of misuse and abuse compared to other **benzodiazepines**.
- *Would I take it?:* No. Avoid this drug.

Diazepam (Valium®)

- *The up side:* Diazepam's effects are apparent rapidly. It is useful for alcohol withdrawal, but lorazepam is likely a better option for this purpose.
- *The down side:* Diazepam accumulates in the body over time, heightening the risk of **cognitive impairment** and falls.
- *Would I take it?:* No, there are better options.

Other treatments for anxiety

Pregabalin (Lyrica®)

- *The up side:* Pregabalin is an **anticonvulsant** with good research evidence demonstrating its benefits for treating anxiety, neuropathic (nerve) pain, fibromyalgia, and **insomnia**. While it is not as effective as **benzodiazepines**, pregabalin can be very useful for patients who have misused **benzodiazepines** in the past or are currently abusing other drugs or alcohol.
- *The down side:* Finding the appropriate dose of pregabalin tends to take more time than it usually does when using **benzodiazepines** for short-term anxiety management. It also costs more, may cause weight gain, and is known to provoke **cognitive** symptoms in some people, most notably a foggy-head sensation. There is some research evidence suggesting that pregabalin can be misused and abused, but it is generally considered a safer option than **benzodiazepines** for patients who have a history of substance abuse.
- *Would I take it?:* Yes.

Buspirone (BuSpar®)

- *The up side:* Buspirone has a **Health Canada** and FDA **indication** for the management of **anxiety disorders** and the short-term relief of the symptoms of anxiety. It is usually well tolerated.
- *The down side:* Buspirone is not nearly as effective as **benzodiazepines**, but it is usually well tolerated and has a very low potential for abuse. The most common side effects are headache, **insomnia**, and upset stomach, which usually resolve quite quickly. Buspirone is frequently under-dosed, which might explain why some patients do not respond adequately.
- *Would I take it?:* Yes.

Atypical antipsychotics (AAPs)

- *The up side:* Some AAPs have a **Health Canada** and FDA **indication** for the treatment of depression and also have data regarding their effectiveness in treating anxiety. Additionally, most have **Health Canada** and FDA **indications** for **bipolar disorder** and **schizophrenia**. Some are more sedating (e.g., quetiapine, olanzapine), which can be helpful for improving sleep in the short term. AAPs have a very low potential for abuse.

- *The down side:* Because AAPs can be associated with serious side effects, including weight gain and movement disorders, they should only be used for the shortest duration possible if they are prescribed for anxiety. Some AAPs may also cause excessive daytime sleepiness, which may negatively impact functioning.
- *Would I take it?:* There are better first-line anxiety treatment choices, mostly due to side effects, especially serious long-term side effects such as weight gain and movement disorders. When possible, other treatments should be employed, but if they are not appropriate, tolerable, or effective, an AAP can be a helpful option.

What treatments are commonly prescribed for depression associated with insomnia?

Lenore, a fifty-year-old emergency department nurse, complained to her family doctor, "If you don't get me to sleep, I think I might take a hammer to my head to knock myself out." After years of shift work, Lenore can't remember having a refreshing sleep, but over the last year, things have gone from bad to worse. She hasn't had a period in over six months and joked to her doctor, "I'm always the hottest person in the room, and by hot, I don't mean sexy!" Her doctor told her that the hot flashes, vaginal dryness, and loss of her regular period suggest she's perimenopausal, and her worsening sleep is likely related to the change in **estrogen** as well. Lenore replied caustically, "Isn't it glorious to be a woman? I'm soaking wet and dry as a bone at the same time. On top of that, I'm awake in bed half the night, but I don't want anyone to touch me!"

As I described in chapter 1, **insomnia** is a common depression symptom and it is also a very common residual symptom of depression, which heightens the risk of **relapse**. Aside from depression, **anxiety**, and other mental illnesses, there are other causes for **insomnia**, with up to 10 percent of adults meeting the **DSM-5** diagnostic criteria for an **insomnia** disorder. **Insomnia** is more common in women and older adults, and it often presents differently depending on age. Young adults tend to have more trouble getting to sleep, while older adults tend to struggle more with staying asleep.

If you ask many perimenopausal women how they're sleeping, you might want to duck! Changes in **estrogen** can completely disrupt normal sleep patterns, especially if **estrogen** is withdrawn suddenly, as would be the case following a total hysterectomy. A partial hysterectomy usually involves removal of all female reproductive organs, excluding the ovaries, while a total hysterectomy involves the surgical removal of the ovaries as well. Ovaries are **estrogen** factories, and when they are removed before a woman is menopausal, that provokes instant **menopause**, rather than the gradual change most women would normally experience. Other hormonal changes, such as thyroid abnormalities, and a range of other medical illnesses and medications can underlie **insomnia**, so it's important to have a medical assessment if **insomnia** becomes **chronic**. One of the most common provocative issues for **insomnia** is shift work. If you ask a perimenopausal shift-worker how she's sleeping, don't just duck, run!

It's important to recognize that **insomnia** is a serious problem that causes or worsens medical and psychiatric illnesses. It has been linked with reduced quality of life, **cognitive** decline and **dementia**, a reduction in driving performance, heart disease, and premature death.

Once the cause for **insomnia** is established, there are many different treatment approaches available that might be helpful. The American Academy of Sleep Medicine recommends psychological and behavioural interventions as well as short-term supplementary medication.

Insomnia can turn any bedroom into a house of horrors, where the inability to sleep becomes an all-consuming concern. Just worrying that they won't sleep is enough to keep some patients from sleeping. There are some important **sleep hygiene** rules below, which are essential first steps for managing **insomnia**. Unfortunately, if you're not sleeping well, you can't pick and choose the ones you like and ignore the rest. If you don't maintain good **sleep hygiene**, your sleep is unlikely to normalize.

My top tips for excellent sleep hygiene

1. **No caffeine after noon.** If you're very sensitive to caffeine, switch to non-caffeinated coffee or tea (note: green tea contains caffeine). Caffeine hangs around in the bloodstream for twelve hours or longer. Be careful with all brown soda pop, which contains caffeine (it's really bad for you anyway, so it's a good time to quit drinking it! While you're at it, consider quitting smoking. It also impairs sleep). Highly caffeinated drinks are very popular, and they are notorious for disrupting sleep.
2. **No alcohol.** Nothing gets you to sleep quite like alcohol, and nothing destroys your sleep quite like alcohol. It really does a number on normal sleep architecture, the phases of sleep everyone goes through every night. If you really want to fix chronically bad sleep, drop the alcohol. Once the sleep problem is fixed, limit alcohol as much as possible and don't drink too close to bedtime. Alcohol's negative impact on sleep tends to worsen with age.
3. **No screen time within an hour of bedtime.** This includes TV, cell phone, and computer screens. What else could you possibly do with your time? Lower the lights, have a bath, read an enjoyable novel, have a pleasant conversation with someone you live with, or meditate. While you're leaving your screens behind for the night, be sure to turn off all unnecessary beeps and notifications from your devices. If possible, store your phone in another room while you sleep.
4. **Sleep in a cool, dark, quiet room.** Warm, loud, well-lit rooms are made for being awake.
5. **Exercise regularly** but not too close to bedtime. While exercise is known to promote a better sleep, if you don't have enough time between exercise and bedtime, you might feel too revved up to settle into sleep. Exercise, even mild to moderate intensity, such as a brisk walk, reduces fatigue and also improves the quality and depth of sleep.
6. **Keep a regular bedtime and wake-up time**, even on weekends. As a serious nap lover, it pains me to say this, but you should avoid naps—they are the enemy of **insomnia** sufferers. However, if it feels impossible to get by without a little shut-eye, a nap should not extend beyond twenty to thirty minutes, and it should happen as early in the day as possible. Set your alarm!

7. **Use your bed for only two things.** If you're not sleeping well, your bed can become an unpleasant, anxiety-provoking place. As such, your time in bed should be reserved only for **sleep and sex**. If you're not doing, or about to do, one of those two things, get out of bed and do something else.

Psychological and behavioural interventions to improve sleep

Psychological and behavioural interventions to improve sleep include **cognitive-behavioural therapy** for **insomnia** (CBT-I), **sleep hygiene** and education, stimulus control, sleep restriction, and relaxation/mindful meditation (see below). CBT-I has the most evidence for its effectiveness and seems to have a broad range of benefits on many aspects of disordered sleep. Along with psychotherapy, other behavioural interventions are the preferred first-line treatments for **insomnia,** but they are not always effective or available.

Stimulus control: What you do while you're in bed impacts your sleep time and quality

If you have **insomnia**, you should use your bed for sleep and sex only: no phone, reading, TV, eating, or other activities that may be stimulating. Go to bed only when you're very sleepy, and, if not asleep within twenty minutes, leave the bedroom, keep the lights low, and do something very boring that does not involve electronics (e.g., read an auto mechanics or knitting magazine, depending on what you find stimulating). Return to bed only when you're very sleepy again, and if you can't sleep within twenty minutes, repeat the above.

Sleep restriction: If you're not sleeping, get out of bed

Limit the time in bed to the time asleep. This time will gradually increase if you follow the stimulus control rules above and by setting a strict wake-up time. Note: it's essential that you get out of bed once your set wake-up time arrives, even if you've had little or no sleep. No napping is also an essential aspect of this approach.

Relaxation training: Improving sleep by reducing physical and emotional tension

Techniques include mindful meditation, progressive muscle relaxation, guided imagery, and breath control.

Cognitive therapy (CT): Changing how we think about sleep

CT includes identifying, challenging, and replacing **dysfunctional** thoughts that create **anxiety** and impair sleep, which leads to a vicious sleepless cycle. CT helps **insomnia** sufferers to understand how much sleep they actually require, recognize those aspects of sleep they cannot control, and address the environmental factors they can control (see **sleep hygiene** tips above).

Cognitive-behavioural therapy for insomnia (CBT-I): The gold standard for high quality sleep

Includes **cognitive** therapy, behavioral interventions (sleep restriction, stimulus control), and education (**sleep hygiene**).

Medications for insomnia

Benzodiazepines are sometimes used to manage **insomnia**, although there are several other available options. I tend to prescribe **benzodiazepines** only for **insomnia** that is related to **anxiety**, which generally involves ruminating on troubling thoughts. Patients will commonly tell me, "I can't turn my brain off when I'm trying to sleep." Anxious patients often report that the worries they might be able to distract themselves from during the day grow exponentially when they try to sleep, and they lose their ability to contain them. Even if during the day they know a worry is excessive and inaccurate, it seems that at night that same thought feels very real and more certain.

In a study published in 2018, nearly 240,000 patients who were prescribed **benzodiazepines** or another sleep medication were monitored for ten years following their initial prescription. At the ten-year mark, very few patients were still taking sleep medications, but of those that were, 0.3 percent of patients were using excessive doses of a prescribed **benzodiazepine**, compared with 0.9 percent of patients prescribed other sleep medications. The study finding that there is a very low risk of escalating to excessive doses of **benzodiazepines** was in line with three other research reports.

Specific benzodiazepines for insomnia

Clonazepam (Rivotril® in Canada; Klonopin® in the USA)

- *The up side:* Clonazepam may be helpful for short-term **insomnia** treatment, as well as anxiety and restless legs syndrome.
- *The down side:* When employed for **insomnia**, short-term use is recommended. Because it has a slower onset of effect, it should be taken at least thirty minutes before sleep. If there is underlying depression or **anxiety disorder**, that must also be treated. Clonazepam poses a risk of excessive morning sedation, **cognitive impairment**, and falls, which is especially concerning for older patients. When **benzodiazepines are prescribed or used inappropriately,** they can be habit forming and **they should never be used in combination with alcohol or opioids.**
- *Would I take it?:* Yes, for the short-term treatment of **insomnia** associated with anxiety.

Lorazepam (Ativan®)

- *The up side:* Lorazepam has a more rapid onset than clonazepam, especially if the sublingual form used. It is also helpful for anxiety and restless legs syndrome.
- *The down side:* When employed for **insomnia**, short-term use is recommended. If there is underlying depression or **anxiety disorder**, that must also be treated.

Lorazepam poses a risk of excessive morning sedation, **cognitive impairment**, and falls, which is especially concerning for older patients. When **benzodiazepines are prescribed or used inappropriately**, they can be habit forming and **they should never be used in combination with alcohol or opioids.**
- *Would I take it?:* Yes, for the short-term treatment of **insomnia** associated with anxiety.

Temazepam (Restoril®) and oxazepam (Serax®)

- *The up side:* These are **benzodiazepines** that were developed for the treatment of **insomnia**. They stay in the blood system for a shorter time than some of the other **benzodiazepines**, so there is less risk of morning hangover. They can be helpful through the night for anxiety and restless legs.
- *The down side:* When employed for **insomnia**, short-term use is recommended. Due to the short time these drugs produce their effect (six to eight hours), they are not as helpful for anxiety during the day. Like all **benzodiazepines**, they pose a risk of excessive morning sedation, **cognitive impairment**, and falls, which is especially concerning for older patients. When **benzodiazepines are prescribed or used inappropriately**, they can be habit forming and **they should never be used in combination with alcohol or opioids.**
- *Would I take it?:* Because I recommend using **benzodiazepines** only when there is associated anxiety, I prefer to prescribe clonazepam or lorazepam. However, if a **benzodiazepine** is being employed solely for the short-term treatment of **insomnia**, these are reasonable choices.

Triazolam (Halcion®) and alprazolam (Xanax®)

- *The up side:* These are **benzodiazepines** that were developed for the treatment of **insomnia**, but due to their potency and greater risk of side effects, I don't believe there is an up side to using these two medications.
- *The down side:* These two medications have a higher risk of side effects, including **cognitive impairment** and falls, when compared to other **benzodiazepines**. They are more likely to be habit forming and are more difficult to discontinue that other **benzodiazepines**.
- *Would I take it?:* No. Avoid these drugs.

Non-**benzodiazepine** sleep treatments include zopiclone (eszopiclone in the United States), zolpidem, and zaleplon (United States only). These are also sometimes known as the z-drugs, perhaps because they all start with the letter z, or maybe because they're supposed to increase your zzz's. While these products have official **indications** for **insomnia** from US and Canadian regulators, their **product monographs** warn of daytime memory loss and **psychomotor impairment** (slowed movements and reaction time), abnormal thinking, and behavioural changes, which may include complex behaviours (e.g., sleep driving—driving after taking the drug but having no recollection of driving), and depression and suicidal thoughts and actions.

The z-drugs, like all sleep medications, are recommended for short-term use only. Patients who have an underlying psychiatric illness that has not been adequately managed may increase the dose over time, which can lead to misuse and abuse. The misuse of sleep medication is a greater risk for non-**benzodiazepine** z-drugs than it is for **benzodiazepines**, although it is the z-drugs that have the official **indication** for sleep.

Specific z-drugs for insomnia

Zopiclone (Imovane® in Canada) or eszopiclone (Lunesta® in the USA)

- ***The up side:*** Lengthy **clinical experience** and usually effective and well tolerated.
- ***The down side:*** Unpleasant metallic taste that can remain through the day and impact the taste of food.
- ***Would I take it?:*** Yes, preferably for short-term use only.

Zopidem (Sublinox® in Canada; Ambien® in the USA)

- ***The up side:*** Very rapid onset (for sublingual form) and generally very well tolerated. Zopidem is less likely than zopiclone to cause a morning hangover. Sublingual zopidem can also be taken in the middle of the night, if three to four hours of sleep time is remaining, with a lower risk of morning hangover. It does not cause an unpleasant metallic taste.
- ***The down side:*** Some patients find the sedating effects do not last long enough.
- ***Would I take it?:*** Yes, preferably for short-term use only.

Zaleplon (Sonata® in USA only)

- ***The up side:*** Very rapid onset and generally very well tolerated. Zaleplon is less likely than zopiclone to cause a morning hangover and it does not cause an unpleasant metallic taste.
- ***The down side:*** Some patients find the sedating effects do not last long enough.
- ***Would I take it?:*** Yes, preferably for short-term use only.

Melatonin is another commonly used sleep treatment that has variable evidence for its benefit. It is a naturally occurring **hormone** that is released from the brain's pineal gland. The release of melatonin from the pineal gland increases in the evening, as the sun goes down, and reduces in the morning, as the sun rises. Its release is impacted by the amount of sunlight in one's environment, but we each have our own **circadian rhythm**, which is also associated with melatonin release. The **circadian rhythm** is the brain's twenty-four-hour internal clock, which determines when we get drowsy and sleep and when we are awake and alert.

Melatonin is considered a natural product, and there is variability in the quality and content of the many available over-the-counter brands. Some products are made from the pineal gland of animals. Melatonin is well tolerated by most patients, although some report daytime sleepiness or drowsiness with a "heavy head" the next morning—headache, dizziness, irritability, and, very rarely, heightened **anxiety** or depression.

Melatonin is used for many types of sleep/wake cycle disturbances, but the usual dose for **insomnia** is 0.5 to 10 mg before bed. That's a wide dose range, but by starting low and increasing the dose slowly over time, you ensure that it is not overdosed, which will result in daytime sleepiness. I usually recommend starting with 3 mg for a week and increasing by 3 mg every one to two weeks to a maximum of 10 mg. However, if there is excessive daytime sleepiness, the dose should be reduced.

In my practice, melatonin tends to work best for shift-workers and for rapid **recovery** from jet lag. Additionally, some peri- and post-menopausal women find it useful, as well as children and adults who have ADHD. As a side note, for jet lag, I'd suggest you take 3 to 9 mg of melatonin at bedtime for a few days before leaving for a trip, for three to five nights after arrival (if it's a longer trip), and for the same length of time upon returning home.

Melatonin

- *The up side:* Melatonin is a natural product that is most useful for **insomnia** associated with **menopause**, ADHD, and shift-work, as well as for the management of jet lag. It is usually very well tolerated.
- *The down side:* Melatonin doesn't work for everyone.
- *Would I take it?:* Yes.

Antidepressants and other medications used for insomnia

Trazodone (Desyrel® in Canada; Oleptro® in the USA)

- *The up side:* Trazodone is an antidepressant that is used primarily for sleep. It is safe for long-term use.
- *The down side:* Trazodone poses a very low risk of priapism (erection lasting longer than four hours that requires medical intervention).
- *Would I take it?:* Yes.

Mirtazapine (Remeron®)

- *The up side:* Mirtazapine is an antidepressant that at very low doses can be used as a sleep aid. At higher doses, it can be helpful for **insomnia** associated with depression and anxiety.
- *The down side:* If taken for longer than a few weeks, mirtazapine can cause significant weight gain.
- *Would I take it?:* No, unless mirtazapine was a necessary and appropriate choice for the treatment of depression. There are other options that do not cause significant weight gain.

Quetiapine (Seroquel®)

- *The up side:* Quetiapine is an **atypical antipsychotic** that may be helpful for **insomnia** associated with depression, anxiety, and other psychiatric disorders. It has official **indications** for the treatment of depression, **bipolar disorder**, and **schizophrenia**.

- ***The down side:*** Unless it is being used for a short time only, quetiapine should not be used for **insomnia** that is not associated with another psychiatric disorder because it can cause serious side effects, including weight gain and movement disorders. Quetiapine may cause excessive daytime sleepiness, which may negatively impact functioning.
- ***Would I take it?:*** No, not as a primary treatment for **insomnia**. There are safer options that do not cause significant weight gain and other serious side effects.

Chapter summary

- When depression symptoms fail to improve after two or more antidepressants are tried—for an adequate time at an adequate dose—the patient is considered to have **treatment-resistant depression (TRD)**.
- Some medications have research evidence demonstrating they are an effective treatment for TRD.
- Failing to manage every depression symptom constitutes the greatest risk for depression **relapse**.
- The research data regarding the effectiveness of sleep medications is, taken as a whole, of low quality. That's why improving **sleep hygiene** and using psychological techniques, like CBT-I and mindful meditation, are highly encouraged.

Don't accept "good enough." Even if the sadness and loss of interest has resolved, if there are remaining symptoms, such as ongoing **insomnia**, fatigue, or **cognitive** symptoms, keep asking for help until they're fully resolved too.

A real patient's story

I CALL THEM THE Bermuda Triangle years: five years of struggling with depression.

I was deeply sad, and I could start sobbing at any moment. I felt deeply ashamed.

I strained to do or plan the simplest of daily tasks. I would find myself in one room forgetting that I had been making breakfast, or sitting on the floor with a pile of mail in my lap, unsure of what to do next. This could go on for minutes or hours.

I lost interest in food and often forgot to eat. I lost weight and felt vaguely uncomfortable with compliments about how "great" I looked, knowing my clothes hung on me but not caring.

I had trouble sleeping and, when I did, had night terrors, waking up almost every night sobbing or desperately calling out, soaked in sweat.

I became hypersensitive to noise, people, and lights.

The **cognitive** symptoms were the worst. It felt like a wasting disease of the brain. I couldn't rely on myself to think through simple things. Making toast to go with cereal was too much at once. My life swirled downwards with a fierce momentum that threw me sideways, disoriented to time and place. The sharp corners of my usual thoughts became murky, like trying to discern shapes from a distance on a rainy November night.

I couldn't reply to a question with a simple answer. My sentences tangled into each other and trailed off into tangents I felt helpless to control. I also experienced **anxiety** to such a degree that it became excruciating to be in my own skin.

I got lost driving home, where I had lived for years. I got lost driving to work. One morning when I was getting ready for work, I forgot to put my blouse on over my undershirt and had to wear my jacket until lunch, when I drove myself home to change. Simple tasks at work became bewildering. Even the basic task of filing papers chronologically left me in a muddle and crying in the bathroom. I couldn't concentrate or make decisions about almost anything.

Eventually, I had to leave work altogether, and that was devastating. I had to face the fact that I could no longer do work that I loved—or any work. Being disabled felt like the biggest failure I had ever had. I no longer belonged anywhere or had a purpose. My upbringing valued being able to work above almost everything. My family couldn't understand, and I couldn't explain it.

My physician of many years had been treating my depression and **anxiety** with medications, but they weren't effective. No one could understand or explain why I was experiencing such severe **cognitive impairment**. I felt tiny and helpless, and I began to feel hopeless. My functioning had deteriorated severely. I had isolated myself from friends and family and was struggling with a huge financial burden without any income. It's hard to think back on those years—they were dark and terrifying times.

I am now in such a different place. I am healthy, even happy. I am in an intimate relationship, have some new acquaintances, have my swimming and my poetry project, and I'm studying wild bees and painting.

“Success is not final; failure is not fatal: it is the courage to continue that counts.”

WINSTON CHURCHILL

13

What are the non-medication treatments for depression?

IN CHAPTER 2, I described how depression is a bio-psycho-social disorder, and the treatment of depression should consider those three factors. While some treatments primarily target the biological aspects of the disorder, the psycho-social treatments are powerful, often essential interventions.

In this chapter, I review non-prescription depression treatments. **Neurostimulation** treatments directly stimulate the brain, which should reinforce the concept of depression as a brain illness. I also describe psychotherapies in this chapter, and they too impact brain function, as do all effective depression treatments. Finally, I will address the complementary and alternative treatments that have evidence demonstrating their effectiveness and tolerability for some patients struggling with depression.

What are treatment guidelines and how can they help when choosing a depression treatment?

In 2016, the Canadian Network for Mood and Anxiety Treatments (CANMAT) published updated treatment guidelines for depression. These well-respected guidelines are considered some of the best in the world, because they evaluate and reflect the highest quality research evidence. Additionally, the **CANMAT guidelines** consider the **clinical experience** of psychiatrists across the country, as well as undergo a careful review by international experts. I refer to the **CANMAT guidelines** in this chapter because they have conducted a thorough and up-to-date review of the available research.

If a treatment is recommended "first-line" by the CANMAT guidelines, that means there is adequate high-quality research evidence and enough clinical experience for it to be a reasonable first choice as a depression treatment. Second-line treatments should be reserved for patients who have not adequately responded to first-line recommendations.

The **CANMAT guidelines** also determine if the evidence supports the use of a treatment in mild to moderate depression or for more severe depression, and whether it should be used on its own or in combination with another antidepressant treatment. Sometimes, based on the evidence, the **CANMAT guidelines** also conclude that a treatment has demonstrated value for the management of **acute** symptoms or for the maintenance of wellness.

While the **CANMAT guidelines** were developed for prescribers, I am referring to them here to lend credibility to my **clinical experience**, because formal psychotherapy, **neurostimulation,** and alternative treatments are not my areas of expertise.

Will psychotherapy help me?

My practice is focused on psychopharmacology, which refers to the treatment of serious mental illnesses with medication. However,

I am a true believer in the value of psychotherapy, also known as talk therapy. I believe every interaction with a patient should be therapeutic and is actually a form of psychotherapy. I also believe that psychotherapy impacts how **genes** are expressed and that, if done well, it is a powerful tool for overcoming depression.

Developing high-quality research studies to evaluate the effectiveness of a psychotherapy treatment is challenging, because of the obvious personality and style differences between every therapist and every study participant. While some forms of talk therapy have more research evidence to support their effectiveness than others, taken as a group, many different forms of talk therapy appear to offer similar benefits.

The success of psychotherapy depends on four core elements:

1. the knowledge and skill of the therapist (see chapter 7),
2. whether there is a good fit with the therapist (see chapter 7),
3. whether the patient is well enough to participate in talk therapy, and
4. whether the patient is motivated and willing to change.

Am I well enough to participate in talk therapy?

Recall that Eloise is a forty-two-year-old woman who was referred to a psychiatrist for treatment of depression. Her family doctor initially recommended talk therapy, but she didn't feel the psychologist was a good fit. Additionally, Eloise said she was unable to focus during her sessions or follow through with homework. She told the psychiatrist, "I used to love reading, but now I can't get past the first page of a novel. I can't even read the newspaper. I keep losing my keys and I had to get my mother to pick me up to drive me to this appointment because I don't trust my driving." Her sadness and anxiety are so severe that she has taken time off work. She feels she might need medication and her family doctor wasn't sure it was necessary.

As you will learn in the pages that follow, psychotherapy has an abundance of scientific evidence supporting its value for the treatment of depression. This is particularly true for mild and moderate depression but also for more severe depression, especially in combination with medication treatments. However, I believe that a brain must be working adequately to benefit from formal psychotherapy. That's because high-quality talk therapy, supported by solid research evidence, is all about learning new information and applying new skills. Whether it's learning to think differently, breathe differently, or behave differently, you need a brain that can consider, practice, and integrate new information. You must be able to, in a word, *learn*.

Recall from chapter 1 that **cognitive** symptoms are very common in depression and include deficits in memory, concentration, thinking speed, and **executive functioning**. Most severely depressed brains are **cognitive**ly impaired, which means the ability to focus, remember, and integrate new information is seriously compromised. For instance, an inability to read a newspaper article and recall at its end how it began reflects **cognitive impairment**. That impairment truly compromises the ability to benefit from psychotherapy, even with the most skilled therapist.

The creation of a therapeutic alliance, the instillation of hope, supportive comments, and helpful direction are still extremely valuable aspects of a therapeutic relationship, but if someone is severely depressed, they need more than a supportive ally. Sometimes medication or another treatment for severe depression is necessary before formal psychotherapy is appropriate and truly beneficial.

It's important to consider these issues because it's possible to spend hundreds or even thousands of dollars on psychotherapy that is not useful, due to a patient's inability to learn. Additionally, if psychotherapy doesn't work due to **cognitive impairment**, it can unfairly cause a loss of faith in what might have been a very helpful intervention, when the time was right.

What are the most common types of talk therapy?

It is beyond the scope of this book to describe every type of psychotherapy in depth, but I will define the most common types and provide some background and evidence for each.

Cognitive-behavioural therapy (CBT)

> Jojo, a thirty-year-old accountant, felt her life was not turning out as she had hoped. She had a plan that by thirty she would be married and have a couple of kids. She also expected to be a partner in her firm by now, but she was recently passed over for a promotion, which was given to a younger colleague. Jojo was devastated. Being passed over confirmed to her that she was a complete failure and that she would never amount to anything. Since that news, she's been in constant conflict with her boss, her parents, and her boyfriend. Her misery was further compounded by the fact that her boyfriend was away on business and missed her birthday. "I know you all hate me. That's probably because you know that I'm a failure," she wrote in a blistering email to family and friends. Those who love her reacted with compassion and wrote her supportive emails in response; however, Jojo felt they were being dishonest and that everyone saw her as she saw herself—a huge disappointment.

Cognitive-behavioural therapy (CBT) is the psychotherapy that has the most abundant, high-quality research evidence to support its effectiveness in the treatment of depression. A substantial body of research evidence has demonstrated the value of CBT for both **acute** depression as well as for the prevention of depression **relapse.** That evidence has included diverse patient populations, such as pregnant and **postpartum** women, adolescents, and the elderly. **The CANMAT Depression Treatment Guidelines recommend CBT as a first-line treatment for depression.**

CBT was developed based on the premise that depression is caused by and continues to be a problem for patients who have

dysfunctional thoughts and behaviours. The thoughts, also called **cognitive** distortions, are inaccurate, irrational, unhelpful, distressing, and negative. Basically, **cognitive** distortions are lies your brain tells you, and because they happen so often, eventually the lies start to feel like the truth. We start to perceive the world through the distorted lens of negative thinking, whether the thoughts are about our self, other people, or situations from the past, present, or future.

The C in CBT refers to identifying those **cognitive** distortions and then confronting them with more accurate interpretations or facts. The B in CBT is the behavioural changes that are undertaken once the **cognitive** distortions are identified and confronted.

A few examples of common **cognitive** distortions:

1. **All-or-nothing or black-and-white thinking:** An inability to see any shades of grey: you're either perfect or the worst person ever. Jojo's black-and-white thinking includes her thought *If I don't get the promotion that means I'm the biggest loser in the world.*

2. **Overgeneralization:** Reaching a conclusion based on one incident or one piece of evidence. Jojo didn't get the promotion, so she concluded, *I'm a failure and I'm never going to amount to anything in life.*

3. **Jumping to conclusions:** Also known as mind-reading, this involves knowing how another person is feeling without asking them to be sure you're right. In Jojo's case, she thought, *My boyfriend missed by birthday. He must hate me and think I'm a disappointment.*

4. **Emotional reasoning:** Whatever I am feeling must be true. *I feel stupid and ugly; therefore I must be stupid and ugly.*

5. **Personalization:** Believing that everything someone else says or does is related to you. *My boyfriend is irritable. He must be angry with me.*

CBT is not a passive process. It is usually time-limited, and the estimated number of sessions should be established early in the **therapeutic relationship.** CBT can also be an intense process, which requires focus, attention, and practice. However, with a skilled therapist, it is generally approached in a hierarchical manner: confronting the least distressing thoughts and changing the less challenging behaviours first and building on each success. In my experience, it's much more difficult to change the way we think than to change the way we behave, but both are important and powerfully influence how we feel. CBT therapists sometimes follow algorithms or have written modules, allowing participants to review the information at home and practice their new skills in between sessions.

CBT's ultimate goal is to help people learn to control their own thoughts and their responses to their thoughts, whether internally or through their behaviour. They feel more confident because their thoughts and behaviours are better aligned with their wishes and needs. As they gradually feel more confident and self-aware, they tend to become more involved at home, school, or socially, which brightens their mood.

Psychotherapy can be expensive, and while it can be a very worthwhile investment, if it's not in the budget, CBT is also available through dozens of books, online programs, and apps. Of course, none of these will work without a motivated user. Doing CBT on your own can be highly effective, but only if you're willing and able to put in the necessary time and effort.

Behavioural activation (BA)

Marco had been severely depressed for a few years. During his illness, he lost his job and became increasingly isolated, spending most of his time alone in his room. He avoided friends and family and stopped playing guitar, which was his passion. When he was most ill, he found it hard to leave home, so he started to have his groceries delivered. With medication, Marco's depression finally started to improve, and he began to feel hopeful and interested

> again, but he was still struggling to do things that used to come easily. He still felt uncomfortable reaching out to friends, telling his doctor, "How do I explain where I've been? They've probably moved on with their lives, anyway." He hasn't cancelled the grocery delivery, and he's not sure where his guitar is, but most importantly, he hasn't been able to even think about finding a job. As soon as the idea enters his mind, he feels a stab of anxiety and immediately tries to think of something else.

Whether it's riding a bike, public speaking, reading, or shaving, with practice we get better at doing things. It's common for patients who are recovering from depression to report they are feeling better but they're still not "doing better." As mentioned in the CBT section, it's usually easier to change behaviour than it is to change thinking, and sometimes pushing oneself to do an activity can provoke more activity and lead to overall functional improvement.

Behavioural activation (BA) is based on the idea that depression is caused and maintained by the avoidance of upsetting or distressing emotions or situations. Initial avoidance leads to prolonged avoidance and eventually withdrawal from all activities and inertia. Much like CBT, BA should follow a hierarchical approach. Patients should work on easier activities to start and then move on to increasingly difficult ones, building on previous successes to expand their functional repertoire.

In Marco's case, after being away from work for a few years, the first step to getting back to life should not be the most stressful, challenging step, such as applying for a job. Marco would benefit from taking small steps towards increasing his activity. Perhaps a good first step would be to find his guitar. Next would be to play for a few minutes just a couple of times a week.

If Marco's place was a mess, after years of poor self-care, perhaps he could slowly work at getting it cleaned up. However, it's best to take this process in small steps as well. I usually suggest my patients write out a flexible schedule (kitchen first, then bathroom, then bedroom, and finally living room) and plan to spend only thirty minutes each day on cleaning. If the plan is to start with the kitchen, it might take a few weeks to get it done, but at least it's getting done. Taking thirty minutes a day is manageable for most people, and once the thirty minutes is over, Marco can stop and not think about it again until the next day. Building in physical activity always starts with a short walk, with the aim to build towards a thirty-minute walk every day.

While there are formal tenants for the use of BA, I believe it is an important aspect of **recovery** for anyone who has struggled with depression, since almost everyone finds it difficult, to some degree, to get back to their old routines and activities. **The CANMAT Depression Treatment Guidelines recommends BA as a first-line treatment for acute depression and as a second-line treatment for the maintenance of wellness following depression.**

Mindfulness-based cognitive therapy (MBCT)

MBCT combines **mindfulness** meditation training and **cognitive** therapy. A great colleague of mine, paraphrasing a Zen saying, described **mindfulness** as "allowing your negative thoughts in the front door and letting them out the back door, but not serving them tea."

Essentially, we all have negative, unpleasant, and distressing thoughts sometimes. Some of us have them much too often, while others only experience them now and again, but they're a normal human experience and we must learn to deal with them. **Mindfulness** teaches acceptance of those thoughts: they're ours, whether they are real or exaggerations or flat-out false, and we must show ourselves compassion, accept that they are our thoughts but not ruminate on them ("don't serve them tea").

In combination with **cognitive** therapy, which teaches skills necessary for confronting or reframing inaccurate or upsetting thoughts, **mindfulness** meditation can be a powerful force for managing depression symptoms. Beyond that, those who are able to learn and incorporate **mindfulness** skills report feeling less anxious and more peaceful.

There are many ways to learn **mindfulness**, whether with a therapist, by reading a book, or through online programs or apps. There are some excellent apps that have **mindfulness** meditations lasting just a few minutes, if that's all the time you've got. I had a patient tell me that when she's feeling overwhelmed at work as a teacher, she'll ask her class to read silently and use her **mindfulness** app to do a five-minute meditation. She's also taught her students **mindfulness**, to the approval of parents and fellow staff members.

Most of the favourable research for MBCT has been in the area of **relapse** prevention or the maintenance of wellness following depression. **The CANMAT Depression Treatment Guidelines have therefore recommended MBCT as a first-line treatment for the maintenance of wellness and as a second-line treatment for acute depression.** Evidence suggests that MBCT is most effective when used in combination with another depression treatment.

Interpersonal therapy (IPT)

IPT is a style of therapy that focuses on how patients relate to others (friends, loved ones, colleagues) as the cause or a factor in the maintenance of depression. There are four key areas of focus for IPT: loss or bereavement, social role changes or transitions (e.g., new life roles may include parenting, retirement, or a job change), social challenges due to excessive sensitivity (e.g., being easily hurt due to perceived slights by others), and disagreements or disputes.

There is a solid body of evidence for the value of IPT in diverse patient populations (e.g., adults, adolescents, and **peripartum** women). **The CANMAT Depression Treatment Guidelines recommend IPT as a first-line treatment for acute depression and as a second-line treatment for the maintenance of wellness, in combination with another depression treatment.**

Should I have group or individual therapy?

Skills based on each form of psychotherapy I have discussed here can be learned one-on-one with a therapist, in a group setting, or by using apps, books, or online programs.

I don't ever recall anyone saying to me, when I broached the subject of group therapy, "Yes, I love the idea!" In fact, I most often receive a stony-faced stare, followed by "No, thank you, that's not for me" or a more colourful "Not in this lifetime." I will admit that I was not an early adopter of the group therapy concept, but I have learned that a very well-organized and skilfully led group can be a highly therapeutic experience. However, a disorganized and poorly led group can be a disaster.

Group therapy is meant to be something of a family experience. While everyone in the group should have at least one thing in common beyond a mental illness, the differences between the individual participants often enhances the value of the group experience. Participants learn from one another, they are urged to see different viewpoints, and they will hear **insights** or experiences from a younger man or an older woman, perhaps someone they wouldn't have heard from before.

For a group to be a valuable and enriching experience, it must have highly skilled and intelligent leaders who guide respectful, open discussions and create a safe, comfortable environment for all participants. Most groups follow a specific psychotherapy program, such as CBT, and many include modules, so group members can follow along, complete homework, and report challenges and progress at the next meeting.

Many patients fear having their confidential, personal information exposed at a group meeting, but it's important to remember that everyone at the meeting is also struggling with some of the same challenges, and they too wish to have their confidentiality maintained. A well-run group starts with very clear ground rules, and breaking those rules should have immediate consequences, in order to protect the health and safety of the group members.

Group therapy has other benefits: it's usually much less expensive, has shorter wait-lists, and is often more available than individual therapy. My patient's preference is paramount, but I urge them not to knock it before they try it.

How many sessions will I need?

Gone are the days, because absent is the evidence, that anyone should spend an hour a day, for six days a week, for years on end on a blank-faced therapist's couch, free-associating and recounting their dreams. Sometimes a cigar is just a cigar.

Scientific evidence has demonstrated the value of short-term psychotherapy interventions: eight sessions of CBT or IPT can be adequate and effective. Of note, there seems to be added value associated with more frequent visits initially and then stretching out sessions over longer periods to allow for follow up to reinforce important information and fine-tune new skills. Of course, some patients do benefit from more visits over a longer period; however, if symptoms have failed to significantly improve over eight to ten sessions, it's time to re-evaluate the situation. If there is no benefit evident, it's important to ask, "Is this the right therapy/treatment?"; "Is this the right therapist?"; and "Are we treating the right diagnosis?"

What are the neurostimulation treatments for depression?

Neurostimulation treatments use electrical or magnetic stimulation to target brain areas known to be involved in the cause or maintenance of depression. Most are non-invasive treatments, because they do not require direct contact with the brain. There are, however, two invasive treatments that require surgery and are reserved for patients who have not benefitted from any other treatment.

In this section, I will describe the two most common **neurostimulation** treatments, **electroconvulsive therapy (ECT)** and repetitive transcranial magnetic stimulation (rTMS). Other non-invasive treatments include transcranial direct current stimulation (tDCS), which is a third-line treatment, and magnetic seizure therapy (MST), which is in the investigational phase of development and not yet readily available. Invasive treatments include vagus nerve stimulation (VNS), which is a third-line treatment reserved for the most chronically ill and treatment-resistant patients, and deep brain stimulation (DBS), which is in the investigational phase of development and has very limited availability.

Electroconvulsive therapy (ECT)

I am sure the movie *One Flew Over the Cuckoo's Nest* did more harm to psychiatric care than any other movie ever made. In that film, patients in a psychiatric unit are punished and their behaviour controlled using ECT. I know that psychiatric practices were not always humane, and I continue to have grave concerns about the treatment of vulnerable individuals who have a mental illness, but my experience and the research evidence clearly demonstrates that ECT is arguably the most effective treatment in psychiatry. While it is surely the most controversial treatment in psychiatry as well, ECT is the **gold standard** treatment for severe depression.

Through this book, I am sharing my twenty years of psychiatric experience and expertise. I am also reflecting and interpreting what I believe to be the highest quality research on the subjects I discuss. While the topic of ECT is handled no differently than any other I have tackled, due to the controversial nature of the treatment, I feel it's important to acknowledge that there are people who would strongly disagree with my pro-ECT stance. Some have gone so far as to suggest that ECT is a crime against humanity.

Like any treatment, ECT doesn't work for everyone, and some patients tolerate it better than others. However, and most importantly, many of my patients believe ECT saved their lives. If my child had a serious depression, and initial treatments were ineffective, I would urge them to consider ECT, and if I had a serious depression, I would have ECT.

Because the vast majority of people would not be excited by the notion of having their brain electrified, and we're taught from childhood that electrocution should be avoided, it will come as no surprise that ECT is likely the most thoroughly researched treatment in all of medicine.

ECT is performed in an operating room setting, usually in the presence of an anesthetist, a psychiatrist, and skilled nurses, who treat hundreds of patients every year. To have ECT, patients receive a general anesthetic and an anesthetist is there to ensure the patient is safely put to sleep and awakened quickly. An intravenous (IV) line is inserted to administer the anesthetic medication along with an agent that relaxes the muscles. The entire process, from IV insertion to awakening, usually takes five to ten minutes.

Once the patient is asleep, one or two electrodes are placed on their head and a pulse of electricity is given that provokes a short seizure. It is the seizure that provides the rapid antidepressant effect, although exactly how an ECT seizure effectively treats depression is not fully understood. However, because the seizure is generalized—which means it affects the entire brain—there are likely many separate effects that lead to its overall benefits.

There are many hypotheses for why ECT is so effective. Compared to other antidepressant treatments, it has the most profound effect on producing and growing healthy new **neurons**, which is necessary to effectively treat depression (see **neurogenesis** in chapter 4). There is also a **hormone** hypothesis, because ECT treatments are associated with normalization of the **hypothalamic-pituitary-adrenal (HPA) axis** in depressed patients (see chapter 4). The most widely accepted hypothesis is the **anticonvulsant** theory, which is based on the observation that ECT changes the brain's seizure threshold, which means it becomes more difficult to have a seizure during the course of treatment. ECT also provokes changes in critical brain **neurotransmitters**, including GABA and **glutamate**.

ECT treatments are usually given two or three times a week for one to two weeks and then with reduced frequency over several weeks. Most people require at least six to eight treatments, and some will require fifteen treatments or more before their symptoms fully remit. Sometimes, because the effect is so remarkable and rapid, and no other treatment has been effective, patients will opt for maintenance ECT once they've responded fully to the treatment. This usually involves having a single treatment at regular intervals, usually every three to six weeks for many months or even for many years.

There are certainly pros and cons associated with ECT, which must be carefully considered when determining if it is the best treatment choice for an individual patient. The pros are its unparalleled effectiveness and the rapidity of its effect. Some patients experience improvement from a devastating depression after only one or two treatments.

Additionally, ECT is an extremely safe treatment. A 2017 study analyzed data from 766,180 treatments across thirty-two countries and found an ECT-related mortality rate of 2.1 per 100,000 treatments. The greatest risk associated with ECT is having a general anesthetic, so most programs require an anesthesia assessment to minimize those risks. Patient's satisfaction, safety, and side effects have improved significantly over the last few decades, due to advances in anesthesia and improvements in the ECT technique.

The cons of ECT may seem minor to patients when their depression is extremely severe, but commonly there is a mounting frustration with the treatment once they start to feel better. This is in part due to the hassles associated with getting the treatment done, which involve visiting a hospital. In many communities, ECT is offered only to those admitted to hospital, although some programs offer out-patient treatments. However, this requires overnight fasting, very early in the morning treatment, and a great deal of support from family or friends, since it is necessary to be accompanied for twenty-four hours following the treatment, because of the risks associated with having a general anesthetic.

The ECT side effect that patients find most frustrating and worrisome is memory loss. While the research evidence demonstrates the risks of memory loss are primarily associated with short-term memories for events that occur during a course of ECT, patients still find it very annoying and fear they are sustaining a brain injury. A very small proportion of patients have reported they experienced permanent memory loss; however, research studies have consistently demonstrated that ECT-related memory impairment is transient and usually resolves within a few months of stopping the treatment.

Seizures are associated with amnesia, so no one remembers what happened when they've had a seizure. By having many seizures over several weeks, it's very difficult for the brain to store new memories. ECT-related memory loss is more pronounced with each treatment and it can take several months for patients to feel that their memory is working well again. While those having ECT maintain their long-term memories, they can forget major events that happen during the time of treatment. For instance, if you host your child's birthday party in the midst of a course of ECT, you might forget everything about the event, including the fact that it happened at all.

Importantly, as I have noted several times throughout this book, severe depression is often associated with significant **cognitive** symptoms. These symptoms are not always recognized by patients until their mood symptoms start to improve. Responding to ECT is no different: as depression starts to get better, patients will notice they are unable to think as clearly, concentrate, or remember as well as they could before they were depressed. While ECT is undoubtedly associated with short-term memory challenges, depression-related **cognitive** symptoms further contribute to the frustrating side effect and tend to recover slowly, regardless of the depression treatment that is employed.

Advances in ECT techniques have reduced the **cognitive** side effects associated with the treatment. In fact, a 2018 study found that elderly patients did not show deleterious **cognitive** effects six months following a course of ECT, most patients tolerated the treatment well, and a small group even experienced **cognitive** enhancement in the months following ECT.

Factors that increase the risk for **cognitive impairment** include advanced age, especially if there is pre-existing **cognitive impairment**, and the use of bitemporal ECT, which means electrodes are placed on both sides of the forehead. Using one electrode, especially if placed on the right side (unless the patient is left-handed), has been shown to result in less **cognitive impairment** but might also result in less robust ECT effects, or at least effects that are evident more slowly.

Over the years, I have learned some great tricks from my patients to mitigate ECT-related memory loss. Firstly, it's essential to write everything down: appointments, yes, but everything else that's important. Otherwise, what you wish to remember may instantly and irrevocably disappear. Additionally, keep a journal of the highlights of important or meaningful events right after they happen and read them occasionally during the course of ECT, so the memories are more likely to be maintained.

The other common ECT side effects include post-treatment headache, anesthesia-related nausea, and feeling exhausted for the day following treatment. The headache and nausea can usually be managed quite easily, sometimes with treatment before the ECT is administered, and the exhaustion requires a day of rest. Otherwise, most patients tolerate the treatment very well, but everyone could do without the short-term memory loss.

It is close to impossible to work during ECT, even if treatments are done as an out-patient. This is especially true early in the course of treatment, when ECTs are given several times a week. While relatively little time is required for the actual treatment, full **recovery** can take twenty-four hours due to the general anesthetic. As treatment progresses, depression symptoms will improve, but memory issues can become frustrating and impact work performance. This constitutes another con: loss of income due to time away from work.

Antidepressant medications are often continued during ECT, unless they might interfere with having a seizure. For instance, because **benzodiazepines** are also **anticonvulsants**, they are commonly discontinued, or at least they are not taken the evening before an ECT treatment. Once the ECT is slowly discontinued, antidepressant medications will often be effective, even though they weren't fully effective before ECT was initiated. In fact, studies have demonstrated lower **relapse** rates when antidepressant medication is continued during a course of ECT compared to studies where medication was begun following the discontinuation of ECT. This may be due to the brain changes provoked by the ECT, which are then maintained by medication. Many people require ongoing antidepressant medication treatment following a course of ECT, unless they opt for maintenance treatments, because medications substantially reduce the risk of **relapse**.

Unfortunately, due to the **stigma** and fear associated with ECT, despite its safety and effectiveness, it is often reserved as a last resort for the most severe, treatment-resistant depressed patients. However, any patient with severe depression that is impairing their ability to function should be offered ECT. Research evidence demonstrates that depression symptoms are more likely to respond robustly to ECT earlier in the course of illness, when there have been fewer medication trials.

Likewise, any patient who has a **psychotic** depression or is intolerant to medication should also be informed that ECT may be a viable option. It has also been demonstrated to rapidly reduce **suicidal ideation** in severely depressed patients. The treatment has been associated with a 20 percent greater reduction in suicide risk when compared with antidepressant medication treatments.

Even some of the most vulnerable patient groups benefit from ECT. Depression in elderly patients tends to be highly responsive to the treatment. The **prevalence** of **cognitive impairment** associated with ECT may be higher in elderly patients, but most experience full resolution of short-term memory loss, and some also notice **cognitive** enhancement. Finally, ECT is considered safe in all trimesters of pregnancy because it has not been found to cause short- or long-term harm to a developing fetus. **Psychotic** depression in pregnancy usually responds well to ECT and is well tolerated. **The CANMAT Depression Treatment Guidelines recommend ECT as a first-line treatment for depression and second-line as a maintenance treatment for depression.**

A 2018 study gathered patients' thoughts regarding their experience with ECT:

- **More likely to accept ECT:** Factors that made participants more likely to choose, agree, or accept having ECT, or enhanced their preparation experience included: the doctor made the decision; a desperate last resort; witnessing others or themselves benefitting; and family support.
- **Less likely to accept ECT:** Factors that made participants less likely to choose, agree, or accept having ECT, and/or negatively impacted on their preparation experience included fear, negative family experiences, and concerns about side effects.
- **What added to the experience:** Numerous aspects enhanced the participants experiences of ECT, including sharing the journey with others; caring and compassionate interactions with staff; being less scary than expected; and rapid mental health improvements.
- **What worsened the experience:** Negative aspects included side effects; aspects of the procedure itself; **stigma** and shame; and having to wait in line for the ECT treatment.
- **What could be done better:** Participants offered many suggestions for how to improve the process of supporting individuals in making decisions related to ECT and the treatment experience itself, including: more information; bringing up the option of ECT earlier; information and support from others who have had ECT; better planning for management of side effects; and greater family involvement.

Repetitive transcranial magnetic stimulation (rTMS)

Repetitive transcranial magnetic stimulation is a non-invasive treatment that involves the generation of electrical currents, using an external magnetic coil, to target specific brain areas responsible for depression. While an awake patient sits or lies down in a comfortable resting position, an electromagnetic coil is held against their scalp, usually on the forehead. No anesthesia is required. The coil passes magnetic pulses that provoke an electrical current within the brain. The electrical current stimulates **neurons**, ultimately reducing depression symptoms. The **mechanism of action** of rTMS is still not fully understood; however, much like ECT, it is thought to impact several different processes that are responsible for the onset and maintenance of depression.

rTMS is usually given by a specialized nurse or trained technician, under the supervision of a psychiatrist. Each session lasts between thirty and sixty minutes, and most programs that offer rTMS follow a protocol that ranges from three to five treatments per week. Less frequent treatments will work more slowly, and ultimately the same number of treatments are generally necessary, in the range of twenty-five to thirty sessions in total. Some protocols are accelerated, where the patient receives several treatments each day over a shorter period (five to ten days).

rTMS is generally reserved for patients who have not responded to medication or psychotherapy, although it is commonly used in combination with antidepressant medication, which might make it more effective. It can be customized for each patient, because it can be adjusted based on the intensity, pattern, frequency, and the site of the stimulation, according to a patient's needs.

rTMS is usually well tolerated, but it is time consuming. The most commonly reported side effects include scalp pain during the treatment and post-treatment headache. These side effects tend to be less bothersome over the course of treatment and are usually managed quickly and completely with an over-the-counter analgesic, such as acetaminophen, and neither side effect tends to result in treatment discontinuation. rTMS is not recommended for patients with a history of seizures or if the patient has any metallic hardware in their brain, including cochlear implants, brain stimulators or electrodes, or aneurysm clips. However, metallic fillings are fine. Extra caution is necessary for patients who have a cardiac pacemaker, implanted defibrillator, or a brain injury (stroke, tumour, or other brain abnormality).

rTMS is not as effective as ECT, especially for patients with **psychotic** symptoms or for those who previously failed to respond to a course of ECT. Therefore, rTMS should be considered prior to trying a course of ECT. While ECT is more effective, its **cognitive** effects are definitely more bothersome. Most rTMS patients have no **cognitive** complaints.

According to the CANMAT Depression Treatment Guidelines, there is adequate research evidence to recommend rTMS as a first-line treatment for depressed patients who have failed at least one antidepressant treatment. After successful rTMS treatment, depression **relapse** is common, so maintenance therapy, which involves less frequent treatments over six to twelve months, is often recommended.

What are the alternative and complementary therapies for depression?

Exercise

Regular physical exercise has been well studied in depression and, likely through a variety of mechanisms, it has been shown to be a beneficial depression treatment. Exercise has a positive impact on several **neurotransmitters** associated with depression (e.g., **serotonin** and **norepinephrine**). It also reduces the **stress hormone cortisol**, and it provokes an increase in **brain-derived neurotrophic factor** (**BDNF**), which is necessary for **neurogenesis** (see chapter 4). In fact, participating in exercise might prevent the onset of depression in vulnerable individuals.

Psychologically, exercise helps garner a sense of personal control, since it is something a patient struggling with depression can do for themselves that will positively impact their symptoms. Exercise can also reduce painful symptoms and having greater stamina and improved muscle tone are rarely experienced as a downer. Exercise can also enormously benefit fatigue, which is a very common residual symptom of depression.

The word "aerobic" literally means "with oxygen," so **aerobic exercises** are energetic and sustained, make you breathe harder and faster, increasing oxygen consumption and strengthening your heart and lungs. **Aerobic exercises** include activities such as vigorous walking or jogging, swimming, soccer, biking, tennis, and dancing.

"Anaerobic" means "without oxygen," although without oxygen we'd all die, so **anaerobic exercises** still require breathing. **Anaerobic exercises** are usually brief bursts of intense activity, such as weight lifting, and your body must rely on energy stored in muscles rather than just oxygen to get the job done. **Anaerobic exercises** build muscle and promote power, speed, and strength rather than endurance. Interestingly, **aerobic exercises** can become **anaerobic exercises** if they are performed at high intensity; for instance, jogging is aerobic, but sprinting is anaerobic.

Both **aerobic** and **anaerobic exercise** have evidence for reducing depressive symptoms. The best news: high-intensity activity is not necessary to benefit from exercise. Getting your heart rate up for thirty minutes, through mild to moderately intense exercise, five days a week has been shown to provide an antidepressant effect. If exercise is beneficial, discontinuing exercise can actually be detrimental, so there is a value to creating a routine that is not excessively strenuous, if exercise hasn't been a usual part of your routine. Sustainability is key. Two major research reviews have demonstrated that exercise can be as effective as medication or talk therapy for mild to moderate depression. Likewise, there is evidence that supervised exercise programs might offer greater benefit. **The CANMAT Depression Treatment Guidelines recommend exercise first-line for the treatment of mild to moderate depression and second-line, in conjunction with other treatments, for moderate to severe depression.**

Light therapy

While there are many reasons why a tropical holiday is so enjoyable, a major factor is related to sunlight. We all seem to feel better when we leave a dark, rainy, cold environment for a winter getaway in the sun, and there is some solid science demonstrating the benefit of sunlight on mental well-being.

Light therapy, also known as phototherapy, is a well-researched treatment that is most often recommended for depression with a seasonal pattern (see page 15). The **mechanism of action** for **light therapy** is not fully understood, but it is thought to impact a patient's **circadian rhythm** and **neurotransmitters** associated with depression. Exposure to natural light has also been found to be effective for the treatment of **seasonal depression.** A 2017 study found, after following nearly 300 patients over six years, that sunshine duration and global radiation were the most significant factors associated with **seasonal depression** symptoms.

Light therapy involves daily exposure to bright light, which is usually administered at home, using a commercially available light box. The standard **light therapy** protocol involves early morning light exposure (no later than noon), using a light with a specific intensity (10,000 lux) for thirty minutes a day. Protocols usually suggest using the light for four to six weeks, but most patients will experience benefit within one to two weeks. If there is no noticeable benefit after two or three weeks, it is unlikely the treatment will be worthwhile. **Light therapy** is generally very well tolerated, with occasional complaints of headache and strained or sore eyes.

While there have been many studies supporting the benefit of **light therapy** for seasonal pattern depression, some recent studies have produced evidence demonstrating **light therapy**'s benefits for non-**seasonal depression** as well. **The CANMAT depression treatment guidelines have endorsed light therapy as a first-line treatment for seasonal depression and as a second-line treatment, alone or in combination with medication, for mild to moderate non-seasonal depression.**

Sleep deprivation

It certainly seems counterintuitive, when **insomnia** is a common and highly distressing depression symptom, that sleep deprivation can have a rapid and significant antidepressant effect. Sleep deprivation therapy requires that patients stay awake for up to forty hours for two or three episodes over a week, interspersed with **recovery** sleep or partial sleep deprivation (only three to four hours per night). Some research has suggested that a week of partial sleep deprivation (a maximum of three hours of sleep per night) may also be effective.

Sleep deprivation appears to impact **neurotransmitters** associated with depression and might also affect how brain **glial cells** communicate (see chapter 4). One large review study demonstrated that sleep deprivation is beneficial for moderate to severe depression when used in combination with antidepressant medication.

Because the benefits of sleep deprivation alone tend to be short-lived, its use in combination with other treatments is more likely to offer a sustained benefit. Not surprisingly, the most common side effect associated with sleep deprivation is daytime sleepiness. Also concerning would be safety-sensitive work situations, because of the risk of exhaustion on the job, and a heightened risk of seizures in sensitive individuals.

The CANMAT Depression Treatment Guidelines do not recommend sleep deprivation except for more severely depressed patients, when used in combination with other treatments, and only after other first-line and second-line treatments have failed. Sleep deprivation should not be undertaken unless it is under a doctor's supervision.

Yoga

I previously mentioned a lovely patient of mine who told me she had to finally accept that she couldn't yoga her way out of her depression, but that doesn't mean that yoga isn't a helpful tool. Yoga practitioners seek physical, mental, and spiritual balance, through improving strength, flexibility, stability, breath control, and body awareness. Meditation is also a critical aspect of yoga practice, which likely plays a role in its depression benefits.

There is evidence that yoga normalizes the **hypothalamic-pituitary-adrenal (HPA) axis** (see chapter 4) and positively impacts **neurotransmitters** associated with depression. There is a great deal of research concluding that yoga benefits depressed patients; however, the data is not of high quality. As such, **the CANMAT Depression Treatment Guidelines recommend that yoga be used second-line, in combination with other treatments, for mild to moderate depression.**

What over-the-counter medications have good evidence for depression treatment?

While there are more than 100 complementary or alternative treatments available to consumers, only three **over-the-counter** (not requiring a prescription) **medications** are recommended as first- or second-line by **evidence-based treatment** guidelines. They are omega-3 fatty acids, S-adenosyl-L-methionine (SAM-e), and St. John's wort. However, it is important to keep in mind that there is very little monitoring of the quality of so-called natural products by regulatory agencies, and much of what is available on store shelves may be of low quality. In fact, some products might not contain any active ingredient at all.

Omega-3 fatty acids

Fish, nuts, and seeds contain the fatty acids eicosapentaenoic acid (EPA) and docosahexaenoic acid (DHA), which have well-established health benefits. There are many large research review papers demonstrating the benefits of omega-3 fatty acids as a treatment for depression; however, other studies have concluded that there is no clinical difference between omega-3 and **placebo.**

The usual dose of omega-3 that is recommended for the treatment of depression is three to nine grams per day. Most patients have no side effects, but mild, usually transient, side effects can occur, including stomach upset (e.g., diarrhea, nausea) and, depending on the formulation, a fishy aftertaste. Combining omega-3 with blood thinners, also called anticoagulants, may require more careful lab monitoring, so it's important to speak to a doctor before adding this treatment.

Because of the contradictory evidence, **the CANMAT Depression Treatment Guidelines recommend omega-3 as a second-line treatment for mild to moderate depression and as a second-line treatment, in combination with another antidepressant, for more severe depression.**

S-adenosyl-L-methionine (SAM-e)

SAM-e is the most natural of the natural products because it is made in the human body. It has been a commonly prescribed treatment for depression in Europe for many years, both as an oral tablet and as an intravenous and intramuscular injection. In North America, it is considered a dietary supplement and is not as commonly prescribed.

SAM-e likely works by positively impacting the **neurotransmitters** associated with depression. The recommended dose of the dietary supplement is 400 to 800 mg twice daily with meals. It is generally well tolerated, although some patients complain of worsening **anxiety**, fatigue, stomach upset (e.g., nausea, diarrhea), sleep disturbance, headache, and irritability. **The CANMAT Depression Treatment Guidelines recommend SAM-e as a second-line add-on treatment for mild to moderate depression.**

St. John's wort (SJW)

St. John's wort, also known as *Hypericum perforatum*, is a plant that has been used medicinally for centuries. SJW has been studied extensively for the treatment of depression, but its commercially available forms can vary widely with respect to dose and purity. The likely **mechanism of action** of SJW is through its effect on **serotonin** receptors, but it might also have other important mechanisms, including impacting the enzyme **monoamine oxidase** (see page 194), as well as **hormones** that influence depression.

SJW is generally very well tolerated, but there are sometimes complaints of stomach upset, headaches, and other side effects commonly associated with **serotonin** antidepressants, such as SSRIs and SNRIs.

Because of the abundance of research evidence, SJW has been **recommended as a first-line treatment for mild to moderate depression by the CANMAT Depression Treatment Guidelines and as a second-line add-on treatment for moderate to severe depression.**

Third-line non-prescription treatments

The following natural products have some research evidence for their value in the treatment of mild to moderate depression; however, that evidence is of lower quality than that of the treatments recommended first- and second-line. They include: acetyl-L-carnitine, *Crocus sativus* (saffron), DHEA, folate, and *Lavandula* (lavender). These treatments are not well regulated, so the quality of the products will vary widely. In fact, some products don't actually contain any active ingredient. I suggest speaking to your doctor if you are thinking about using one of these treatments, since some have been associated with side effects, might not be appropriate during pregnancy, or might interfere with other prescription medication.

Chapter summary

- There is strong scientific evidence demonstrating the value of talk therapy for the treatment of depression.
- **Electroconvulsive therapy (ECT)** is the **gold standard** treatment for severe depression.
- Exercise, yoga, and **light therapy** have scientific evidence supporting their benefit as depression treatments and for the maintenance of wellness.

- A limited number of non-prescription treatments have demonstrated antidepressant benefit, including omega-3 fatty acids, SAM-e, and St. John's wort.

Depression treatment decisions are based on the severity of the symptoms, the safety and tolerability of a treatment, and, most importantly, a patient's wishes. While some treatments are reserved for the most severely ill patients, some are beneficial for every depressed individual—most notably, exercise.

A real patient's story

DEPRESSION ENCOMPASSES EVERY facet of my life. It's always there, and I can't escape or ignore its barrage of negative notions. Although its fruition was a result of cumulative traumatic events, it seems as if in a single day my world turned upside down. Despite having done hours upon hours of work, with a fantastic support system, most days I still feel depression's shroud darkening my thoughts. It seems as if any bump in the road can trip me up and I slide backwards a little bit. Most days I feel like a fake, presenting a strong exterior, but in truth that is not at all what I feel. While I do believe that there have been traumatic events that I can attribute these feelings to, I also realize that in my perception of life's normal struggles I find them to be catastrophic. My mantra was always "look back, but don't stare." However, even that is too hard, so I am trying to follow the more realistic approach of just living in the present moment.

14

What are some myths about depression?

THERE IS A great deal of harm that can be done by perhaps well-meaning yet utterly uninformed mental health "experts." Their lack of scientific training is often merely a preamble ("I'm not a doctor, but..."). They speak with enthusiasm and authority as they peddle supplements, homeopathic tinctures, detox enemas, and antioxidant smoothies, with the goal of liberating patients from their **evidence-based treatments** and dollars from their wallets.

There is little regulatory oversight hindering those who claim that costly, completely useless products are beneficial for serious illnesses. These charlatans take advantage of ailing, vulnerable patients and their families to enrich themselves, and **Health Canada** and the FDA are doing little or nothing to protect consumers.

Myth: Detoxifying treatments have antidepressant benefits

Despite claims from some "expert" celebrities, detoxifying drinks, enemas, and foot baths have absolutely no credible scientific evidence to support their cost or use. In fact, there is more credible evidence describing the serious potential risks associated with these unregulated treatments. We already have a built-in natural detox system: our liver! It's our chief detoxifier, working in concert with the digestive tract, spleen, and kidneys. We also have urgent detox mechanisms, such as vomiting and diarrhea. Our bodies remove waste, fight infections, and regulate nutrients, oxygen, water, and whatever else the detox promises to normalize or equalize. Using pseudoscientific mumbo-jumbo, purveyors of detoxification treatments are modern-day snake-oil salesmen.

Myth: Dietary supplements are all you need

There is emerging evidence highlighting the importance of diet in the development, treatment, and prevention of mental illnesses. How gut flora (microorganisms that live in our intestines) could act as both a cause and treatment for serious mental illnesses is an exciting area of research. However, whether particular foods are protective or heighten the risk of mental illness has yet to be established with high-quality scientific research.

As mentioned in chapter 5, mental illnesses increase the risk of obesity, and some psychiatric medications heighten that risk. Regrettably, fad dieting is rarely an effective means of weight control, and diet myths abound. It's difficult to stick to a structured, healthy diet when perfectly well. It's close to impossible when also trying to cope with the symptoms of a mental illness.

Seeking guidance from a skilled dietitian or other informed healthcare provider or reading information from a reputable website can help to create a dietary plan that is both tolerable and sustainable. Foods that are high in sugar, as well as bread, cereal, rice, and pasta, are major culprits for excessive weight gain and associated **inflammation.**

Most of us get all the vitamins and nutrients we need from our diet, even if it's not perfect, so supplements are usually expensive and unnecessary. However, using specific supplements in psychiatry is an active area of research. Occasionally, a specific vitamin or mineral is deficient and needs to be supplemented. For instance, low iron or vitamin B_{12} can result in anemia, which is associated with severe fatigue, and lab work to rule this out should be part of a psychiatric assessment. High doses of water-soluble vitamins (including B and C) don't accumulate in the body, so getting more than you need generally means you're feeding the fishes your expensive vitamins. However, fat-soluble vitamins (A, E, D, and K) can accumulate and be toxic, leading to harmful effects. Additionally, some minerals are also dangerous in high doses; for instance, iron is highly toxic in overdose.

Myth: Homeopathy works

Homeopathy is hogwash, but don't take my word for it. Ben Goldacre's book *Bad Science* skilfully debunks the myth of **homeopathy**. Aisles in pharmacies dedicated to homeopathic treatments give it undeserved and dangerous credibility. It greatly distresses me that pharmacists, who are generally acknowledged to be the most trusted of health professionals, would have anything to do with the sale of these bogus treatments. Sadly, it will take the deaths of innocents before these treatments are removed from pharmacy shelves. Pharmacies that carry these products are doing so solely for financial gain, since there is no credible evidence that supports the recommendation of homeopathic treatments.

Myth: Cannabis is an effective depression treatment

I have included cannabis in this section because of the widely held belief that it is a cure-all treatment for many mental illnesses, including depression. However, I am not aware of any reputable treatment guidelines anywhere in the world that recommend cannabis as a treatment for any psychiatric disorder.

A local Vancouver newspaper's most recent count tallied ninety-five cannabis dispensaries. In Colorado, an independent newspaper reported, "There are 698 storefronts you can walk into to buy medical or retail marijuana... more than triple the number [of] Starbucks (216) in the state." You'll also note that apparently cannabis is a wonder drug that effectively treats everything from fungal toes to brain tumours. However, a careful review of the evidence does not back up the claims these purveyors make regarding the usefulness of cannabis for the treatment of mental illnesses.

There are few high-quality studies for medicinal cannabis in any area of medicine. Studies often differ in terms of the type, source, and dose of cannabis, making them difficult to compare. Most cannabis studies are open-label, lack a **placebo** or another drug comparator, or have too few subjects to demonstrate the value of the treatment. This makes it extremely difficult for doctors to determine whether cannabis is a safe or effective treatment to offer patients.

The best quality evidence for medicinal cannabis is for chemotherapy-induced nausea. Pain management evidence is less robust and there is some evidence for the use of cannabis in epilepsy and for muscle spasticity. For mental illnesses, there is poor quality data supporting cannabis treatment and more evidence demonstrating its harms.

Physicians have not consistently or effectively confronted cannabis-related myths, nor have we adequately educated our patients. When I tell parents about the risks associated with cannabis use, especially for the developing brain (e.g., for their children), they often express shock. Many believe it's like oregano—a safe, natural product that adds a little spice to life.

There are about 100 different types of cannabinoids, but the two best known and studied are tetrahydrocannabinol (THC) and cannabidiol (CBD). Tetrahydrocannabinol (THC) is responsible for the high associated with cannabis, but what is available on the schoolyard is not your grandparent's pot anymore. Over the last fifty years, street pot has been bred to heighten its potency, from 1 to 4 percent THC to 20 to 40 percent or more, depending on the product.

Concentrated products, such as shatter, are produced by extracting THC using solvents like butane and can contain more than 80 percent THC. These high-potency THC products have made cannabis more impairing, more addictive, and more dangerous for the developing brain. THC is not benign and there's a mountain of scientific evidence, compiled over decades, to prove it poses serious risks, particularly for young brains.

Cannabidiol (CBD) is another cannabis ingredient, which reduces the impact of THC and likely contributes to its medicinal benefits. CBD has been demonstrated to have **anti-inflammatory**, analgesic, **anticonvulsant**, and anti-**anxiety** properties. Cannabis has been shown to worsen **anxiety** when it contains low CBD and high THC and improve **anxiety** when it contains low THC and high CBD.

Most studies assessing the relationship between depression and cannabis use demonstrate a high **prevalence** of depression among cannabis users and vice versa. A 2018 study followed 307 subjects for one year and found that cannabis use, especially non-medical use, among patients with depression may impede symptom improvement while reducing the likelihood they will seek appropriate depression treatment. Additionally, cannabis use among adults with depression is associated with high rates of **suicidal ideation** and an increased risk of severe psychiatric symptoms.

A 2017 study found that cannabis users and non-users had similar rates of depression, however several other studies found there was a far higher risk of **anxiety** and depression among cannabis users compared with non-users. Depression and **anxiety** are associated with more frequent cannabis use and a higher rate of problem use. Several studies have found that alterations in the brain's endocannabinoid system, which includes brain structures affected by cannabis use, can provoke the onset of depression.

There is research evidence demonstrating that THC-induced changes in brain structure and function, found in regular users of high-potency cannabis, may be inherited by subsequent generations through **epigenetic** modification (see chapter 3). The **chronic** use of high-potency THC is postulated to result in altered **gene expression.** The modified **gene**, which causes brain changes in a cannabis-smoking parent, may be passed on to their child, resulting in the same brain changes, even if the child never smokes cannabis.

There is no single cause for **schizophrenia.** THC alone is not responsible, but there is an abundance of evidence that the frequent use of high-potency THC can provoke the earlier onset of **schizophrenia** by up to six years. While similar associations have not been established with any other illicit drugs or alcohol, there is solid evidence to suggest a causal link between THC and **schizophrenia.** Of note, CBD might offer some significant antipsychotic benefits for patients with **schizophrenia.** High quality research trials are necessary to better understand these promising early research findings.

Despite the clear lack of evidence supporting its value in the treatment of depression, and more data demonstrating its harms, several studies have reported that medical cannabis is currently being used as a treatment for depression, even being prescribed by physicians.

Prescribers must thoughtfully consider the evidence and share it with their patients. It is not acceptable to prescribe a drug simply because it helped another patient (this is called anecdotal evidence). Drugs that lack high-quality evidence, like cannabis, should be reserved for patients who are suffering and for whom the appropriate use of conventional treatments have failed. While some patients who haven't responded to conventional treatments will benefit from cannabis, we need more evidence before widespread medicinal use for the treatment of mental illnesses is defensible. **Clinicians** require better education and **evidence-based treatment** guidelines in order to develop confidence when discussing the potential benefits and harms associated with cannabis.

If your healthcare professional is recommending mega-dosed vitamins, kale enemas (or, for that matter, anything that includes depression and enema in the same sentence), homeopathy, or cannabis to treat depression, I implore you to consider finding someone else to ask for help. Depression is a serious illness, and anyone claiming to be able to cure depression, cancer, or any other serious illness with unproven treatments isn't a real health professional. You deserve better.

A real patient's story

I WAS CONFUSED BY what was happening to me—both my mind and body. What would a person like me have to be anxious about? I had severe headaches, lack of appetite, was frequently vomiting, and crying uncontrollably. My thoughts were scattered, unclear, and foggy. I continued going to school and tried to keep a smile on my face, hoping that no one would notice, so I could push my way through my final exams.

After completing my finals, I flew back home to live with my parents. The following day, my family doctor gave me my first diagnosis of major depression, and I was forced to take a medical leave of absence from school. The diagnosis was alarming. I thought people who were depressed were sad, and I was far from sad. My doctor went on to tell me this illness was quite prevalent in my family (he had treated a lot of our relatives), and I needed to limit my **stresses.**

I did not know how I felt about my diagnosis, let alone having to ingest these pills I was prescribed into my "healthy" body I worked so hard on. I had never taken prescription or over-the-counter drugs, let alone experimented with street drugs or alcohol.

I felt all the control I once had over my life was slipping away. Negative thoughts would enter my mind a mile a minute and nothing would make them stop. Logically I knew they were not true, but they continued to manifest. These dark thoughts consumed me and for the next six months, they set the tone for my mood and behaviour.

The hardest thing to come to terms with was the diagnosis of depression and now being labelled as a "depressed person." The **stigma** I associated with depression was that depressed people are always sad. They do not have motivation, willpower, or strength. Perhaps they had a difficult childhood and are unhappy or miserable. But I learned that depression does not *look* a certain way or affect a certain kind of person. People's experiences with depression are often different. Some go through it just once, during a tough period in their life, while others battle the condition for years. What helps one person get better may not be what helps another get better. Depression knows no bounds and can affect anyone: a close friend or family member, a colleague, or someone you see walking on the street. You have no idea that this person is suffering from this debilitating illness and, more often than not, suffering alone.

During my third major depressive episode, my mom had a theory that my body was becoming reliant on these pills. So I tried alternative methods such as naturopathic medicine, acupuncture, **CBT (cognitive-behavioural therapy)**, and met numerous psychiatrists and psychologists, but nothing seemed to get me better. In fact, I got worse. I became so hopeless with my diagnosis and felt like *this* was now my life: I was an on-and-off-again depressed person. If I did too much, I would get sick. If I pursued my dreams in life, which meant working hard and taking on **stresses**, I would get sick.

My last depressive episode was definitely my lowest point—I was ready to quit and leave this planet. I was hospitalized for one month so I could have access to a treatment called **electroconvulsive therapy (ECT)** as an in-patient. Although debilitating, ECT saved my life. I went on to have it for over two years of maintenance therapy where I was unable to work consistently and remember things (a side effect of ECT is short-term memory loss).

My message to anyone suffering is this: you are not alone and you are not damaged. This is absolutely not your fault, so please talk to someone and get help. Everyone's depression and cause for depression are different, and what helps them get them better is also different. Some do well with medication, some do well with psychotherapy, or a combination. Do not allow anyone to judge you and your struggles, and, most importantly, do not judge yourself.

Today, with the help of all my support systems and educating myself about my illness, I am proud to say it has been four years since my last episode—the longest period since my first episode.

People who have beaten cancer are considered survivors. I see myself as a survivor of depression. With both cancer and depression, the patient is fighting for their life. I no longer see myself as weak or damaged but the opposite—resilient and strong. I have flipped the **stigma** I once felt with my illness and instead see it as my gift.

15

What depression treatments are available for special populations?

WHILE IT IS outside the scope of this book to be the definitive resource for the use of psychiatric treatments for special populations—such as children and adolescents, pregnant women, and the elderly—I will touch on some of the major issues that should be considered if you or someone you love is in one of these groups.

Peripartum and postpartum depression

As I described in chapter 6, in the **DSM-5**, the **peripartum** period includes the time during pregnancy and four weeks **postpartum.** However, doctors and researchers commonly extend the time to include up to twelve months after delivery, which is referred to as the **postpartum** period. There are definitely special considerations when managing depression in women who are pregnant or **postpartum.** Most expectant or new moms wish to avoid all medications; however, it is important to remember that depression can be very serious and have long-term effects on both the mother and her child (see chapter 6).

Whenever possible, depending on the severity of her symptoms, pregnant or breastfeeding mothers should be offered psychotherapy (see chapter 13), and other non-medication depression treatments, such as exercise. However, following a careful assessment, if a woman and her doctor determine that medication treatment is necessary, research evidence strongly supports the importance of diagnosing and appropriately treating depression in pregnancy. The top concern should always be the safety of the mother and her developing or breastfeeding child.

Drugs known to harm a developing fetus are referred to as teratogens. Many of us remember the tragic outcomes associated with the drug thalidomide, which was taken by many Canadian mothers during pregnancy to manage morning sickness. Unbeknownst to the mothers and their doctors, thalidomide was a teratogen, and many children were born with missing or malformed limbs. Other teratogens can lead to miscarriage, physical malformations (of the limbs, heart, brain, or spinal cord), or developmental delay.

Malformations occur in 3 percent to 6 percent of pregnancies worldwide, often with no known cause. The highest risk period for medication-related malformations is during the first trimester (the first three months of pregnancy) when major organs are formed, but some drugs can pose risks during the second and third trimester as well. Additionally, almost all medications can be passed to an infant, to varying degrees, through breast milk, and some can pose a risk for a breastfed child.

Any study assessing the effect of a drug on pregnant women would struggle to recruit subjects, so it is very difficult to gather evidence regarding the safety of new treatments in that population. This is where studies on rodents and other animals have been used extensively. However, because up to 45 percent of pregnancies are unplanned, medication use during an unexpected pregnancy is one way by which we better understand drug safety. **This highlights**

the importance of discussing contraception and the safety of medications during pregnancy with all child-bearing-age patients.

There are very few medications used in psychiatry that carry a risk of teratogenicity. If possible, those treatments should be avoided entirely in women of child-bearing age, whether they are using contraception or not. This is because most psychiatric medications should be taken long term, and it's difficult to ensure effective contraception is maintained over extended periods.

Beyond teratogenicity, a medication's impact on neonatal adaptation, which refers to how a newborn adapts to life in the outside world, is also an important consideration. Immediately following birth, a newborn must adapt rapidly to the chilly environment outside Mom's cozy, fluid-filled *casa del uterus*. At birth, infants suddenly discontinue any medication their mother was taking that crossed the placenta. If Mom is prescribed an antidepressant that has a high risk of **discontinuation symptoms** (see page 212), such as paroxetine or venlafaxine XR, her baby will be at risk of those symptoms following birth. While not considered dangerous, **discontinuation symptoms** can make the infant uncomfortable and difficult to settle. As such, those antidepressants that have a higher risk for causing **discontinuation symptoms** are best avoided in pregnant or child-bearing-age women.

A 2018 paper in the *Clinical Obstetrics and Gynecology* journal reviewed the most up-to-date research regarding the safety of psychiatric medication for pregnant and lactating mothers and their babies. Happily, the great majority of research demonstrates that SSRIs, SNRIs, TCAs, and other antidepressants, such as bupropion and mirtazapine, do not pose a significant risk to moms or their babies. Less medication is shared with the baby through breast milk than there is during the pregnancy, so if a medication is working and well tolerated, it should be continued after delivery, even if Mom is breastfeeding.

Until recently, no medications were specifically indicated for the treatment of **postpartum** depression, so doctors prescribed the same antidepressants employed to treat depression at other times of life. For mothers suffering from the most severe **postpartum** depression symptoms, **electroconvulsive therapy** (ECT) is considered a very safe and rapidly effective option, especially if there are associated **psychotic** symptoms, **acute** suicidal thoughts, or if Mom is unable to care for herself or her child. However, the FDA recently approved brexanolone (Zulresso®), which is given intravenously over several days and works very quickly, usually within forty-eight hours, to provide nearly immediate relief for new mothers who are experiencing severe depression. Brexanolone is available in the United States only, and is provided through a restricted program that requires the drug be administered by a healthcare provider in a certified facility because the mother must be monitored very carefully due to possible serious side effects. It is unclear if or when brexanolone will be available in Canada.

A patient, her family, and her doctor must weigh the risks and benefits when deciding whether to take a medication and determining which medication should be employed. While each patient must make her own decision, it's important to continue to maintain contact with a healthcare provider if she decides against medication, in case the situation changes and medication becomes unavoidable.

It's common for women who unexpectedly become pregnant to stop their medication immediately, without consulting a physician, for fear of harming their child. However, if she is prescribed a medication with good evidence for its safety in pregnancy, her symptoms are well managed, and she's tolerating it well, most specialists recommend the medication be continued at the current dose. If she insists on stopping the medication, discontinuing it slowly (referred to as a slow **taper**) will help to avoid any **discontinuation symptoms** (see page 212).

If a woman experiences a depression **relapse** during pregnancy, it's usually a good idea to try a medication that worked previously first, so long as it is safe during pregnancy. Sometimes dose adjustment is required during pregnancy and then again after delivery, but this is usually based on each individual woman's experience.

A mother who has a previous history of **postpartum** depression is at high risk of **relapse** during subsequent pregnancies and should be monitored very closely. If possible, measures should be put in place before delivery that might help to prevent a **relapse**, such as ensuring extra help at home so she gets adequate sleep.

And now a few words about breastfeeding... *you are not a bad mother if you don't breastfeed*! I am certain that there are very intelligent, well-adjusted people, including Nobel laureates, astronauts, and even some psychiatrists who were not breastfed, and their brains still developed and allowed them to be successful, contributing members of society. **While breast milk is undoubtedly a good thing, and breastfeeding can make life easier, and it's a nice, cozy thing to do, if it hurts too much, it's too difficult, you hate it, or you just don't want to do it, that's up to you.**

If you're suffering from a mental illness and you can't breastfeed, please don't feel bad. More than anything, your baby needs you to be well. Please don't let anyone shame you into breastfeeding because *they* think it's the best thing you can possibly do. You own your body. You decide. Breast is only best if it's best for *both* you and your baby.

The ultimate goal here is a healthy mom and a healthy baby. Mom and baby need to bond, both during the pregnancy and after delivery. An exhausted, harried, guilt-ridden mother, especially one who is depressed, won't be in top bonding form. Breastfeeding does not equal bonding. Skin-to-skin contact in a safe, low-**stress** environment, where the mom feels a sense of calm and control, promotes bonding.

If you do decide to breastfeed, be sure to pump milk so a partner, friend, or loved one can help with the feeding whenever possible, and you can get some sleep. Again, you'll hear from some "breastfeeding warriors" that you will provoke "nipple confusion" and your child will, as a result, fail to get into Harvard, but I can assure you that a hungry baby will learn to eat. It's a life skill, and you can't start too early building those, can you, breastfeeding warriors?

The best way to feel comfortable with ongoing psychiatric medication during pregnancy and when breastfeeding is to be armed with information. Start with your prescriber, but there are also some great websites you can visit to get the most up-to-date information regarding medication safety in pregnancy and for lactation.

Youth depression

Today, young people have so much "future pressure": they're told by school counsellors in grade nine that every breath they take for the remainder of their high school years will irrevocably determine whether they'll be able to feed, clothe, and shelter themselves in the future. For some, their preparation for university starts in utero. I was an oblivious kid, which extended well into my thirties, and upon reflection I've decided it's not the worst thing to be unaware of all the crap that swirls around you as you grow up. It seems we're not allowing kids to be kids for very long. Perhaps that's why so many young people today struggle with depression and **anxiety**. Social media drives an awareness of *everything*.

According to the CDC, in 2015, suicide was the second-leading cause of death among people between the ages of fifteen and twenty-nine years old. Boys between the ages of fifteen and nineteen have a completed suicide rate that was three times greater than girls the same age, but suicide attempts are twice as high among girls than among boys, likely because girls tend to choose less lethal methods. More than 90% of adolescent suicide victims met the criteria for a psychiatric diagnosis before their death. Other important risk factors include agitation, drug or alcohol intoxication, and a serious, recent stressful life event.

Concerningly, evidence suggests that young people are at much greater risk from media exposure than adults and may imitate suicidal behaviour seen online or on television. In fact, adolescent "cluster suicides" have been associated with media coverage of a youth suicide, and the risk has been correlated with the amount, duration, and prominence of the coverage. While more research is needed to better understand the risks of media and suicide clustering, the National Institute of Mental Health (NIMH) has published suggested guidelines for media and online reporting of deaths by suicide.

Whenever possible, depressed children or adolescents should be offered psychotherapy (see chapter 13), as well as other non-medication depression treatments depending on the severity of the symptoms. However, following a careful assessment, if a young person (and perhaps their family, depending on the child's age) and their doctor determine that medication treatment is necessary, research evidence supports the importance of diagnosing and appropriately treating depression.

Few antidepressant medications have received a formal **indication** from regulators (see page 161) for their use in young people. Much like the challenges posed by recruiting pregnant women as subjects for research studies, parents aren't usually keen to allow their children to try experimental drug treatments. Medications that have received an official **indication** for depression in young patients are often limited to a range of ages that reflect the studies completed by the drug company. For instance, a drug might have an **indication** for depression in twelve- to sixteen-year-old children, but what about severely depressed children who are aged ten or eleven?

When a depression is severe enough to require an antidepressant treatment, most doctors will stick closely to the medications that have received an official **indication**; however, there are no antidepressant medications officially indicated for young patients in Canada, and only two in the United States. If a child in Canada is severely depressed, what should their prescriber do? Most specialists use off-label antidepressant treatments for depression for their young patients, because of the substantial evidence of the harm associated with under-treated or untreated depression, including the risk of completed suicide.

One of the major concerns regarding the use of antidepressants in young patients is whether these medications increase the risk of suicidal thoughts and behaviours. In 2004, the FDA added a **black-box warning** regarding suicide risk for children taking antidepressants on all antidepressant **product monographs**, which in 2006 was extended to include young people up until age twenty-five. **Health Canada** has a similar warning in all of their antidepressant **product monographs.** The warning states that children and adolescents taking antidepressant medications should be closely monitored for any worsening depression symptoms, the emergence of suicidal thinking or behaviour, or unusual changes in behaviour, such as sleeplessness, agitation, or withdrawal from normal social situations. The close monitoring is most important during the first month of treatment, although ongoing monitoring is prudent.

Comprehensive reviews of pediatric trials have demonstrated the benefits of antidepressant medications likely outweigh their risks to young patients with severe depression and **anxiety disorders.** In a 2007 FDA review, no completed suicides occurred among nearly 2,200 children treated with SSRI medications. However, about 4 percent of those taking antidepressant medications experienced suicidal thinking or behaviour, including suicide attempts, compared to 2 percent of those taking **placebo.**

SSRI medications are usually well tolerated by children and adolescents, but for some children, they can trigger agitation and abnormal behaviour. Although it has been shown that suicidal thoughts and behaviours increase in some individual youths taking SSRIs, on average, when depression is treated, suicide risk substantially declines. Large and more representative community-based studies have suggested that higher rates of SSRI prescribing are associated with lower suicide rates, and that suicide attempts are more common before an SSRI is prescribed.

After the addition of the **black-box warning**, researchers noticed some worrisome trends. Specifically, the rates of depression treatment and the diagnoses of new cases of depression substantially declined. One study included data from 1.1 million adolescents, 1.4 million young adults, and 5 million older adults, collected between

2000 to 2010 from eleven health plans in the United States. Within two years of the FDA warning, the study found antidepressant use plummeted by 31 percent for adolescents, 24.3 percent in young adults, and 14.5 percent in adults. While the FDA advisory focused on youth, it appears it impacted the appropriate treatment of adults with depression as well.

Likewise, there was also a reduction in new depression diagnosis. One US study found that depression diagnosis by primary care doctors decreased by 44 percent for children, 37 percent for young adults, and 29 percent for all adults in the years following the addition of the **black-box warning.** The **prevalence** of depression has not changed, so this reduction is associated with a failure to make the diagnosis. It was troubling that researchers did not find a compensatory increase in the use of other depression treatments, such as psychotherapy.

In addition to the decreased diagnosis and prescribing rates, researchers identified a marked increase in psychiatric-drug poisoning, which was used in one study as an indicator of attempted suicide. Two years after the **black-box warning** was issued, psychiatric drug poisonings increased by 21.7 percent among ten- to seventeen-year-olds and by 33.7 percent among those aged eighteen to twenty-nine. Furthermore, completed suicide between the ages of ten and thirty-four increased between 1999 and 2010. It is not possible to directly link the **black-box warning** and the rate of suicide attempts and completed suicides, although it seems clear the intended mission of the warning, which was to reduce the risk of suicide, was not successful.

Recent exposure to an antidepressant medication is rare (1.6%) for young people who die by suicide, which demonstrates that most youths do not have access to treatment. Several studies showed a negative correlation between antidepressant prescribing and completed adolescent suicide: better access to treatment reduces suicide risk. In fact, the 28% decrease in completed suicides in the ten- to nineteen-year-old age group from 1990 to 2000 has been attributed to an increase in youth antidepressant prescribing over the same time period. A 2009 paper demonstrated that treating depressed youth with antidepressants reduces suicides by 31.9%, which is similar to the reductions seen in adult and elderly populations (32.2% and 32.3%, respectively). A large US survey found a significant decrease in adolescent suicide with every 1% annual increase in antidepressant prescribing. Another study found that prescribing SSRIs significantly lowered suicide rates among children and adolescents between the ages of five and fourteen.

It is impossible to predict a child's risk of suicidal behaviour associated with antidepressant treatment with any degree of certainty, because depression increases the risk for suicide, completed suicide among young people is rare, and research studies usually exclude patients who are considered at high risk for suicide.

There are more than twenty published and unpublished high-quality research studies evaluating SSRIs in children and adolescents suffering from depression. More recent comprehensive reviews of the research evidence have determined that the SSRIs fluoxetine, escitalopram, and sertraline were significantly better than **placebo** for young depressed patients. The SSRI fluoxetine has the most robust evidence demonstrating that its benefits outweigh the risks for patients aged eight to eighteen. Fluoxetine has received the official **indication** for depression in that age group from the FDA but not from **Health Canada**. In 2009, the FDA approved the SSRI escitalopram for treatment of adolescent depression. The FDA also determined that the SSRI paroxetine should not be used in children and adolescents.

Most importantly, prescribers must know that the risk posed by untreated depression has always been far greater than the very small risk associated with antidepressant treatment. I urge my fellow prescribers to engage young patients and their parents and to thoughtfully consider these risks; have open, direct discussions about suicide; and monitor for suicidal thoughts and behaviours very carefully. But, for heaven's sake, please diagnose and treat depression.

Depression in the over sixty-five set

Depression effects about 5 percent of those over the age of sixty-five, but it can be difficult to diagnose in older adults because of the overlap between depression symptoms, non-specific symptoms related to aging, and the symptoms of many common medical problems. Research has demonstrated that depression in old age doubles the risk of all-cause death; for severe depression, the mortality rate triples compared to elderly adults who are not depressed.

In many countries, rates of completed suicide increase with age, which is likely to become a more prominent issue as our population ages. White males between the ages of forty-four and sixty-five and over the age of eighty-five have the highest rates of completed suicide. To read more about suicide, see chapter 16.

There does not appear to be any difference between how older and younger adults respond to antidepressant treatments, but older patients are at greater risk of depression **relapse.** Several large studies have found that all classes of antidepressant medications were more effective than **placebo** in achieving depression response and **remission**, even for elderly patients with severe depression symptoms. However, studies indicate that older patients tend to be more sensitive to antidepressant side effects, including a greater risk of falls and fractures, abnormal bleeding, and low sodium levels. ECT and psychotherapy have also been shown to be effective in older depressed patients.

Of great concern for many of my patients is whether depression might heighten their risk of **dementia.** This comes up often because of how frequently **cognitive** symptoms are associated with depression (see chapter 1), especially in older patients. **Cognitive** symptoms associated with depression in the elderly is sometimes referred to as **pseudo-dementia**, because patients can appear to have marked **dementia** that is actually attributable to depression. Their concerns appear to be well founded: research has demonstrated that a recent episode of depression later in life increases the risk of **dementia** by four- to six-fold, and that risk is especially high in those who have persistent depressive symptoms.

In a 2018 study, nearly 42 percent of individuals with both mild **cognitive impairment** (MCI) and active or recent depression progressed to Alzheimer's disease within two years, while 31.6 percent of those with a more remote history of depression progressed to Alzheimer's. The usual annual conversion rate from MCI to Alzheimer's disease is about 15 percent. The authors suggested that individuals with a combination of MCI and recent depression are at particularly high risk of Alzheimer's and should be considered for preventive treatment.

Research suggests that aggressively treating depression in older adults might mitigate the risk of **dementia**. Interestingly, a medication that is sometimes used as an add-on treatment for severe depression, lithium, might be a worthwhile strategy for protecting a vulnerable depressed brain from progressing to **dementia**. Lithium is neuroprotective, which means it protects brain cells from harm. It also reduces the production of the protein amyloid, which is associated with Alzheimer's disease. Furthermore, lithium increases the removal of Alzheimer's-associated proteins from the brain, which improves the survival of **neurons**.

Older patients often need the same doses of antidepressant medications to experience their full benefit, but because they may be more sensitive to side effects, it's generally important to initiate treatment at a lower dose and increase the dose more slowly. Rather than the usual, "start low, go slow" for antidepressant dosing, for older patients I tend to "start lower and go slower" and still aim for the dose that works best and is well tolerated, just like I do for younger patients.

Chapter summary

- Evidence clearly demonstrates that the treatment of depression and anxiety in pregnant and **postpartum** women protects the health and safety of both the mother and her child.
- Children and adolescents treated with an antidepressant should be closely monitored for worsening depression symptoms, the emergence of suicidal thinking or behaviour, or unusual changes in behaviour. However, it is important that depressed young people be diagnosed and treated, because untreated depression is associated with completed suicide.
- Elderly depressed men are the highest risk group for suicide and all elderly depressed individuals are at high risk for **cognitive** symptoms, which are sometimes misattributed to the onset of **dementia**.

If you or someone you love is a member of one of these special groups of individuals struggling with depression, please be aware that there is strong scientific research supporting the importance of identifying and treating depression, even for the oldest, youngest, and most pregnant among us. If a healthcare professional is refusing to offer treatment, it's essential to find someone who reads and follows the scientific research and will provide evidence-based treatment to anyone in need.

A real patient's story

SOME PEOPLE DESCRIBE suicide as selfish. To me, it is the exact opposite of being selfish. I thought of suicide as being the only thing I could do to make other people happy. I thought I would be doing them a favour. Other people would be glad when I was no longer around. They would wonder what took me so long.

Some people describe suicide as a cry for help. I don't believe suicide is a cry for help, because I knew "help" existed, but I also knew that it could not help me. I also knew that treatment would not help me because I believed I was permanently and irreparably flawed, and I could not overcome these flaws no matter how much help I received or how hard I tried. When treatment failed, it simply proved my original point, namely that I am personally and permanently flawed.

16

What is the connection between depression and suicide?

ACCORDING TO 2016 data published by the Government of Canada:

- An average of ten people die by suicide each day in Canada.
- Of the approximately 4,000 deaths by suicide each year, more than 90 percent were living with a mental health problem or illness.
- Suicide is the ninth-leading cause of death in Canada but the second-leading cause among ten- to twenty-nine-year-olds (though still a rare occurrence).
- For every one suicide death, there are five self-inflicted injury hospitalizations, twenty-five to thirty attempts, and seven to ten people profoundly affected by suicide loss.

According to the American Foundation for Suicide Prevention:

- For every suicide, there are twenty-five attempts.
- On average, there are 123 suicides per day in the United States.
- Each year, 44,965 Americans die by suicide.

- Suicide is the tenth-leading cause of death in the United States.
- Suicide costs the economy $69 billion annually.
- Men die by suicide 3.53 times more often than women. Women make more attempts.
- The rate of suicide is highest in middle age and older men.
- White males accounted for seven out of ten suicides in 2016.
- Firearms accounted for 51 percent of all suicides in 2016.

When should I be concerned?

Low risk of suicide:

- An older person focusing on normal end-of-life issues, especially those with severe and advanced medical illness.
- Anyone having occasional thoughts about their own mortality.
- Those who do not feel they would be better off dead.

Plan: These thoughts are not indicative of suicidal risk, but anyone who is depressed should be monitored for increasing suicidal thoughts.

Moderate risk of suicide (passive suicidal thoughts):

- Those who are wondering if they'd be better off dead.
- Those who wonder if life is worth living.
- No plans of suicide.

Plan: Anyone having these thoughts should be encouraged to talk to a mental health professional.

High risk of suicide:

- Those who feel completely hopeless and worthless and feel sure they'd be better off dead.
- Those who have considered how they might kill themselves, even if they have not taking steps to put the plan in place (e.g., search the internet for how much medication to take, considering seeking out a lethal means (weapon, drugs)).

Plan: Anyone experiencing these thoughts or exhibiting these behaviours should be immediately referred to a mental health professional and monitored closely.

Immediate risk for suicide:

- Those who have access to lethal means and an active plan in place (e.g., "I plan to overdose tomorrow").
- Those who can see no reason to continue being alive.

Plan: Anyone experiencing these thoughts or exhibiting this behaviour requires immediate assessment and support. Call 9-1-1 or take to emergency services.

Suicide is a major and growing public health issue. Recent data from the US Centers for Disease Control and Prevention (CDC) reported a 30 percent increase in suicide across all age groups between 1999 and 2016. Suicide risk is most often viewed as a symptom of a mental illness, which conveniently explains the individual's wish to die. However, understanding suicide risk is much more complicated than one plus one equals two (depression plus hopelessness/divorce/financial strain equals suicide). The risk for suicide often festers over months or even years, as the individual comes to terms with the concept and grows increasingly comfortable with suicide as an option and then determines it is the only possible choice.

As I described in chapter 1, depression is commonly associated with thoughts of suicide as a possible escape from emotional pain. Those with passive **suicidal ideation** wish to die but do not have a specific plan. **Active suicidal ideation** means there is a desire to die as well as a plan to act on suicidal thoughts. Suicidal behaviour is defined as self-injury with the intent of ending one's life, whether these are unsuccessful attempts or completed acts.

The continuing **stigma** regarding suicide must end, including the commonly held belief that suicide is, at its core, a selfish act. In my experience, patients with suicidal thoughts express a wish to escape from their constant emotional or physical pain but also wish to set their loved ones free. They view themselves as a massive burden on their friends, family, and even society, and suicide becomes the best option to free everyone.

While it is absolutely necessary to diagnose and treat serious mental illnesses, which will certainly reduce suicide risk, another very important consideration is empathy. Empathy is too often missing from the delivery of psychiatric services. Reducing suicidality to just another symptom of mental illness is not appropriate, nor is it helpful to patients. Caregivers must learn to listen to their patients' expressions of emotional pain and distress and offer an empathic response. **When a patient feels heard, believed, and understood, they are more inclined to see a path forward, a path that doesn't involve suicide.**

In 2015, suicide was the second-leading cause of death among people between the ages of fifteen and twenty-nine years old. According to research from the CDC, more than 1 million high school students are treated for a suicide attempt each year. Thoughts of suicide are common in adolescents and are considered an important risk factor for attempted suicide.

Suicide capability, or the degree to which a person feels they are able to make a suicide attempt, heightens the risk of a completed suicide. Factors that increase suicide capability include growing fearlessness about death, exposure to others who are self-harming, access to lethal means, and previous self-harm, even if the harm was not for suicidal intent. Exposure to others who are self-harming appears to be the factor that most reliably distinguishes between young people with **suicidal ideation** and those who go on to have suicidal behaviour.

In many countries, including Canada and the United States, completed suicide rates increase with age. Because the proportion of the elderly is increasing worldwide, due to increased life expectancy and falling birth rates, suicide rates are likely to increase in countries with aging populations.

There has also been a recent spike in the frequency of **suicidal ideation** among older patients, whether or not they have depression. A study of 1,226 older adults found that 29 percent of subjects with severe depression symptoms, 11 percent with mild depression symptoms, and 7 percent with no depression said they had a wish to die. This highlights the fact that **suicidal ideation** is not only associated with depression. In fact, in 2016, the CDC reported that 54 percent of people in twenty-seven US states who died by suicide had no diagnosis of a mental illness. A history of serious **suicidal ideation**, severe life **stress** (e.g., loss of spouse, financial strain), drug or alcohol abuse, and physical disability or severe illness are also important risk factors for suicide. The risk of suicide is significant when it is related to a serious physical illness, especially early in the course of treatment (for instance, soon after cancer chemotherapy or renal dialysis is initiated).

Although **suicidal ideation** is a risk factor for completed suicide, thoughts of death can be common among older adults. If an older adult is thinking about death, it's important to understand whether these are normal thoughts regarding their own mortality or whether they are passive suicidal thoughts or **active suicidal ideation**, reflecting an imminent intention to commit suicide.

While suicide is considered a tragic, preventable outcome, it is unclear how best to support those who are at greatest risk. Most **clinicians**, faced with a concerning patient, look to the most up-to-date scientific evidence to guide our offers of assistance. Unfortunately, most research on suicide prevention focuses on whether an intervention worked and not on the factors that increased or reduced the likelihood that an intervention was helpful.

There are universal suicide prevention programs, which target broad populations regardless of their risk, such as high school or university suicide reduction programs. There are also selective prevention programs, which target groups that are at higher risk for suicide, such as those with psychiatric illnesses or first-responders. Finally, there are indicated suicide prevention programs, which target those who have already had **suicidal ideation** or an attempt.

Not much data is available to inform decisions regarding the best fit for a specific program. We need more research to better understand if age, sex, gender, race, ethnicity, socioeconomic status, level of social support, or mental or physical health are important determinates for a program's success. Likewise, some programs can be effectively offered face-to-face, online, over the phone, through peer support, with a professional, in a group, or in a one-on-one interaction. These are called moderating factors, and they are the keys to more effective suicide prevention.

The following are the greatest risk factors associated with suicide:

- White males between the ages of forty-four and sixty-five and over the age of eighty-five;
- having a psychiatric diagnosis—especially major depression, **bipolar disorder**, **schizophrenia**, PTSD, substance abuse or dependence, and eating disorders—and a history of treatment noncompliance;
- a history of physical, sexual, or emotional abuse;
- recent loss of a loved one, financial **stress**, or a serious medical illness; and
- access to lethal means (e.g., guns, drugs for overdose).

The most protective factors are:

- a strong support system;
- religious or spiritual beliefs (e.g., that suicide is a sin);
- family/children;
- a fear of death.

If you are worried that your loved one or anyone else is at imminent risk of serious harm or death, call 9-1-1 immediately. The police are accustomed to managing situations that involve mental illness. Don't ignore your gut when it's telling you to call police. Explain the situation to the emergency operator and follow their instructions.

Chapter summary

- Rates of suicide have increased substantially over the last decade for reasons that are not fully understood.
- Suicide is associated with depression and other mental illnesses, but suicide is not always associated with a mental illness.
- Suicide is the second-leading cause of death among people between the ages of fifteen and twenty-nine years old, but those at greatest risk of completed suicide are men between the ages of forty-four and sixty-five and those over the age of eighty-five.

If you are having suicidal thoughts, ask a professional for help. If you don't receive it, please ask someone else. Likewise, urging your loved one to seek help from a professional (e.g., family doctor, psychologist, psychiatrist) and ensuring they attend or accompanying them to that appointment is an essential first step. Suicide helplines offer an immediate empathic ear for someone who is suffering. They are also equipped to offer options for urgent community support. Suicide helplines and suicide and depression resources for each province and territory can be found in appendix 1.

Conclusion
The gifts we give ourselves

MUCH OF WHAT I write in this section you will have read before, but I think it bears repeating. My clinical experience (and research backs it up) is that when a patient leaves my office, they almost instantly forget at least 80 percent of what I said during our meeting. Sometimes that's because I talk too much, but there are other reasons for their forgetfulness, including the fact that many of my patients are struggling with **cognitive** symptoms that make memory and concentration difficult. As well, some patients are constantly confronted with negative messages from friends, family, other health professionals, and the media about mental illness and psychiatric treatments. Doubt and fear tend to push aside my positive, encouraging suggestions.

While this book has focused mostly on my **clinical experience** and the science of depression, I spend much of my time with patients talking about life. Whether it's about relationships, work, school, or finances, we don't really understand another person's life without listening to their stories. There is more to providing education about mental illnesses, whether to my patients or my colleagues, than science.

I am often asked how I can listen to sad, painful stories every day and not get depressed myself. There are probably several reasons why, but chief among these are the incredible people in my life that have helped me to be all the different Dianes I need to be to have a healthy, productive, contented life. I have a wonderful husband and caring in-laws, perfect (of course!) children, a highly supportive mother, loving brothers, great colleagues, and hilarious, loving friends. I also have many inspiring patients who have overcome great adversity and continue to fight every day to recover or to stay well. They treat me with respect and appreciation. These people—my family, friends, colleagues, and patients—are gifts I cherish, and I feel incredibly grateful for every one of them.

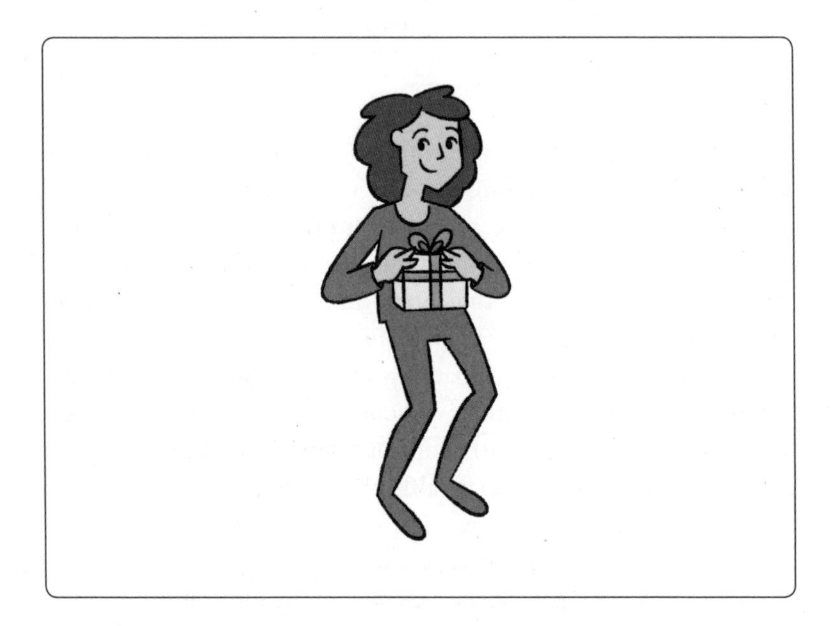

In my humble opinion, some of the greatest gifts in life are the gifts we give ourselves. I have given myself three essential, life-altering mental gifts. I think these gifts have helped me to protect my mental health and care for many very ill patients without losing myself. Regrettably, these gifts didn't suddenly arrive in my brain at age eighteen and work for me through my adult life. I had to learn them through the challenges I have faced as an adult, and some of these gifts only came to me over the last decade. I didn't know how important they were when I was younger, but now I know that they are critical for finding emotional peace and contentment as an adult.

One mental gift is the complete belief that the only person on earth I can control is me. It's one thing to think and say this, but once I truly incorporated this belief into my DNA, it changed my life. If you have children, you'll know this is the case: these helpless little beings pop out of the womb and scream and poop and do whatever they want immediately! As a parent, we have zero control. We can comfort them with love, food, warmth, and a clean diaper, but for some babies, even with a full tummy, the coziest blanket, and the cleanest diaper, they're still inconsolable. Likewise, we can't control our partner, children, friends, extended family members, patients, or anyone else on earth. Knowing this set me free.

As a psychiatrist, I can try to help, guide, console, and encourage my patients, but ultimately they will decide what they think, feel, and do. Add to that concept the fact that we each have the power to control and change ourselves personally, including what we think, how we feel, and how we behave, and that should help us to feel some sense of control over our destiny.

My next mental gift is my desire to seek forgiveness. I forgive, and every time I do, I know it's a gift I've given myself. I forgive so I can feel better. It doesn't always happen quickly, and I don't always forget what caused the problem, but I do seek to forgive. In my experience, hatred, fear, and anger corrode the container they're in: carrying those emotions hurts me more than anyone. When I forgive, I take a heavy weight off my shoulders. I also apologize. It's very Canadian of me to seek forgiveness for just about everything, but if I appreciate the gift of forgiveness, I'm sure others benefit from my apology if I've hurt them, even unintentionally, which I hope will help them to forgive me.

My final mental gift is gratitude. I have so much to be grateful for, and I try to think about that every day. When I feel frustrated, angry, or at my wit's end, I force myself to think of something I feel grateful for, and I feel a sense of relief. It's very sad to think that when someone is depressed, it's nearly impossible to feel positive emotions, including gratitude. Feeling grateful when depressed is perhaps an oxymoron, but during **recovery**, as positive thoughts slowly creep back, finding gratitude in small things (e.g., a bird singing outside the window, sunshine peeking through the clouds, taking a shower) can become a source of strength and **recovery**.

I write about these mental gifts because I feel it's important to remind my readers that depression is a complicated illness. It's so much more than a diagnosis, a crappy childhood, genetics, a drug, or a therapy. What we think and how we feel about ourselves, others, and our circumstances powerfully influence our resiliency and, when depressed, our **recovery**.

The statement "I am depressed" really says it all. When depressed, people believe the illness defines them. In fact, a depressed person is a person who has an illness called depression, and, as I wrote many times throughout this book, that illness is a personal journey. It looks and feels different for every individual, and the route to **recovery** is different for every individual as well.

On the other side of depression, many people find they are more resilient, kinder, more grateful, and more loving. I have had many patients tell me, "I would never have asked to be depressed, but I know it made me a better person." Most importantly, please know that if you're struggling with depression, while it can take time and sometimes tremendous patience, **there is always a path ahead**.

Sixteen essential milestones on the path to recovery

1. If you see yourself or someone you love in the words and stories describing the depression diagnosis, you've already taken the first step towards **recovery.**
2. One might never know *exactly* why they developed depression, but by understanding what factors we can control, and those factors we cannot control, we can shift our focus away from assigning blame towards finding solutions.
3. We have an enormous capacity to change, if we wish to, simply by deciding to take control of the one person we *can* change: ourselves. That said, you can't will yourself out of a serious depression, and a kick in the pants doesn't work either. Sometimes taking control of yourself means accepting help.
4. We have the ability to grow new brain cells and rewire our brain every day of our lives. In fact, **recovery** from depression depends on it.
5. If you or someone you love has physical symptoms that are not explained by a medical cause, it's important to consider whether

depression or another mental illness might be the cause or a contributor.

6. Depression in women and men may differ in terms of lifetime risk, symptoms, and response to treatment, yet too often both doctors and patients fail to consider the power of **estrogen** and how it can impact both body and mind.
7. The first line of depression defence is a family doctor, who can diagnose and provide treatment or, based on an individual's needs, refer for appropriate treatment. If you don't have a family doctor, reach out to the mental health services in your community.
8. Seeking professional help for depression, surrounding yourself with supportive, understanding people, and keeping your distance from those who are unsupportive are all essential aspects of depression **recovery**.
9. Depression treatment must be personalized to meet each individual's needs. There are many options available, and while there is no one perfect treatment, there is one that is best for you.
10. The key to finding the right medication for depression is communication. It's important to listen carefully to your prescriber and ask questions if you have concerns, as well as to report symptom changes and side effects. When all team members are fully and honestly engaged, **recovery** is not just possible but likely.
11. Any treatment can cause unwanted effects, including psychotherapy and exercise (unless you've never rolled your ankle taking a brisk walk). By taking the time to find the depression treatment that's best for you, you'll protect both your mental and physical health.
12. Don't accept "good enough." Even if the sadness or loss of interest has resolved, if there are remaining symptoms, such as ongoing **insomnia**, fatigue, and **cognitive** symptoms, keep asking for help until they're fully resolved too.

13. Depression treatment decisions are based on the severity of the symptoms, the safety and tolerability of a treatment, and, most importantly, a patient's wishes. While some treatments are reserved for the most severely ill patients, some are beneficial for every depressed individual—most notably, exercise.

14. If your healthcare professional is recommending mega-doses of vitamins, kale enemas (or, for that matter, anything that includes depression and enema in the same sentence), **homeopathy**, or cannabis to treat depression, I implore you to consider finding someone else to ask for help. Depression is a serious illness, and anyone claiming to be able to cure depression, cancer, or any other serious illness with unproven treatments isn't a real health professional. You deserve better.

15. If you or someone you love is a member of one of a special group of individuals struggling with depression, please be aware that there is strong scientific research supporting the importance of identifying and treating depression, even for the oldest, youngest, and most pregnant among us. If a healthcare professional is refusing to offer treatment, it's essential to find someone who reads and follows the evidence and will provide treatment to anyone in need.

16. If you are having suicidal thoughts, ask a professional for help. If you don't receive it, please ask someone else. Likewise, urging your loved one to seek help from a professional (e.g., family doctor, psychologist, psychiatrist) and ensuring they attend or accompanying them to that appointment is an essential first step. Suicide helplines offer an immediate empathic ear for someone who is suffering. They are also equipped to offer options for urgent community support.

Acknowledgements

THIS BOOK HAS lived in my brain for a very long time, so it was a labour of love to get it onto these pages. As with all labour, it was also a pain in the butt sometimes and definitely a relief when it was done. As such, I must first thank my mother, Barbara, who endured a very long and painful labour (I was nearly ten pounds!) to bring me into the world. My mom is a big Diane fan—she read my manuscript again and again and only told me how much she loved it, as a mother should. I dedicated this book to my mom and my brothers because we've stuck together and loved each other, despite many, *many* ups and downs, and I am grateful for them every day.

Another huge and heartfelt thanks to my husband, Stuart, and the fruits of our (well, my) labour, Robert and Shannon, for putting up with my travel, writing, and general craziness. Kathy, my daughter from another mother (and father), thank you for your support. To my friends and colleagues who reviewed the manuscript, I am truly grateful for you and for your thoughtful feedback. A huge thank-you to my incredibly patient editor, Amanda; and to Mike Lipkin, for introducing me to Jesse and her outstanding Page Two team. My heartfelt thanks and appreciation for my peer-editors and contributors, Charbel, Annette, Brian, Tim, Kelly, Ian, Amy, Megan, Jane, AA, and Milena, for your stories, support, and encouragement.

Finally, I want to thank my patients, whose bravery inspires me every day. Just walking into a pharmacy where everyone knows your name is enough to put anyone off their treatment, yet you persist and endure. It is a privilege to be invited into your lives and to help you to navigate your path to wellness.

Appendix 1
Canada-wide resources for mental illness support and treatment

Suicide crisis helplines

- Crisis Services Canada—Canada Suicide Prevention Service (CSPS)
  Toll-free: 1-833-456-4566 (available 24/7)
  For residents of Quebec: 1-866-APPELLE (1-866-277-3553)
  Text 45645 between 4 p.m. and 12 a.m. ET
- Crisis Text Line (Powered by Kids Help Phone) Canada Wide
  Kids Help Phone
  Text Services: Text CONNECT to 686868 (also serves adults)
  Chat Services: (6 p.m.–2 a.m. ET): kidshelpphone.ca
  Youthspace.ca (NEED2 Suicide Prevention, Education & Support)
  Youth Text (6 p.m.–12 a.m. PT): 778-783-0177
  Youth Chat (6 p.m.–12 a.m. PT): youthspace.ca

Alberta

Suicide helplines

- Alberta's Mental Health Helpline (available 24/7)
  Phone: 1-877-303-2642
  Kids Help Phone: 1-800-668-6868
- Distress Line for Mental Health Crisis
  Phone: 780-482-HELP (4357)

Depression resources

- Provincial Health Information Line
  Toll-free: 8-1-1 (available 24/7)
  Web: myhealth.alberta.ca
- Information and referral specialist
  Phone: 2-1-1
  Web: ab.211.ca
- Kids Help Phone (Youth Counselling Line)
  Phone: 1-800-668-6868
- The Organization for Bipolar Affective Disorders Society (OBAD)
  Phone: 403-263-7408; 1-866-263-7408 (toll-free)
- Momentum Walk-In Counselling Society
  #706, 5241 Calgary Trail NW, Edmonton, Alberta, T6H 5G8
  Phone: 780-757-0900
- Postpartum Depression Support Group—Alberta Parenting for the Future Association
  Phone: 780-963-0549
- Child and Youth Mental Health: Suicide Prevention, Mindfulness
  24/7 Crisis Line: 780-743-HELP (4357)
  Phone: 780-743-8605
- Calgary Counselling Centre: Assisting individuals dealing with depression
  Phone: 403-691-5991

- Canadian Mental Health Association (Alberta Division)
  Phone: 780-482-6576
  Web: alberta.cmha.ca

British Columbia

Suicide helplines

- The Crisis Intervention and Suicide Prevention Centre of BC (BC-Wide Crisis Centre)
  Phone: 1-800-SUICIDE (1-800-784-2433) (available 24/7 in up to 140 languages)
- Mental Health Support Line (BC-wide)
  Phone: 310-6789 (no area code needed; free and available twenty-four hours a day)
  One-on-one online chats: crisiscentrechat.ca
- Suicide Attempt Follow-up, Education & Research (S.A.F.E.R.)
  To refer yourself to S.A.F.E.R., contact the Access and Assessment Centre
  Phone: 604-675-3700

Depression resources

- bc211: Vancouver-based nonprofit organization that specializes in providing information and referral regarding community, government and social services in BC
  Web: redbookonline.bc211.ca
- Mental Health Support Line (BC-wide)
  Phone: 310-6789 (no area code needed; free and available twenty-four hours a day)
- Call HealthLink BC
  Toll-free: 8-1-1 (available 24/7 in over 130 languages)
  Deaf and hearing-impaired: 7-1-1

- Seniors' Distress Line
  Phone: 604-872-1234

- The BC Children's Kelty Mental Health Resource Centre
  Toll-free: 1-800-665-1822
  Email: keltycentre@cw.bc.ca
  BC Children's Hospital, Mental Health Building, 4555 Heather Street, Vancouver, BC, V6H 3N1, Room P3-302 (3rd floor)

- The KUU-US Crisis Line: First Nations– and Indigenous-specific crisis and mental health issues line
  Phone: 1-800-588-8717
  Youth line: 250-723-2040
  Adult line: 250-723-4050

- The Mood Disorders Association of BC (MDABC)
  Phone: 604-873-0103
  (Option 1 for Psychiatric Clinic and option 2 for the Counselling and Wellness Office)
  Email: info@mdabc.net
  Web: mdabc.net
  480–789 Pender St. W., Vancouver, BC, V6C 1H2

- Pacific Post Partum Support Society
  Phone: 604-255-7999; 1-855-255-7999 (toll-free)

- HeretoHelp/Mental Health and Substance Use Information BC
  Web: heretohelp.bc.ca/get-help

- MindHealthBC
  Web: mindhealthbc.ca

- Canadian Mental Health Association (British Columbia Division)
  Phone: 604-688-3234; 1-800-555-8222 (toll-free)
  Suite 905, 1130 West Pender Street, Vancouver, BC, V6E 4A4
  Web: cmha.bc.ca

Manitoba

Suicide helplines

- Manitoba Suicide Prevention and Support Line (available 24/7) "Reason to Live"
  Phone: 1-877-435-7170 (1-877-HELP170)
- Klinic Crisis Line
  Phone: 204-786-8686 or 1-888-322-3019; 1-877-435-7170 (toll-free)
  TTY: 204-784-4097
- Kids Help Phone (national line available to Manitoba youth)
  Phone: 1-800-668-6868

Depression resources

- The Mood Disorders Association of Manitoba
  Toll-free: 1-800-263-1460
  Peer Support: 204-786-0987
  Postpartum Warmline: 204-391-5983
- Mindfulness Based Stress Reduction courses: offered through CMHA Manitoba and Winnipeg
  Phone: 204-982-6100
  Web: mbwpg.cmha.ca
- Canadian Mental Health Association (Manitoba and Winnipeg Division)
  Phone: 204-775-6442

New Brunswick

Suicide helplines

- Suicide Prevention CHIMO Helpline (province-wide)
  Phone: 1-800-667-5005 (available 24/7; bilingual)

Fredericton area: 450-HELP (4357)
Web: gnb.ca/0055/index-e.asp

Depression resources

- Provincial Health Information Line
  Phone: 8-1-1
  Web: gnb.ca/0217/Tele-Care-e.asp

- Moncton: Vitalite Mental Health Moncton
  Phone: 506-862-4144
  81 Albert St, 4th Floor, Moncton, NB, E2C 1B3

- Richibucto: Community Mental Health Centre
  Phone: 506-523-7620
  Place Cartier, Unit 153, Richibucto, NB, E4W 5R5; P.O. Box 5001

- Saint John: Community Mental Health Centre
  Phone: 506-658-3737
  55 Union Street, 3rd floor, Saint John, NB, E2L 5B7

- Sussex: Community Mental Health Centre
  Phone: 506-432-2090
  30 Moffett Avenue, Sussex, NB, E4E 1E8

- St. Stephen: Community Mental Health Centre
  Phone: 506-466-7380
  41 King Street, St. Stephen, NB, E3L 2C1

- Fredericton: Community Mental Health Centre
  Phone: 506-453-2132
  P.O. Box 5001, 65 Brunswick Street, Fredericton, NB, E3B 5G6

- Woodstock: Community Mental Health Centre
  Phone: 506-325-4419
  200 King Street, Woodstock, NB, E7M 5C6; P.O. Box 5001

- Edmundston: Community Mental Health Centre
  Phone: 506-735-2070
  Carrefour Assomption, 121 Église Street, 3rd Floor, Suite 331;
  P.O. Box 5001

- Grand Falls: Community Mental Health Centre
  Phone: 506-475-2440
  131 Pleasant Street, Grand Falls, NB, E3Z 1G1; P.O. Box 5001

- Campbellton: Community Mental Health Centre
  Phone: 506-789-2440
  6 Arran Street, Campbellton, NB, E3N 1K4

- Bathurst: Community Mental Health Centre
  Phone: 506-547-2038

- Caraquet: Community Mental Health Centre
  Phone: 506-726-2030

- Miramichi: Community Mental Health Centre
  Phone: 506-778-6111
  1780 Water Street, Suite 300, Miramichi, NB, E1N 1B6

Newfoundland and Labrador

Suicide Helplines

- Mental Health Crisis Centre
  Phone: 1-888-737-4668 (toll-free); 709-737-4668 (local)

Depression resources

- Provincial Health Information Line
  Phone: 8-1-1
  TTY: 1-888-709-3555

- Mental Health Crisis Line
  Phone: 709-777-3200; 1-888-737-4668 (toll-free)

- CHANNAL Peer Support
  Phone: 753-2560; 1-855-753-2560 (toll-free)

- Mental Health Adult Services: central intake for the St. John's area
  Phone: 752-8888

- Blomidon Place: mental health services for children, youth, and their families
  Phone: 709-634-4171
  133 Riverside Drive, Corner Brook, NL, A2H 6J7; P.O. Box 2005

- DoorWays: mental health and addictions walk-in service
  - Bonne Bay: Bonne Bay Health Centre—Cow Head Medical Clinic
    Phone: 458-2381, ext. 266
  - Burgeo: Calder Health Care Centre
    Phone: 886-1550 or 886-2185
  - Corner Brook: Phone: 634-4506; 35 Boone's Road
  - Deer Lake: Phone: 635-7830; 20 Farm Road
  - Port aux Basques: Phone: 695-6250
  - Port Saunders: Phone: 861-9126
  - Stephenville: Phone: 643-8740

Northwest Territories

Suicide helplines

- NWT Helpline
  Phone: 1-800-661-0844

Depression resources

- NWT Community Counselling Program (CCP): find community counsellors by region
  Web: nwthelpline.ca

- Canadian Mental Health Association (NWT Division)
  Phone: 867-873-3190

Nova Scotia

Suicide helplines

- Mental Health Mobile Crisis Team (MHMCT)
  Phone: 1-902-429-8167; 1-888-429-8167 (toll-free)

Depression resources

- Provincial HealthLink
  Phone: 8-1-1

- Mental Health and Crisis Response Services—AVH (self-referral)
  Middleton: 902-825-4825
  Kentville: adult/older adult: 902-679-2870;
  child/youth: 902-679-2873

- Mood Disorders Clinic
  Phone: 902-473-2585
  Abbie J. Lane Memorial Building, Room 3089, 5909 Veterans' Memorial Lane, Halifax, NS, B3H 2E2

- Centre for Emotions and Health
  Phone: 902-473-7172
  Abbie J. Lane Memorial Building, 7th Floor, Suite 7101B, 5909 Veterans' Memorial Lane, Halifax, NS, B3H 2E2

- IWK Health Centre: Children and Youth Mental Health
  Phone: 1-902-470-8888; 1-888-470-5888 (toll-free)

- Beacon Program: for young adults eighteen to thirty-five living with mental illness
  Phone: 902-678-8361 (available 24/7)

- Seniors Mental Health Services (65+): For those suffering from feelings of depression, anxiety, grief, memory loss, and various types of dementia or other mental health problems
  Phone: 1-855-273-7110 (Chipman Building)
  Phone: 1-855-273-7110 (Soldier's Memorial Hospital)

- Other centre mental health resources:
    - Bayers Road Centre: Phone: 902-454-1400
    - Belmont House: Phone: 902-466-1830
    - Cobequid Community Health Centre: Phone: 902-865-3663
    - Cole Harbour Place: Phone: 902-434-3263
    - Hants Community Hospital: Phone: 902-792-2042

Nunavut

Suicide helpline

- Kamatsiaqtut Helpline
  Phone: 1-800-265-3333; 1-867-979-3333
  (12 a.m.–7 p.m. English; 7 p.m.–12 a.m. local language)

Depression resources

To access mental health services, call or visit your local health centre to book an appointment.

Ontario

Suicide helplines

- Call the Mental Health Helpline
  Phone: 1-866-531-2600

- Toronto Distress Centre
  Phone: 416-408-4357

Depression resources

- Mood Disorders Association of Ontario: Managing Depression and Anxiety
  Phone: 1-866-363-MOOD (6663)
  36 Eglinton Ave. West, Suite 602, Toronto, ON, M4R 1A1

- Mental Health Helpline: Referral Specialists
  Toll-free: 1-866-531-2600 (available 24/7)
  Web: mentalhealthhelpline.ca
- TeleHealth Ontario: Contact TeleHealth Ontario when you have health-related questions or concerns about depression, suicide, or other mental health concerns
  Toll-free: 1-866-797-0000
  Toll-free TTY: 1-866-797-0007
- BounceBack Ontario: Free skill-building program designed to help adults and youth (fifteen-plus) manage symptoms of depression and anxiety
  Toll-free: 1-866-345-0224
- Ontario Psychological Association: Confidential, free referral service
  Phone: 416-961-5552
- Psychotherapy Referral Service Toronto: Matches your unique needs and personality with a trained and experienced psychotherapist
  Immediate help call 416-920-0655 at any time and leave a message. Someone will get back to you within twenty-four hours to arrange an interview.
- Equilibrium-Oakville: Peer support group for individuals and families who are affected by a mood disorder.
  Phone: 905-693-4270; 1-877-693-4270 (toll-free)
  Email: info@equilibrium-oakville.com
- Canadian Mental Health Association (Ontario Division)
  Web: cmha-yr.on.ca

Prince Edward Island

Suicide helpline

1-800-218-2885 (twenty-four-hour province wide bilingual service)

Depression resources

- Changeways Core Program: for dealing with low mood and depression
  - Montague: Phone: 902-838-0960
  - Charlottetown: Phone: 902-368-4430; 902-368-4911
  - Summerside: Phone: 902-888-8380
  - O'Leary: Phone: 902-859-8781

- Mental health walk-in clinics:
  - Montague: Community Mental Health: Phone: 902-838-0960
  - Charlottetown: Richmond Centre (for individuals sixteen and older): Phone: 902-368-4430; McGill Centre (for individuals sixteen and older): Phone: 902-368-4911
  - Summerside: Prince County Hospital: Phone: 902-888-8180
  - Lennox Island: Lennox Island Health Centre (for Lennox Island residents only): Phone: 902-831-2711
  - O'Leary: O'Leary Health Centre: Phone: 902-853-8670

- Canadian Mental Health Association (PEI Division)
  Phone: 902-566-3034
  Email: division@cmha.pe.ca

Quebec

Suicide helpline

- Centre de prévention du suicide de Québec
  Phone: 1-866-APPELLE (1-866-277-3553); 1-866-277-3553 (bilingual)

Depression resources

- Quebec Anxiety Depressive BiPolar Disorders Support Association: Support groups; self-management support program for anxiety, depression and bipolar disorder J'avance! program; discussion forums
  Phone: 1-866-REVIVRE (738-4873) (toll-free support line available across Canada)
  5140 Saint-Hubert Street, Montreal, QC, H2J 2Y3
  Discussion forum (French only): revivre.org/forum

- AMI-Quebec–Action on Mental Illness: Workshops, support groups, counselling, events, hospital support, library with literature resources
  Phone: 514-486-1448; 1-877-303-0264 (toll-free)
  Outside Montreal: 1-877-303-0264
  5800 Boul. Décarie, Montreal, QC, H3X 2J5
- Information and Referral Centre of Greater Montreal
  Phone: 514-527-1375 or 2-1-1
- AMI-Quebec-Action on Mental Illness: Support for families of patients affected by mental illness
  Phone: 514-486-1448; 1-877-303-0264 (toll-free)
  5800 Boul. Décarie, Montreal, QC, H3X 2J5

Saskatchewan

Suicide helplines

- St. Paul and District Crisis Centre
  Phone: 1-800-263-3045; 780-645-5195 (serving Alberta and Saskatchewan)
- Regina Mobile Crisis Service Suicide Line
  Phone: 306-525-5333; 306-757-0127 (available 24/7)
- Saskatoon Mobile Crisis
  Phone: 306-933-6200 (available 24/7)
- Prince Albert Mobile Crisis Unit
  Phone: 306-764-1011
- Rural Saskatchewan: Farm Stress Line
  Toll-free: 1-800-667-4442

Depression Resources

- HealthLine: Provincial Health Information Line
  Phone: 8-1-1
  Web: health.gov.sk.ca/healthline

- Mobile Crisis Services: mental health walk-in service
  1646 11th Ave, Regina, SK, S4P 0H4

Saskatoon

- Centralized Intake & Mental Health & Addictions Services
  Centralized Intake: 306-655-7777
  Adult Services: 306-655-410
  Children's Mental Health Services: 306-655-7800
  Youth Community Counselling: 306-655-7802
  - Depression Support Group
    Phone: 306-270-9181
  - Anxiety & Mood Disorders Program
    Phone: 655-7777
  - Peer Support Program—Mental Health
    Phone: 655-4590
  - After Suicide Support Saskatoon: Ages sixteen to twenty-four
    Phone: 306-249-5666; 933-6200
  - Friends and Relatives of People with Mental Illness (FROMI): Support group for families, relatives and caregivers of people with mental illnesses
    Phone: 306-249-0693; 933-2085; 242-7670

- Kids Help Phone
  Phone: 1-800-668-6868

- Canadian Mental Health Association (Saskatchewan Division)
  Phone: 1-800-461-5483; 306-525-560

Yukon

Suicide helpline

- Yukon distress and support line
  Phone: 1-844-533-3030 (7 p.m.–3 a.m. PT)

Depression resources

- Provincial Health Information Line—Yukon HealthLine
  Phone: 8-1-1
  From satellite phone: 1-604-215-4700
  Web: hss.gov.yk.ca/811.php

Appendix 2
Mood tracker

- Keeping track of your mood and other aspects of your life for a few months can help you to better understand what important factors are impacting your mood (e.g., alcohol, hours of sleep, and menses).
- You may wish to photocopy this page and fill it in each evening before bed (best to keep beside your bed so you remember).
- If you start using your mood tracker on the fourth of the month, fill in the chart starting on the corresponding date.
- If you're feeling fine for part of the day, but in the evening your mood is worse, fill in one-half of the "stable" circle and one half of the "mild," "moderate," or "severe" circle, depending on how you're feeling.
- Sharing your mood tracker with your doctor/therapist will help them to better guide your recovery.

Month: **Year:** **Weight:**

Fill in the circle that best describes your mood each day:

Days	1	2	3	4	5	6	7	8	9	10	11	12	13	14	15	16	17	18	19	20	21	22	26	27	28	29	30	31
Mood (e.g., Today, I was not depressed or I felt mildly/moderately/severely depressed)																												
Not depressed	○	○	○	○	○	○	○	○	○	○	○	○	○	○	○	○	○	○	○	○	○	○	○	○	○	○	○	○
Mild	○	○	○	○	○	○	○	○	○	○	○	○	○	○	○	○	○	○	○	○	○	○	○	○	○	○	○	○
Moderate	○	○	○	○	○	○	○	○	○	○	○	○	○	○	○	○	○	○	○	○	○	○	○	○	○	○	○	○
Severe	○	○	○	○	○	○	○	○	○	○	○	○	○	○	○	○	○	○	○	○	○	○	○	○	○	○	○	○
Rate out of 10. 10 = severe symptoms 0 = no symptoms																												
Anxiety	○	○	○	○	○	○	○	○	○	○	○	○	○	○	○	○	○	○	○	○	○	○	○	○	○	○	○	○
Irritability	○	○	○	○	○	○	○	○	○	○	○	○	○	○	○	○	○	○	○	○	○	○	○	○	○	○	○	○
Sleep	○	○	○	○	○	○	○	○	○	○	○	○	○	○	○	○	○	○	○	○	○	○	○	○	○	○	○	○
Fill in circle if the following applies today:																												
Alcohol	○	○	○	○	○	○	○	○	○	○	○	○	○	○	○	○	○	○	○	○	○	○	○	○	○	○	○	○
Cannabis	○	○	○	○	○	○	○	○	○	○	○	○	○	○	○	○	○	○	○	○	○	○	○	○	○	○	○	○
Menses	○	○	○	○	○	○	○	○	○	○	○	○	○	○	○	○	○	○	○	○	○	○	○	○	○	○	○	○
Did you take you medications today?	○	○	○	○	○	○	○	○	○	○	○	○	○	○	○	○	○	○	○	○	○	○	○	○	○	○	○	○
Where you physically active today?	○	○	○	○	○	○	○	○	○	○	○	○	○	○	○	○	○	○	○	○	○	○	○	○	○	○	○	○

Here is an example of a completed mood tracker:

Month: November **Year:** 2019 **Weight: 187 lbs (November 3)**

Fill in the circle that best describes your mood each day:

Days	1	2	3	4	5	6	7	8	9	10	11	12	13	14	15	16	17	18	19	20	21	22	26	27	28	29	30	31
Mood (e.g., Today, I was not depressed or I felt mildly/moderately/severely depressed)																												
Not depressed	○	○	○	○	○	○	○	○	○	○	○	○	○	○	○	○	○	○	○	○	○	○	○	○	○	○	○	○
Mild	●	○	○	○	○	○	○	○	○	○	○	○	○	○	○	○	○	○	○	○	○	○	○	○	○	○	○	○
Moderate	○	●	●	○	○	●	○	○	○	○	○	○	○	○	○	○	○	○	○	○	○	○	○	○	○	○	○	○
Severe	○	○	○	●	●	○	○	○	○	○	○	○	○	○	○	○	○	○	○	○	○	○	○	○	○	○	○	○
Rate out of 10. 10 = severe symptoms 0 = no symptoms																												
Anxiety	④	④	⑥	⑥	⑨	⑨	⑦	○	○	○	○	○	○	○	○	○	○	○	○	○	○	○	○	○	○	○	○	○
Irritability	②	②	④	④	⑥	⑥	⑤	○	○	○	○	○	○	○	○	○	○	○	○	○	○	○	○	○	○	○	○	○
Sleep	⑥	⑥	④	③	③	③	⑤	○	○	○	○	○	○	○	○	○	○	○	○	○	○	○	○	○	○	○	○	○
Fill in circle if the following applies today:																												
Alcohol	○	○	○	●	●	●	○	○	○	○	○	○	○	○	○	○	○	○	○	○	○	○	○	○	○	○	○	○
Cannabis	○	○	○	●	○	○	○	○	○	○	○	○	○	○	○	○	○	○	○	○	○	○	○	○	○	○	○	○
Menses	○	○	○	○	○	○	●	●	○	○	○	○	○	○	○	○	○	○	○	○	○	○	○	○	○	○	○	○
Did you take you medications today?	⊗	○	○	⊗	⊗	⊗	○	○	○	○	○	○	○	○	○	○	○	○	○	○	○	○	○	○	○	○	○	○
Where you physically active today?	○	○	○	⊗	○	○	○	○	○	○	○	○	○	○	○	○	○	○	○	○	○	○	○	○	○	○	○	○

Glossary

Active suicidal ideation A wish to die as well as a plan to act on that wish.

Acute Of a sudden or unexpected beginning, or of a rapid or short duration. Referring to the onset and progression of a disease. For instance, acute depression might refer to a recent onset of depression, as opposed to chronic depression, which suggests the symptoms of depression are longstanding.

Adrenal gland Endocrine glands located at the top of each kidney. They are responsible for the production and release of cortisol, the body's most important stress hormone.

Adrenocorticotropic hormone (ACTH) A hormone released from the pituitary gland in response to stress. ACTH is a hormone messenger that plays an important role in the functioning of the hypothalamic-pituitary-adrenal (HPA) axis. In response to stress, the hypothalamus releases corticotropin-releasing factor (CRF) and it in turn provokes the release of ACTH. ACTH then causes the adrenal gland to produce and release cortisol, the body's most important acute and chronic stress hormone.

Adverse childhood event (ACE) Usually defined as a highly stressful life event that has the potential to impact a child's mental and physical health. ACEs are defined by the research study that is assessing their impact but might include parental divorce; death of a loved one; physical, sexual, or emotional abuse; living in extreme poverty; or a child's or close loved one's diagnosis of a life-threatening illness.

Adverse effects Another term for the undesired effects, or side effects, of a medication.

Aerobic exercise Energetic and sustained physical activity associated with increased oxygen consumption, leading to strengthening of the heart and lungs. Aerobic exercises include vigorous walking or jogging, swimming, soccer, biking, tennis, and dancing. Aerobic exercises can become anaerobic exercises if they are performed at high intensity; for instance, jogging is aerobic, but sprinting is anaerobic.

Affect One's expression of their emotional tone. An appropriate affect would be displayed as a smile when happy or a serious expression when engaged in a business meeting. An inappropriate affect is described when an individual is unable to show a normal range of emotions, which might be associated with schizophrenia or severe depression (flat or blunted affect) or an excessive expression of emotions, which might be seen when an individual is experiencing symptoms of mania or hypomania.

Affective disorder Another term for mood disorders, affective disorders include depression and bipolar disorders.

Akathisia From the Greek meaning "not to sit," akathisia is an extremely uncomfortable, highly distressing physical feeling of restlessness and a need to move. Most often, patients experiencing akathisia complain of a desperate need to move their legs. Akathisia is a side effect most often caused by the use of antipsychotic medications.

Amygdala As the brain's anxiety centre, the amygdala is the brain structure responsible for receiving and processing sensory information predominately related to fear and anxiety. The amygdala then sends fear-related information to the hypothalamus and other brain structures, which causes a behavioural response to the threatening or anxiety-provoking situation, such as running away or fighting back.

Anaerobic exercise Brief bursts of intense activity that build speed and power rather than endurance. This includes activities such as weight lifting that cause the body to rely on energy stored in muscles rather than oxygen. Aerobic exercises can become anaerobic exercises if they are performed at high intensity; for instance, jogging is aerobic, but sprinting is anaerobic.

Anhedonia An emotional state in which a person is unable to feel pleasure or receive enjoyment from activities that they usually find gratifying and fulfilling.

Anticonvulsant A medication that helps control convulsions (seizures); however, they are also very good mood stabilizers and are often used in treatment of bipolar disorder to help regulate extreme mood fluctuations.

Anti-inflammatory The prefix "anti-" means "against or opposite." To reduce or relieve inflammation (see also "inflammation").

Antipsychotics These medications are used to oppose psychotic symptoms (e.g., hallucinations, delusions). Antipsychotic medications are used to treat disorders such as schizophrenia, bipolar disorder, and delusional disorder. However, a new generation of antipsychotics, referred to as atypical antipsychotics, are useful antidepressants as well, especially for difficult-to-treat depression. The oldest antipsychotics are also called conventional or typical antipsychotics.

Anxiety Excessive, unwarranted, inappropriate fear. It is an unpleasant, sometimes highly distressing emotional experience, which might include worry, rumination, or feeling on edge. Anxiety is very often associated with physical symptoms as well, such as a racing heart, muscle tension, pressure in the chest, sweating, or feeling light-headed, dizzy, or nauseated. Anxiety is often experienced as excessive worry about common, everyday things (e.g., health, work, safety, finances) with a common theme of *What if… ?* People struggling with anxiety usually recognize their worries are excessive but constantly worry, *What if X happens?*

Anxiety disorders Clusters of symptoms where anxiety is the most prominent symptom. The anxiety disorders found in the DSM-5 include generalized anxiety disorder, panic disorder, separation anxiety disorder, specific anxiety disorder, agoraphobia, and social anxiety disorder. Post-traumatic stress disorder is no longer a member of this group but is included in the trauma and stressor related disorders group. Likewise, obsessive-compulsive disorder is no longer a member of the anxiety disorders group but is included in the obsessive-compulsive and related disorders group.

Anxious distress specifier A recent addition to its depression and bipolar diagnoses, the DSM-5 included the anxious distress specifier to encourage clinicians to look for anxiety symptoms and grade their severity when diagnosing depression or bipolar disorder. This is because anxiety very commonly co-occurs with depression and bipolar, its presence often impacts treatment choice, and it significantly heightens suicide risk.

Astrocytes *Astron* is the Greek word for "star," which describes the shape of this glial cell, and its form contributes to its function. Astrocytes are the glial cell responsible for, among other things, feeding and protecting neurons. Its star-shaped form and its many arms enable an astrocyte to reach and support a greater number of neurons and perform its many tasks simultaneously. Astrocytes produce an essential neuron growth factor called brain-derived neurotrophic factor (BDNF), which is required to grow and maintain healthy neurons. Astrocyte dysfunction and reduced BDNF are associated with severe depression.

Attention deficit hyperactivity disorder (ADHD) A disorder of attention, hyperactivity, and impulsivity. ADHD may affect all age groups: preschool through adulthood. The diagnosis is made if difficulty sustaining attention, hyperactivity, and impulsivity are associated with functional impairment at home, school, or work.

Atypical antipsychotics (AAPs) Also known as second-generation antipsychotics, these drugs block dopamine in the limbic area of the brain, which provides an antipsychotic effect. However, they also impact other neurotransmitters, including serotonin and norepinephrine. It is their affinity for serotonin that makes these newer antipsychotic medications so different from the older conventional or typical antipsychotics. These additional effects also make atypical antipsychotics useful for the treatment of disorders other than schizophrenia and bipolar disorder, including depression. Atypical antipsychotics are less likely to worsen negative symptoms of schizophrenia. The older medications in the atypical antipsychotic class may cause serious weight gain and changes in cholesterol and blood sugar. Newer atypical antipsychotics carry a much lower risk (see also "antipsychotics").

Atypical depression features Characteristic atypical depression features include reversed vegetative symptoms (sleeping too much, or hypersomnia) and excessive eating with associated weight gain, severe fatigue, and feeling physically weighed down or leaden paralysis (legs feel like lead). The mood associated with atypical depression can brighten for short periods in response to a positive experience but quickly dips again, and patients might be highly reactive to slights or interpersonal conflicts.

Augmentation The literal definition of this word is "to make larger, increase in size or amount, or to make an addition." When used in the context of psychiatric treatment, it refers to the combination of two or more drugs or treatment modalities in an attempt to better manage symptoms.

Behavioural activation (BA) A form of psychotherapy (talk therapy) employed to treat depression. Based on the idea that it's easier to change behaviour than it is to change thinking, BA encourages participants to increase their activity level, especially activities they might have been avoiding due to depression. By increasing their activity, the patient is allowing the behaviour to influence and modify their emotions, feelings, and thought processes. With time and repetition, the goal of BA is to improve functioning and to begin deriving pleasure from the activities.

Benzodiazepine Sometimes referred to as benzos, benzodiazepines are a group of medications that may be used to treat anxiety but also have muscle relaxant, sedation, mood stabilization, anti-agitation, and anticonvulsant (anti-seizure) properties. They are also frequently employed to aid in alcohol withdrawal. The generic names of these medications most often ends in the suffix "-pam" (e.g., lorazepam, clonazepam, diazepam).

Bipolar depression Depression that occurs in association with bipolar disorder (the "low pole"). Bipolar depression may be indistinguishable from unipolar depression, frequently leading to misdiagnosis. A current or previous manic or hypomanic episode is required for a bipolar diagnosis, but if the high is not reported, was not recognized, or has not yet occurred, it is difficult to differentiate unipolar from bipolar depression. It is extremely important to differentiate these two types of depression because they are treated differently.

Bipolar disorder A mood disorder characterized by two mood poles: a low (depressed) pole and a high (manic or hypomanic) pole. The most common bipolar diagnoses include bipolar I disorder, bipolar II disorder, and "soft" bipolar (in the DSM-5 referred to as specified or unspecified bipolar). Bipolar I disorder requires an episode of elevated mood (mania), while bipolar II disorder requires a hypomanic episode. A low pole is required only for a bipolar II diagnosis. Depression, while commonly experienced, is not required for the diagnosis of bipolar I disorder.

Black-box warning This is a warning issued by the US Food and Drug Administration (FDA) for serious or life-threatening risks associated with prescription medications. Health Canada also requires serious safety hazards to be highlighted in a "serious warnings and precautions box" in the product monograph.

Blood-brain barrier A protective barrier between the blood in the body and the blood delivered to the central nervous system (CNS), which includes the brain and the spinal cord. Tiny blood vessels, called capillaries, are made up of cells that are very tightly bound together. The microscopic gaps between the capillary cells act as filters, allowing in oxygen, glucose, and some medications. The filter keeps other larger and often harmful products out of the CNS, such as bacteria, some medications, and other toxins that might be harmful to the brain.

Brain-derived neurotrophic factor (BDNF) A protein produced by the glial cells called astrocytes, BDNF is brain cell fertilizer, which helps nourish and grow neurons (neurogenesis) and helps them to effectively and appropriately connect with other neurons (neuroplasticity). Adequate levels of BDNF are required to maintain brain health. Low BDNF concentrations are found in the brains of depressed suicide victims and has been associated with depression and chronic stress.

Candidate gene A gene that is likely associated with the onset of a disease. The candidate gene may be located in a chromosome region that scientists suspect is involved in the disease, or the product of the gene (a protein or enzyme) is associated with the onset and maintenance of a disease.

CANMAT guidelines The Canadian Network for Mood and Anxiety Treatments, or CANMAT, is an organization composed of psychiatrists and other health professionals who focus on research, treatment, and education regarding mood (e.g., depression and bipolar) and anxiety disorders. By uniting academic knowledge, research, and clinical experience, CANMAT provides prescribers with evidence-based recommendations to guide treatment choices when managing mood and anxiety disorders.

Cardiovascular "Cardio" means heart and "vascular" refers to blood vessels. Cardiovascular diseases refer to diseases affecting the heart and blood vessels and include high blood pressure (hypertension), heart attacks (myocardial infarction [MI]), stroke, and many other disorders.

Central nervous system (CNS) The part of the nervous system that consists of the brain and spinal cord. The nervous system in the other parts of the body is referred to as the peripheral nervous system.

Chromosome Our DNA, which carries our unique genetic code, is attached to proteins and wound into X formations called chromosomes. All humans have twenty-three chromosome pairs (forty-six total). Males and females have the same chromosomes except for the twenty-third pair, which are sex chromosomes. Males have an X and a Y sex chromosome (XY); females have two X sex chromosomes (XX).

Chronic Lasting for a long time, spanning over an extended period, in reference to a disease or condition. Chronic depression refers to depression symptoms that have been present for a long time.

Circadian rhythm From the Latin *circa* ("around") and *dies* ("day"), the circadian rhythm refers to the natural changes that take place in our body throughout the day. They are referred to as a rhythm because they occur at approximately the same time each day. The times of day when we are hungry and sleepy are controlled largely by our circadian rhythms. Many hormones, such as cortisol, estrogen, and melatonin, are released following a circadian rhythm.

Class effect Similar drugs are grouped into classes. Like in a family, all members of the class are related in some way, either by their chemical structure, pharmacology, therapeutic effects, or side effects. When drugs have a class effect, this indicates that as a group they may have a similar mechanism of action, they might be useful for the treatment of a specific disorder, or they have similar side effects, such as weight gain.

Clinical experience A health professional's experience related directly to work with patients, as opposed to theoretical education and laboratory studies. To provide a patient with the best care possible, a health professional will draw from their academic/theoretical knowledge and their clinical experience.

Clinical rating scales When a disorder cannot be diagnosed using objective tests such as blood work or imaging, clinicians must find alternative means, other than relying solely on their own clinical experiences, to correctly diagnose and judge the severity of such disorders. Clinical rating scales are a tool that can help to guide diagnosis and treatment. (See also "depression rating scale.")

Clinician A health professional who works directly with patients, as opposed to one specializing in research, laboratory, or educational/theoretical work.

Cognitive (cognition) Mental processes that involve the acquisition of knowledge and rational judgment. A cognitively intact brain has the ability to focus, retain information (remember), and use newly acquired information.

Cognitive-behavioural therapy (CBT) A form of psychotherapy employed for the treatment of depression and many other psychiatric disorders. CBT is based on the notion that psychiatric disorders result from a patient's cognitive and behavioural distortions (dysfunctional thoughts, beliefs, and behaviours). CBT aims to identify dysfunctional thoughts and then to confront those thoughts and replace them with more accurate interpretations or facts.

Cognitive impairment When the brain is incapable of carrying out some of its most vital and necessary duties related to knowledge, conscious awareness, and judgment. This includes deficits in memory, concentration, thinking speed, and executive functioning. Cognitive symptoms are commonly associated with depression and anxiety. In the elderly, cognitive symptoms associated with a mental illness may be mistaken for dementia.

Collateral information Information regarding a patient that is received from a source other than the patient. Collateral sources may include family members, close friends, work colleagues, or others who have personal knowledge regarding the patient. In some cases, especially when a patient has lost insight, for instance when psychotic or with severe dementia, collateral information can be essential for the health professional to appropriately assess a patient.

College of Nurses A professional licensing organization that registers and regulates the professional activities of nurses (and often nurse practitioners). The main goal of a professional college is the protection of the public. As such, they accept and investigate complaints made by the public.

College of Physicians A professional licensing organization that registers and regulates the professional activities of doctors. The main goal of a professional college is the protection of the public. As such, they accept and investigate complaints made by the public.

College of Psychologists A professional licensing organization that registers and regulates the professional activities of psychologists. The main goal of a professional college is the protection of the public. As such, they accept and investigate complaints made by the public.

Co-morbidity "Morbidity" means "disease or illness," while the prefix "co-", in this context, means "jointly"; co-morbidity is just that: two or more disorders that occur at the same time.

Conventional antipsychotic These first-generation or typical antipsychotics were the first antipsychotic medications to be used for the treatment of psychotic symptoms (e.g., hallucinations, delusions). They work by blocking dopamine receptors in the brain. While the first antipsychotics provided incredible benefits for many patients, they also came with some serious, sometimes irreversible, side effects. For instance, by blocking dopamine in other brain areas, conventional antipsychotics can provoke movement disorders, including tremors and stiffness, severe restlessness (akathisia), and a serious, sometimes irreversible movement disorder called tardive dyskinesia. (See also "antipsychotics.")

Corticotropin-releasing hormone (CRH) A hormone released by the hypothalamus in response to stress. CRH is released as part of the hypothalamic-pituitary-adrenal (HPA) axis and drives the stress response by stimulating the release of adrenocorticotropic hormone (ACTH) from the pituitary gland, which, in turn, triggers the release of cortisol, our most important stress hormone.

Cortisol The body's most important stress hormone. Released by the adrenal glands (endocrine glands located at the top of each kidney), cortisol regulates our body's acute and chronic responses to stress. It also has crucial anti-inflammatory properties that play an important protective role in the prevention of widespread tissue and nerve damage associated with stress and inflammation.

Cytochrome P450 enzymes (CYP) A collection of enzymes that are necessary to break down (metabolize) many medications. Only six of the more than fifty CYP enzymes are responsible for metabolizing 90 percent of medications. How effectively CYP enzymes work is dependent on genetic variability (known as gene polymorphisms). Furthermore, the activity of the CYP enzymes can be inhibited (reduced) or induced (increased) by certain medications. The effects of CYP enzymes are commonly the cause of drug-drug interactions that may lead to problematic side effects or treatment failures.

Delusions A symptom of psychosis. Delusions are false beliefs that are firmly fixed. Patients are unable to see that their delusional belief is false, even when presented with concrete evidence to the contrary. Delusions most often occur in association with schizophrenia and bipolar mania but may also feature in severe depression. A persecutory delusion is a false belief that one is being persecuted (e.g., the false belief that others are trying to harm the individual). A grandiose delusion is a false belief that one is all-powerful or has special powers or gifts (e.g., a false belief that you are a god).

Dementia A disorder associated with gradually advancing impairment of cognition. Symptoms include an inability to focus attention or understand simple concepts, memory deficits, and language difficulties, such as trouble finding words.

Deoxyribonucleic acid (DNA) Found in every cell, DNA carries an individual's genetic code. Our genetic code is like a recipe book, providing precise instructions that regulate an individual's growth, development, reproduction, and all other functions necessary for life.

Depression rating scale A clinical rating scale that is designed to determine depression severity, and quantifying severity can help a clinician decide whether exercise, talk therapy, or medication might be the appropriate treatment to suggest to their patient. It can also help to show the impact of treatment over time.

Diabetes A disease that is characterized by high levels of glucose (sugar) in the blood and urine. Diabetes is caused by the inability to produce insulin (type I diabetes) or the inability of cells to respond appropriately to insulin (type II diabetes). Insulin is a hormone, released from the pancreas, that is responsible for regulating blood sugar levels.

Discontinuation symptoms (syndrome) Sometimes referred to as discontinuation syndrome, a constellation of symptoms associated with the discontinuation of certain medications. Discontinuation symptoms are unpleasant and non-specific and may include flu-like symptoms (nausea, vomiting, diarrhea, body aches, headaches, dizziness, sweating), restlessness, jitteriness, sleep disturbance, anxiety, depressed mood, and electric shock–like feelings. There is a great deal of inter-individual variability related to discontinuation symptoms. Two people discontinuing the same medication may have very different experiences; while one might have no symptoms, the other might have very severe symptoms.

Dopamine A neurotransmitter (chemical messenger) that, along with serotonin and norepinephrine, is linked to the onset and maintenance of depression. As such, dopamine is a target of some antidepressants and all antipsychotic medications. Excessive dopamine in the limbic region of the brain is associated with psychotic symptoms (e.g., delusions and hallucinations). Conversely, a deficit of dopamine in the prefrontal cortex (PFC) at the front of the brain is associated with lack of motivation, apathy, and other negative symptoms of schizophrenia. Dopamine also plays a critical role in motivation, pleasure (e.g., love, lust), and reward seeking, including addiction, as well as attention, learning, and fluidity of movements.

DSM-5 The *Diagnostic and Statistical Manual of Mental Disorders* (DSM-5) is the most recent update of the manual that mental health professionals use to formally diagnose psychiatric disorders.

Dysfunction Not functioning in the expected way or manner; functioning abnormally. Often used to refer to impairment in function of a specific organ or system of the body (for instance, sexual dysfunction).

Electroconvulsive therapy (ECT) A type of neuro-stimulation therapy. Based on an abundance of research evidence, ECT is considered the gold standard treatment for severe depression. ECT involves the administration of a pulse of electricity to the brain through the skull that provokes a short seizure, which is believed to be responsible for its rapid and robust antidepressant effect.

Endocrine glands A network of nine glands that make up the body's endocrine system. The endocrine system consists of glands and organs that regulate and control various body functions by producing and releasing hormones into the blood.

Epigenetics The science of gene expression. Unlike DNA, which cannot be altered, how genes are expressed can be altered by various factors, including one's developmental stage (e.g., puberty, pregnancy) and one's environment, including exposure to toxins (e.g., cigarette smoke) and exposure to childhood adversity (e.g., abuse or neglect).

Estrogen Produced by the ovaries, estrogen is a hormone required for normal female sexual development and reproduction. Estrogen is thought to be responsible for women's heightened risk of depression, as compared to men.

European Medicines Agency (EMA) The European Union agency responsible for protecting consumers by regulating the production, marketing, and sale of medications. The EMA provides an official indication and product monograph for the medications it approves. The product monograph includes all pertinent details regarding a medication's safety and general use.

Evidence-based treatment These are treatments that have been demonstrated to be safe and effective by evidence acquired through high-quality scientific research.

Executive function Cognitive functions including organizing, planning, forward thinking (thinking ahead), and critical thinking. The brain's prefrontal cortex (PFC) is primarily responsible for executive functioning. However, the PFC might not be fully mature until age twenty-five. You might wonder if your teenager's brain is working properly... in fact, for many it isn't and won't be until they're well past their teen years. That's why it's necessary to repeat yourself so often when parenting a teen. Their working memory, another PFC function, likely isn't fully functional yet either. Therefore, it's hard for them to use and retain new information, especially if the information doesn't particularly interest them.

Flat affect Loss of emotional expression. Despite having a reason to respond, those experiencing a flat affect provide little or no emotional response or reaction. This is referred to as a negative symptom of schizophrenia. Blunted affect is diminished emotional expression and may be associated with depression and other psychiatric illnesses.

Food and Drug Administration (FDA) A federal agency of the US Department of Health responsible for protecting consumers by regulating the production, marketing, and sale of medications. The FDA provides an official indication and product monograph for the medications it approves. The product monograph includes all pertinent details regarding a medication's safety and general use.

Gene A section of DNA. Genes contain the information required for cellular differentiation. When specific genes are turned on (expressed) or turned off (suppressed), they direct what a cell will become. How and when genes are expressed makes each of us a unique individual.

Gene expression An expressed gene is a gene that is turned on and is producing the products (proteins, enzymes) that it is programmed to generate.

Generalized anxiety disorder (GAD) An anxiety disorder characterized by excessive, pervasive, difficult-to-control anxiety/worry about a variety of situations that occurs on more days than not for at least six months. For adults, symptoms of GAD include at least three of the following (only one required for children): restless/edgy/keyed-up feeling, easily fatigued, sleep disturbance (falling/staying asleep; restless/unsatisfying sleep), problems concentrating/mind going blank, irritability, and/or muscle tension.

Glial cells These cells make up the bulk (90 percent) of the cells in the brain and include microglia, oligodendrocytes, and astrocytes. These cells play a number of critical roles in maintaining a healthy, functional brain. Depressed brains have been found to have a decreased number of glial cells.

Glutamate A neurotransmitter. Glutamate is the most abundant excitatory messenger of the central nervous system. Depression is associated with abnormal levels of glutamate and, as such, it is the target of some new anti-depressant treatments.

Gold standard The best diagnostic methods or treatments available for a condition.

Gut motility Refers to the movement of the gastrointestinal tract, bowel, intestine.

Hallucination False sensory experiences that occur despite the lack of any external stimulation. Hallucinations may be auditory, olfactory, tactile, or visual. To see, hear, feel, or smell something that is not really there.

Health Canada The Canadian government regulatory body responsible for protecting consumers by regulating the production, marketing, and sale of medications. Health Canada provides an official indication and product monograph for the medications it approves. The product monograph includes all pertinent details regarding a medication's safety and general use.

Heritability Heritability in depression means the extent to which genetic individual differences contribute to individual differences in behaviour (or whether someone will have depression symptoms). Heritability is a proportion: its numerical value ranges from zero (genes do not contribute at all to individual differences) to one (genes are the only reason for individual differences).

Hippocampus Structure found in the temporal lobe of the brain. The hippocampus, a component of the limbic system, is responsible for some aspects of memory and learning, particularly the storage of an individual's emotionally meaningful memories, such as a wedding day, an important graduation, or the birth of a child. For example, there is no calculus in my hippocampus. Because I dislike calculus and it plays no role in my ability to navigate day-to-day life, the moment I completed my final calculus exam, everything I learned was forgotten. Scientists have discovered that severe and chronic depression is associated with a reduction in the size of the hippocampus.

Homeopathy Homeopathy draws its name from *homos*, Greek for "same," and *pathy*, Greek for "feeling," which translates into "similar feeling or similar experience." Homeopathy was developed in eighteenth-century Germany. It was founded on the concept that "like cures like." The German physician who founded homeopathy claimed that if a certain medical substance, when taken by a healthy individual, always causes a set of specific symptoms, then that same substance will cure those symptoms when taken by a person who is ill. As an example, a substance that causes hallucinations in a well person will cure them when taken by a patient who has hallucinations. Homeopathy has been completely debunked and should not be regarded as legitimate science.

Hormone Chemical messenger of the body's endocrine system that travels by blood to distant (target) organs and relays regulatory messages that control our physiology (e.g., hunger, reproduction) and behaviour, as well as our mood and emotions.

Hypersomnia Excessive daytime sleepiness, need for sleep, or time spent in bed. A common atypical depression feature. Despite sleeping much more than they normally would, individuals who experience hypersomnia do not awaken feeling refreshed and have trouble staying awake during the day.

Hypertension Abnormally elevated blood pressure.

Hypertensive crisis A potentially life-threatening increase in blood pressure, which may be accompanied by symptoms including headache, heart racing, chest pain, sore or stiff neck, nausea, vomiting, and sweating. A hypertensive crisis might result when an individual prescribed a MAOI antidepressant ingests certain foods or drugs that increase tyramine.

Hypothalamic-pituitary-adrenal (HPA) axis The brain's stress response command centre. Through the release of the hormones ACTH, CRF, and cortisol, the hypothalamus, pituitary gland, and adrenal glands interact to manage the body's response to stress.

Hypothalamus Brain structure that regulates hormone levels, the wake/sleep cycle, hunger, thirst, body temperature, sexual behaviour, and emotions.

Through its communication with the pituitary and adrenal glands, the hypothalamus is part of the hypothalamic-pituitary-adrenal (HPA) axis and links the nervous system and the endocrine system.

Indication Once research data provided by a drug's manufacturer has been evaluated by a country's medication regulatory agency (e.g., Health Canada, FDA), it may be approved for use to treat a specific disorder, which is the drug's official indication. For instance, antidepressants are indicated for depression. They might also be approved for other indications (e.g., anxiety).

Inflammation Derived from the Latin word *inflamare*, meaning "to set on fire." Inflammation is the body's defence mechanism to manage irritating or harmful stimuli (a toxic or irritating substance, a microorganism like bacteria or virus, or a physical injury). Inflammation allows the body to localize and remove the aggravating agent, as well as any damaged tissue, which allows the body to begin the healing process. However, chronic inflammation is a harmful process.

Insight May be defined several ways, but essentially insight means being able to see or understand something clearly. In psychiatry and psychology, insight may be defined as an individual's understanding of their illness and their understanding of how their illness affects how they interact with others. If one lacks insight, that generally means they are so unwell that they don't realize how seriously ill they are. A loss of insight is most commonly associated with psychotic illnesses.

Insomnia An inability to get to sleep, stay asleep, or awakening too early. A very common symptom of depression. Early insomnia refers to the inability to fall asleep in a usual or acceptable time. Middle insomnia occurs when an individual cannot stay asleep. They awaken during the night and have difficulty or an inability to get back to sleep. Terminal insomnia refers to the inability to fall back to sleep after awakening too early in the morning.

Inter-individual variability Inter-individual variability is the differences that are observed between people. Some examples of inter-individual variability include differences in gender, ethnic background, resiliency, and response to treatments. One person might take an antidepressant medication and experience a robust reduction in depression symptoms and no side effects, while another person might experience no benefits and intolerable side effects.

Interpersonal therapy (IPT) Type of talk therapy that focuses on how patients relate to others (friends, family, work associates) as the cause or a factor in the maintenance of depression.

Light therapy Also known as phototherapy. A therapeutic modality used to treat depression with a seasonal pattern.

Malingering Faking or exaggerating an illness or symptoms of illness for secondary gain (e.g., time off work, financial compensation).

Mast cell White blood cells (also referred to as mastocytes) that are members of the body's immune system. They are found in the gastrointestinal tract and many other areas of the body. Mast cells are small sacks that contain granules of histamine. Depending on where in the body histamine is released, it can alter gut motility or cause sneezing and a runny nose, symptoms that tend to benefit from antihistamine medications.

Mechanism of action Describes how a medication achieves its desired effect.

Melancholic depression Hippocrates used the term *melan* (Greek for "black") *-cholic* to refer to depression. Melancholic refers to the darkness of depression. The main features of melancholic depression are a profoundly depressed, despondent mood that is typically worse in the morning, anhedonia, loss of appetite and weight loss, early morning awakening, and excessive guilt.

Menopause A natural phase in a woman's life marked by the cessation of menstrual periods. Menopause reflects the substantial drop in estrogen due to the loss of ovarian function associated with aging. A woman is considered to be menopausal when she has not had a menstrual period for twelve months. Perimenopause, or the time leading up to the full cessation of menstrual periods, usually begins sometime between the ages of forty-five and fifty-five, with the average age of fifty-one.

Metabolism Regarding medications, metabolism refers to breaking a drug down into other compounds. Metabolism might be necessary to make the drug active or effective or metabolism might be necessary before the drug can be excreted (removed) from the body. We have a system of enzymes that are necessary for drug metabolism, called the cytochrome P450 enzymes (CYP).

Microglia A type of glial cell. Microglia are immune cells of the central nervous system that remove old and damaged neurons and prevent neurotransmitters from accumulating, which is harmful to neurons. Chronic stress and chronic depression is associated with an activation of microglia, resulting in their release of pro-inflammatory cytokines and subsequent damage to neurons.

Mindfulness The awareness and acceptance of one's thoughts, including those that are negative, unpleasant, or distressing. Learning mindfulness skills may help individuals to manage those thoughts so they do not negatively impact their functioning and the quality of their day-to-day lives.

Monoamine oxidase (MAO) An enzyme that metabolizes (breaks down) neurotransmitters, such as serotonin, norepinephrine, and dopamine.

Monoamine oxidase inhibitors (MAOIs) An older group of antidepressants. These medications block the monoamine oxidase (MAO) enzyme, which leads to an increase in the neurotransmitters serotonin, norepinephrine, and dopamine.

Mood disorder Also known as affective disorders, a group of psychiatric illnesses that include major depression and bipolar disorders.

Myocardial infarction (MI) A heart attack.

Nerve terminal The end of a neuron, which contains the chemical messengers (neurotransmitters) used to relay messages across a synapse. Neurotransmitters are released from the nerve terminal into the synaptic cleft in response to an electric impulse.

Neurogenesis The production and growth of neurons.

Neuron Nerve cell. Neurons receive data gathered by our senses from the external environment and send commands to other neurons and cells throughout the body.

Neuroplasticity The ability of the brain to remodel itself, change, and adapt to changes such as stress, trauma, disease, and new situations, behaviours, and skills that take place throughout an individual's life.

Neurostimulation Stimulation of the nervous system, which may be invasive or non-invasive and is used in psychiatry for the treatment of various mental illnesses. Two such treatments are electroconvulsive therapy (ECT) and repetitive transcranial magnetic stimulation (rTMS).

Neurotransmitters Chemicals released from a neuron's nerve terminal in response to an electrical impulse. Neurotransmitters transmit a chemical message across a synapse to an adjacent neuron or cell. By attaching to receptors on the neuron or cell receiving the message, neurotransmitters may excite (agonist) or inhibit (antagonist) the cell. The neurotransmitters most commonly associated with depression are serotonin, dopamine, norepinephrine, GABA, and glutamate.

Norepinephrine A neurotransmitter (chemical messenger). It is one of the most important neurotransmitters linked to depression and a target of many antidepressant medications. Among other activities, norepinephrine is the body's "flee, freeze, or fight" neurotransmitter, necessary to appropriately respond to a stressful, anxiety-provoking situation.

Novel antidepressant "Novel" meaning "new," novel antidepressants are newly developed medications for depression.

Obsessive-compulsive disorder (OCD) A disorder characterized by the presence of obsessions and/or compulsions. Obsessions are recurrent and persistent thoughts, urges, or images that are experienced as inappropriate, intrusive, and unwanted, and cause anxiety or distress. Attempts are made to ignore, suppress, or neutralize the obsessions by a thought or action. Compulsions are repetitive behaviours or mental acts an individual feels driven to perform. They usually follow rigid rules and are meant to neutralize the distress of obsessions or to prevent a dreaded event from occurring. Compulsions are usually time consuming, onerous, clearly excessive, or senseless. While compulsions usually reduce distress, they are not inherently pleasurable. Symptoms of OCD produce distress, are time consuming (>1 h/d), and interfere with function.

Oligodendrocytes Glial cells found in the central nervous system. These cells play a protective, supportive, and insulating role for axons, which are projections of the neurons. The primary role of oligodendrocytes is to help electrical messages to move very quickly along the nerve axon.

Over-the-counter treatments/medications Treatments that do not require a prescription.

Panic attack Also called anxiety attacks, they are sudden, severe, and terrifying experiences (attacks) of anxiety, which reach their peak in a matter of minutes. When in the midst of a panic attack, people commonly report that they're afraid they're going to die, they're "going crazy," or they're having a life-threatening medical event, such as a heart attack or stroke. Panic attacks are usually accompanied by physical symptoms that can mimic heart problems, such as a racing heart rate; pressure or pain in the chest; feeling faint, weak, or dizzy; and shortness of breath.

Panic disorder (PD) A DSM-5 anxiety disorder. Panic disorder is associated with recurrent, sudden, unexpected panic attacks that are usually followed by the fear of having another attack or concern about the possible consequences of having another attack. As a result, patients tend to avoid situations or locations that might provoke another attack.

Perimenopause As the prefix "peri-" indicates, this is the period in a woman's life around or near menopause. It is a transitional phase, during which a woman's ovaries begin to decrease estrogen production, gradually leading to menopause. While the exact timing is highly variable, the perimenopausal period usually starts in the late forties or early fifties and lasts for one to three years.

Peripartum The time around childbirth, including the time of birth and the four weeks postpartum.

Persecutory/paranoid delusion A firmly held, fixed, false belief that others are trying to cause an individual harm. This might include thoughts that they are being monitored, spied on, or conspired against.

Personality disorder A disorder characterized by rigid, firmly established, dysfunctional, and maladjusted patterns of thought and behaviour. Personality disorders are commonly misdiagnosed and should not be diagnosed by a doctor or another health professional that has not known the patient for an extended period of time. Severe psychiatric illnesses can look very much like a personality disorder, and thus personality disorder diagnoses should not be made in the midst of an acute mental illness.

Pharmacogenomics Combines the study of how drugs work (pharmacology) and how genes function (genomics) to understand how a patient's genes can affect their response to medications.

Pituitary gland A pea-sized gland that controls the majority of the endocrine glands in the body. Along with the hypothalamus and adrenal glands, the pituitary is part of the hypothalamic-pituitary-adrenal (HPA) axis, which is a central player in the body's stress management system.

Placebo A substance or treatment that does not contain an active (medicinal) ingredient, such as a sugar pill or a saline injection. In drug research, a placebo is used to demonstrate the effectiveness and tolerability of a new treatment. Placebos used in drug research are made to resemble the active medication, so the study subject and researcher don't know which treatment the subject is receiving. "Placebo-controlled trials" are conducted during new drug development because if the subject or researcher knows the subject is taking the study medication, that can influence how the treatment works. If a study subject experiences a benefit from taking a placebo, that benefit is called a placebo response.

Point prevalence The proportion of a population that has the condition at a specific point in time. For instance, a twelve-month prevalence refers to the number of people expected to have the condition in the next twelve months.

Polymorphism *Poly* means "multiple" and *-morph* means "forms." Gene polymorphism refers to how different forms of a gene can exist in a population and also in each person, since everyone has two copies of each gene.

Postpartum The twelve-month period following a birth.

Post-synaptic neuron The space between two neurons or between a neuron and a target cell is called the synaptic cleft. A post-synaptic neuron refers to the neuron that receives the chemical signal (neurotransmitter) after it has moved across the synaptic cleft. Neurotransmitters interact with receptors on the post-synaptic cell, and that interaction leads to a physiological effect if the neurotransmitter is an agonist or halts the passage of a message if the neurotransmitter is an antagonist.

Post-traumatic stress disorder (PTSD) A disorder that results from experiencing, witnessing, or being confronted with an event or events that involve actual or threatened death or serious injury, or a threat to the physical integrity of one's self or others. The individual's response to the traumatic event is to feel intense fear, helplessness, or horror. Patients experiencing PTSD have re-experiencing symptoms (re-living the event), avoid situations that remind them of the event, feel hyper-aroused (always keyed-up or on edge), and their beliefs and feelings change and often become negative.

Prefrontal cortex (PFC) The area of the brain located directly behind the forehead. The PFC is the executive of the brain, responsible for organizing, planning, thinking ahead, and critical thinking. It is also involved in other important cognitive functions, such as working memory (the ability to remember and use new information rapidly). Low levels of the neurotransmitters norepinephrine and dopamine in the PFC can cause an inability to feel intense emotions (reduced or blunted emotions), low motivation, and apathy, which may be related to depression but may also be a side effect of antidepressant medications that increase serotonin.

Premenstrual dysphoric disorder (PMDD) A psychiatric diagnosis characterized by severe mood swings, irritability, and other physical and emotional symptoms and associated functional impairment present in the days before the menstrual period begins. Approximately 5 percent of women suffer from PMDD.

Premenstrual syndrome (PMS) Mild mood changes that some woman experience in the days before their menstrual period begins that do not impair functioning. PMS is not a psychiatric disorder.

Presenteeism When an employee reports to work despite being sick but is incapable of completing their tasks in a timely, effective manner.

Pre-synaptic neuron The space between two neurons or between a neuron and a target cell is called the synaptic cleft. The pre-synaptic neuron refers to the terminal end of the neuron that releases the chemical signal (neurotransmitter) into the synaptic cleft in response to an electrical impulse.

Prevalence Lifetime prevalence is the proportion of people in a particular population found to be affected by a medical condition (such as depression). The prevalence is calculated by comparing the number of people found to have the condition with the total number of people studied and is usually expressed as a fraction, as a percentage, or as the number of cases per 10,000 or 100,000 people.

Product monograph A document developed by a regulatory agency (see also "regulatory agency") that describes all the critical information regarding an approved medication. It must contain the drug's indications, doses, side effects, and mechanism of action.

Pro-inflammatory cytokines (PICs) Inflammation promoting immune proteins released by activated microglia in the brain. In chronically depressed brains, increased PICs are associated with chronically high concentrations of cortisol and can cause damage to neurons.

Pseudo-dementia Derived from the prefix "pseudo-" (meaning false), it literally means false dementia. One of the most common and persistent symptoms of depression is cognitive impairment, which may include difficulty with concentration and memory, slowed thinking, and impaired organizational and planning skills. However, because these symptoms are also commonly associated with dementia, patients struggling with severe depression may become concerned that they are actually developing dementia. This is a particularly common concern for elderly depressed patients. However, if the cognitive symptoms are determined to be associated with the depression only, the term pseudo-dementia may be applied.

Psychomotor impairment The experience of being mentally or physically slowed down. This is a very prominent feature of depression.

Psychosis Severe psychiatric symptoms associated with thinking that is so impaired that an individual is unable to separate illness from reality. Psychotic symptoms include delusions (false beliefs) and hallucinations (false sensory experiences) and many other symptoms. Psychosis is often associated with a loss of insight (a failure to recognize that the symptoms are a product of the mind and are related to illness). Psychosis is a cardinal feature of schizophrenia and is often associated with bipolar mania. It can also be a feature of severe depression, referred to as psychotic depression. When an individual is experiencing psychosis, they may be referred to as psychotic.

Psychotic Experiencing psychotic symptoms (see also "psychosis"). When an individual is experiencing psychosis, they may be referred to as psychotic.

Puberty A period of sexual maturation that usually occurs between the ages of ten and sixteen. When sexually mature, one is capable of reproduction. During this time, hormone-induced physical changes (e.g., breast enlargement, growth of pubic hair) and emotional changes occur.

Receptor agonist Receptor agonists are substances that activate a receptor, leading to a physiological response.

Receptor antagonist Receptor antagonists are substances that work against, oppose, block, or inhibit a receptor. When a receptor is antagonized, it is unable to cause a physiological effect.

Receptor down-regulation A reduction in the number of receptors present on a neuron. This occurs when there is an increase or accumulation of available neurotransmitters, such as serotonin or norepinephrine, in the synaptic cleft.

Recovery Sustained remission of symptoms and return to functioning. The timeline for recovery is still debated. Commonly, one is considered recovered from depression if they remain asymptomatic and are functioning well for three to six months.

Recurrence A new episode of depression after a complete recovery from a previous episode.

Refractory A disease, disorder, or condition that is unyielding to the treatment being used. This does not label the illness as untreatable but rather that it might just require an alternative treatment plan.

Regulatory agency A government agency responsible for protecting consumers by regulating the production, marketing, and sale of medications. Health Canada, the FDA, and EMA are examples of government regulatory agencies, which assess the safety and efficacy of new treatments before granting approval for their production and distribution. These agencies also monitor the quality of existing medications and gather information about the safety of treatments after they are available to consumers. Regulators determine the official indication(s) and a product monograph for the medications they approve.

Relapse A return of depression symptoms before a depression has fully resolved.

Remission A state of minimal to no symptoms and a return to normal functioning.

Residual symptoms Symptoms that persist after the core depression symptoms, such as depressed mood and anhedonia, have resolved. The most common residual symptoms include fatigue, insomnia, and cognitive symptoms. There is clear evidence that the presence of residual symptoms is the most powerful predictor of relapse; thus, every single depression symptom should be treated to prevent depression from returning.

Reversed vegetative symptoms Common symptoms of atypical depression, including hypersomnia (excessive daytime sleepiness, need for sleep, or time spent in bed) and increased appetite, often associated with weight gain. These symptoms are referred to as "reversed" because they are the opposite of the usual vegetative symptoms of depression, namely insomnia and decreased appetite, as well as a reduction in sexual interest and functioning.

Schizophrenia A chronic psychotic disorder that alters an individual's thinking, emotions, and behaviour. Schizophrenia is characterized by psychotic symptoms, such as hallucinations and delusions, and negative symptoms, which include diminished emotional expression (flat affect), feelings of indifference, and lack of motivation. Schizophrenia also affects cognition; for instance, difficulty with focus and making decisions.

Seasonal depression Refers to recurrent depression episodes that reliably occur and fully resolve at a particular time of the year. Most often commences in the fall or winter and resolves with the "return of the sun" in the spring or summer.

Serotonin A neurotransmitter (chemical messenger). It is one of the most important neurotransmitters linked to depression and a target of many antidepressant medications.

Serotonin receptor agonist Substances that activate serotonin receptors, leading to a conformational change in the receptor (a change in the structure of the receptor) and causes a physiological effect.

Serotonin receptor antagonist Substances that block the usual physiological effect of a serotonin receptor.

Serotonin syndrome A syndrome caused by toxic concentrations of serotonin in the blood. Serotonin syndrome occurs rarely and is highly unlikely to occur in association with antidepressants, even when taken at high doses. The cluster of symptoms that constitute this syndrome can range from mild (diarrhea, agitation, shivering, overactive reflexes) to severe and life-threatening (fever, high temperature, rigid muscles, seizures) and must be diagnosed and treated promptly.

Serotonin transporter Transports serotonin from the synaptic cleft back into the presynaptic neuron.

Sleep hygiene Practices and behaviours that help an individual to achieve quality (healthier) sleep. Good sleep hygiene improves the likelihood of experiencing restorative sleep.

Social anxiety disorder (SAD) An anxiety disorder characterized by a marked fear of performance or social interaction situations, excessive fear of scrutiny or negative evaluation, or a fear of acting in a way (or showing anxiety symptoms) that will be humiliating or embarrassing, which results in avoidance or enduring the situation with distress.

Somatic From the Greek *soma* (meaning "body"). In relation to the body. The physical part of the human body, versus the mind.

Somatic symptoms Refers to the physical symptoms of a disorder, such as pain, nausea, vomiting, sweating, as opposed to emotional symptoms.

Stigma According to *Merriam-Webster*, a mark of shame or discredit. Stigma usually reflects a stereotype of inferiority. Stigma and discrimination are not the same thing. Discrimination is unfair treatment due to a person's identity, whether it is due to race, ethnicity, age, sexual orientation, illness or disability, or other factors. Regarding mental illness, stigma is the negative stereotype or belief that people who have a mental illness are, among other things, dangerous, weird, "messed up," or untrustworthy. Discrimination is the behaviour that results from these negative stereotypes.

Stress A circumstance, condition, or situation that disrupts an individual's normal physical or emotional functioning. What is considered stressful and how we react to stress differs from person to person and is greatly influenced by an individual's mental and physical health. Stress can be necessary and worthwhile; for instance, while in school, we need some stress to encourage us to complete our work in a timely manner. However, severe and prolonged stress can result in mental and physical illness.

Suicidal ideation Suicidal thoughts or ideas. Suicidal ideation can be passive—where there is a wish for death, but no specific suicidal plan is in place—or active, an implicit wish to die along with a plan of how to act on the wish.

Synapse The meeting point between two neurons or a neuron and a target cell.

Synaptogenesis The development of new connections, or synapses, between neurons.

Taper When a physician is reducing or discontinuing a patient's medication, they usually do so in a gradual manner. This gradual reduction of dose is referred to as tapering. Weaning a patient off a certain medication is done in this way to minimize the risk of discontinuation symptoms, which are unpleasant symptoms associated with rapidly discontinuing some medications.

Tardive dyskinesia (TD) A serious, sometimes irreversible, movement disorder brought on by blocking dopamine in specific brain areas. This side effect is most commonly associated with conventional antipsychotics, but all antipsychotics carry some risk of TD.

Thalamus A brain structure that receives all sensory information (sight, touch, hearing, and taste) which is then forwarded to other brain structures, where it is further analyzed and an appropriate response is initiated.

Therapeutic relationship The relationship between a professional from any field of medicine and the patient. A successful therapeutic relationship involves shared responsibilities and includes creating and maintaining appropriate and respectful boundaries, developing trust, and empathy. This relationship is invaluable for the success of a patient's treatment.

Titration A term used to define the process by which a physician adjusts the dose of a medication in order to achieve the desired effect. The doctor titrates the dose to find the amount that is both effective and well tolerated.

Treatment-resistant depression (TRD) When depression symptoms don't improve following an adequate trial (e.g., an optimized dose for four to six weeks) of at least two different antidepressants, the depression is considered treatment resistant.

Tyramine An amino acid involved in blood pressure regulation. It occurs naturally in the body, as well as being found in certain medications and food (e.g., beer, wine, aged cheeses, and cured meat). Tyramine is broken down by the enzyme monoamine oxidase (MAO). Patients prescribed a monoamine oxidase inhibitor (MAOI) antidepressant are unable to properly break down tyramine, leading to its accumulation, which can cause extremely high blood pressure, called a hypertensive crisis. To avoid a hypertensive crisis, patients who are prescribed MAOIs must avoid ingesting anything that may contain significant amounts of tyramine.

Vegetative symptoms Vegetative functions are processes that the body carries out in order to maintain life: sleeping, eating, bowel/bladder function, menstruation, and sexual drive. Depression alters the usual patterns of these activities, resulting in vegetative symptoms of the disorder: sleep disturbances (early awakening), increased appetite, constipation, loss of periods, and reduced libido.

References

Chapter 1

American Psychiatric Association. *Diagnostic and statistical manual of mental disorders, fifth edition*. Arlington, VA: American Psychiatric Association, 2013.

Bromet, E., et al. "Cross-national epidemiology of DSM-IV major depressive episode." *BioMedCentral Med* 9 (2011 Jul 26): 90.

Global Burden of Disease 2013 Collaborators. "Global, regional, and national incidence, prevalence, and years lived with disability for 301 acute and chronic diseases and injuries in 188 countries, 1990–2013: a systematic analysis for the Global Burden of Disease Study 2013." *Lancet* 386 (2015): 743–800.

Greenberg P.E., et al. "The economic burden of adults with major depressive disorder in the United States (2005 and 2010)." *J Clin Psychiatry* 76 2 (2015): 155–62.

Greenberg, P.E., et al. "The economic burden of depression in the United States: how did it change between 1990 and 2000?" *J Clin Psychiatry* 64 12 (2003): 1465–75.

Kessler, R.C., et al. "Lifetime and 12-month prevalence of DSM-III-R psychiatric disorders in the United States. Results from the National Comorbidity Survey." *Arch Gen Psychiatry* 51 1 (1994): 8–19.

Key substance use and mental health indicators in the United States: results from the 2016 National Survey on Drug Use and Health Substance Abuse and Mental Health Services Administration. Rockville, MD: Center for Behavioral Health Statistics and Quality, Substance Abuse and Mental Health Services Administration, 2017. Retrieved from https://www.samhsa.gov/data/.

Lojko, D., Rybakowski, J.K. "Atypical depression: current perspectives." *Neuropsychiatr Dis Treat* 13 (2017 Sep 20): 2447–56.
Pae, C.U., Tharwani, H., et al. "CNS Drugs. Atypical depression: a comprehensive review." *CNS Drugs* 23 12 (2009 Dec): 1023–37.
Parker, G. "Atypical depression: a valid subtype?" *J Clin Psychiatry* 68 3 (2007 Mar): e08.
Parker, G. "Classifying depression: should paradigms lost be regained?" *Am J Psychiatry* 157 (2000): 1195–203.
Parker, G., Fink, M., et al. "Issues for DSM-5: whither melancholia? The case for its classification as a distinct mood disorder." *Am J Psychiatry* 167 7 (2010 Jul): 745–7.
Parker, G., Fletcher, K., et al. "Inching toward Bethlehem: mapping melancholia." *J Affect Disord* 123 1–3 (2010 Jun): 291–8.
Parker, G., Roy, K., et al. "Atypical depression: a reappraisal." *Am J Psychiatry* 159 9 (2002 Sep): 1470–9.
Parker, G., Roy K., et al. "The nature of bipolar depression: implications for the definition of melancholia." *J Affect Disord* 59 3 (2000 Sep): 217–24.
Patten, S.B., Williams, J.V., Lavorato, D.H., Wang, J.L., McDonald, K., Bulloch, A.G. "Canadian Community Health Survey–Mental Health (CCHS-MH)." *Can J Psychiatry* 60 1 (2015 Jan): 23–30.
Perugi, G., Fornaro, M., Akiskal, H.S. "Are atypical depression, borderline personality disorder and bipolar II disorder overlapping manifestations of a common cyclothymic diathesis?" *World J Psychiatry* 10 1 (2011 Feb): 45–51.
Silverstein, B., Angst, J. "Evidence for broadening criteria for atypical depression which may define a reactive depressive disorder." *Psychiatry J* (2015): 575931.
Sramek, J.J., Murphy, M.F., Cutler, N.R. "Sex differences in the psychopharmacological treatment of depression." *Dialogues Clin Neurosci* 18 (2016): 447–57.
Stewart, J. "Atypical depression: history and future." *Psychiatr Ann* 44 12 (2014): 557–62.
Stewart, W.F., Ricci, J.A., Chee, E., et al. "Cost of lost productive work time among US workers with depression." *JAMA* 289 23 (2003): 3135–44.
Taylor, M.A., Fink, M. "Restoring melancholia in the classification of mood disorders." *J Affect Disord* 105 1–3 (2008 Jan): 1–14.
Thase, M.E. "Recognition and diagnosis of atypical depression." *J Clin Psychiatry* 68 Suppl 8 (2007): 11–6.

Chapter 2

Aranda, M.P., Chae, D.H., Lincoln, K.D., Taylor, R.J., Woodward, A.T., Chatters, L.M. "Demographic correlates of DSM-IV major depressive disorder among older African Americans, Black Caribbeans, and non-Hispanic

Whites: results from the National Survey of American Life." *Int J Geriatr Psychiatry* 27 9 (2012 Sep): 940–7.

Bagdy, R.M., Quilty, L.C., Ryder, A.C. "Personality and depression." *La Rev De Psychiatr* 53 1 (2008): 14–25.

Balzer, B.W., Duke, S.A., Hawke, C.I., Steinbeck, K.S. "The effects of estradiol on mood and behavior in human female adolescents: a systematic review." *Eur J Pediatr* 174 (2015): 289–98.

Birmaher, B., Dahl, R.E., Williamson, D.E., et al. "Growth hormone secretion in children and adolescents at high risk for major depressive disorder." *Arch Gen Psychiatry* 57 (2000): 867–72.

Burcusa, S.L., Lacono, W.G. "Risk for recurrence in depression." *Clin Psychol Rev* 27 8 (2007): 959–85.

Byers, A.L., Yaffe, K., Covinsky, K.E., Friedman, M.B., Bruce, M.L. "High occurrence of mood and anxiety disorders among older adults: the National Comorbidity Survey replication." *Arch Gen Psychiatry* 67 (2010): 489–96.

Caspi, A., Sugden, K., Moffitt, T.E., et al. "Influence of life stress on depression: moderation by a polymorphism in the 5-HTT gene." *Science* 301 5631 (2003): 386–9.

Fanous, A.H., Neale, M.C., Aggen, S.H., Kendler, K.S. "A longitudinal study of personality and major depression in a population-based sample of male twins." *Psychol Med* 37 (2007): 1163–72.

Ferrari, A.J., Charlson, F.J., et al. "Burden of depressive disorders by country, sex, age, and year: findings from the global burden of disease study 2010." *PLoS Med* 10 11 (2013 Nov): e1001547.

Fischer, M. "Psychoses in the offspring of schizophrenic monozygotic twins and their normal co-twins." *Br J Psychiatry* 118 (1971): 43–52.

Foley, D.L., Neale, M.C., Gardner, C.O., et al. "Major depression and associated impairment: same or different genetic and environmental risk factors?" *Am J Psychiatry* 160 12 (2003 Dec): 2128–33.

Fredriksen-Goldsen, K.I., Kim, H.J., et al. "The cascading effects of marginalization and pathways of resilience in attaining good health among LGBT older adults." *Gerontologist* 57 Suppl 1 (2017 Feb): S72–83.

Galvao, T.F., Silva, M.T., et al. "Pubertal timing in girls and depression: A systematic review." *J Affect Disord* 155 (2014): 13–19.

González, H.M., Vega, W.A., et al. "Depression care in the United States too little for too few." *Arch Gen Psychiatry* 67 1 (2010): 37–46.

Gressier, F., Calati, R., Serretti, A. "5-HTTLPR and gender differences in affective disorders: a systematic review." *J Affect Disord* 190 (2016): 193–207.

Griffith, J.W., Zinbarg, R.E., et al. "Neuroticism as a common dimension in the internalizing disorders." *Psychol Med* 40 7 (2010): 1125–36.

Haber, M.G., Cohen, E.J.L., Lucas, E.T., Baltes, B.B. "The relationship between self-reported received and perceived social support: a meta-analytic review." *Am J Commun Psychol* 39 (2007): 133–44.

Herek, G.M. "A nuanced view of stigma for understanding and addressing sexual and gender minority health disparities." *LGBT Health* 3 6 (2016 Dec): 397–9.

Herek, G.M., Garnets, L.D. "Sexual orientation and mental health." *Annu Rev Clin Psychol* 3 (2007): 353–75.

Herek, G.M., McLemore, K.A. "Sexual prejudice." *Annu Rev Psychol* 64 (2013): 309–33.

Hill, J., Holcombe, C., et al. "Predictors of onset of depression and anxiety in the year after diagnosis of breast cancer." *Psychol Med* 41 7 (2011): 1429–36.

Hyde, J.S., Mezulis, A.H., Abramson, L.Y. "The ABCs of depression: integrating affective, biological, and cognitive models to explain the emergence of the gender difference in depression." *Psychol Rev* 115 (2008): 291–313.

Janzen, B., Karunanayake, C., Rennie, D., Katapally, T., et al. "Racial discrimination and depression among on-reserve First Nations people in rural Saskatchewan." *Can J Public Health* 108 5–6 (2018 Jan 22): e482–7.

Kendler, K.S., Gardner, C.O., Prescott, C.A. "Personality and the experience of environmental adversity." *Psychol Med* 33 7 (2003 Oct): 1193–202.

Kendler, K.S., Gatz, M., Gardner, C.O., Pedersen, N.L. "Personality and major depression: a Swedish longitudinal, population-based twin study." *Arch Gen Psychiatry* 63 (2006 Oct): 1113–20.

Kendler, K.S., Myers, J., Prescott, C.A. "Sex differences in the relationship between social support and risk for major depression: a longitudinal study of opposite-sex twin pairs." *Am J Psychiatry* 162 (2005): 250–6.

Kendler, K.S., Ohlsson, H., et al. "The genetic epidemiology of treated major depression in Sweden." *Am J Psychiatry* (2018 Jul 19): appiajp201817111251.

Kuehner, C. "Gender differences in unipolar depression: an update of epidemiological findings and possible explanations." *Acta Psychiatr Scand* 108 (2003): 163–74.

Kuehner, C. "Why is depression more common among women than among men?" *Lancet Psychiatry* 4 (2017): 146–58.

Lewinsohn, P.M., Rohde, P., Seeley, J.R., Klein, D.N., Gotlib, I.H. "Natural course of adolescent major depressive disorder in a community sample: predictors of recurrence in young adults." *Am J Psychiatry* 157 10 (2000 Oct): 1584–91.

Lincoln, K.D. "Personality, negative interactions and mental health." *Soc Serv Rev* 82 2 (2008 Jun 1): 223–51.

Luppa, M., Sikorski, C., Luck, T., et al. "Age- and gender-specific prevalence of depression in latest-life—systematic review and meta-analysis." *J Affect Disord* 136 (2012): 212–21.

Martel, M.M. "Sexual selection and sex differences in the prevalence of childhood externalizing and adolescent internalizing disorders." *Psychol Bull* 139 (2013): 1221–59.

McCrae, R.R., Costa Jr., P.T. "Personality trait structure as a human universal." *Am Psychol* 52 5 (1997 May): 509–16.

McEwen, B.S., Akama, K.T., et al. "Estrogen effects on the brain: actions beyond the hypothalamus via novel mechanisms." *Behav Neurosci* 126 (2012): 4–16.

Munafò, M.R. "The serotonin transporter gene and depression." *Depress Anxiety* 11 (2012 Nov 29): 915–7.

National Women's Law Center. "Health care refusals harm patients: the threat to LGBT people and individuals living with HIV/AIDS." (2014) Retrieved from https://nwlc.org/wp-content/uploads/2015/08/lgbt_refusals_factsheet_05-09-14.pdf

Noteboom, A., Beekman, A., Vogelzangs, N., Penninx, B. "Personality and social support as predictors of first and recurrent episodes of depression." *J Affect Disord* 190 (2016 Jan 15): 156–61.

Office of Disease Prevention and Health Promotion. "Lesbian, gay, bisexual, and transgender health." (2016) Retrieved from https://www.healthypeople.gov/2020/topics-objectives/topic/lesbian-gay-bisexual-and-transgender-health.

Papakostas, G.I. "Cognitive symptoms in patients with major depressive disorder and their implications for clinical practice." *J Clin Psychiatry* 75 1 (2014 Jan): 8–14.

Rao, S., Mason, C.D. "Minority stress and well-being under anti-sodomy legislation in India." *Psychol of Sexual Orient and Gender Div* 5 4 (2018): 432–44.

Ripke, S., Wray, N.R., Lewis, C.M., et al. "A mega-analysis of genome-wide association studies for major depressive disorder." *Mol Psychiatry* 18 (2013): 497–511.

Sarason, I.G., Sarason, B.R., Shearin, E.N., Pierce, G.R. "A brief measure of social support: practical and theoretical implications." *J Soc Pers Relatsh* 4 (1987): 497–510.

Sharpley, C.F., Palanisamy, S.K., et al. "An update on the interaction between the serotonin transporter promoter variant (5-HTTLPR), stress and depression, plus an exploration of non-confirming findings." *Behav Brain Res* 273 (2014): 89–105.

Steiner, M., Dunn, E., Born, L. "Hormones and mood: from menarche to menopause and beyond." *J Affect Disord* 74 (2003): 67–83.

Stice, E., Ragan, J., Randall, P. "Prospective relations between social support and depression: differential direction of effects for parent and peer support?" *J Abnorm Psychol* 113 (2004): 155–9.

Streed, C. "Association between gender minority status and self-reported physical and mental health in the United States." *JAMA Intern Med* 177 8 (2017): 1210–2.

Sullivan, P.F., Neale, M.C., Kendler, K.S. "Genetic epidemiology of major depression: review and meta-analysis." *Am J Psychiatry* 157 (2000): 1552–62.

Travis, L.A., Lyness, J.M., et al. "Social support, depression, and functional disability in older adult primary-care patients." *Am J Geriatr Psychiatry* 12 3 (2004): 265–71.

Uher, R., McGuffin, P. "The moderation by the serotonin transporter gene of environmental adversity in the etiology of depression: 2009 update." *Mol Psychiatry* 15 (2010): 18–22.

Williams, D.R., González, H.M., Neighbors, H. "Prevalence and distribution of major depressive disorder in African Americans, Caribbean Blacks, and non-Hispanic Whites results from the National Survey of American Life." *Arch Gen Psychiatry* 64 3 (2007): 305–15.

Chapter 3

Bredy, T.W., Grant, R.J., Champagne, D.L., Meaney, M.J. "Maternal care influences neuronal survival in the hippocampus of the rat." *Eur J Neurosci* 18 10 (2003 Nov): 2903–9.

Champagne, F., Diorio, J., Sharma, S., Meaney, M.J. "Naturally occurring variations in maternal behavior in the rat are associated with differences in estrogen-inducible central oxytocin receptors." *Proc Natl Acad Sci USA* 98 22 (2001 Oct 23): 12736–41.

Champagne, F., Meaney, M.J. "Like mother, like daughter: evidence for non-genomic transmission of parental behavior and stress responsivity." *Prog Brain Res* 133 (2001): 287–302.

Champagne, M., Virbel, J., et al. "Impact of right hemispheric damage on a hierarchy of complexity evidenced in young normal subjects." *Brain Cogn* 53 2 (2003 Nov): 152–7.

Chen, Y., Baram, T.Z. "Toward understanding how early-life stress reprograms cognitive and emotional brain networks." *Neuropsychopharmacol* 41 1 (2016 Jan): 197–206.

Danese, A., Moffitt, T.E., et al. "Adverse childhood experiences and adult risk factors for age-related disease: depression, inflammation, and clustering of metabolic risk markers." *Arch Pediatr Adolesc Med* 163 12 (2009 Dec): 1135–43.

Danese, A., Moffitt, T.E., et al. "Dysfunctional nurturing behavior in rat dams with limited access to nesting material: a clinically relevant model for early-life stress." *Neuroscience* 154 3 (2008 Jun 26): 1132–42.

Lucassen, P.J., Naninck, E.F., et al. "Perinatal programming of adult hippocampal structure and function; emerging roles of stress, nutrition and epigenetics." *Trends Neurosci* 36 11 (2013 Nov): 621–31.

Lucassen, P.J., Oomen, C.A., et al. "Regulation of adult neurogenesis and plasticity by (early) stress, glucocorticoids, and inflammation." *Cold Spring Harb Perspect Biol* 7 9 (2015 Sep 1): a021303.

Lucassen, P.J., Pruessner, J., et al. "Neuropathology of stress." *Acta Neuropathol* 127 1 (2014 Jan): 109–35.

Molet, J., Maras, P.M., Avishai-Eliner, S., Baram, T.Z. "Naturalistic rodent models of chronic early-life stress." *Dev Psychobiol* 127 1 (2014 Dec): 1675–88.

Naninck, E.F., Hoeijmakers, L., et al. "Chronic early life stress alters developmental and adult neurogenesis and impairs cognitive function in mice." *Hippocampus* 25 3 (2015 Mar): 309–28.

Pan, P., Fleming, A.S., Lawson, D., et al. "Within- and between-litter maternal care alter behavior and gene regulation in female offspring." *Behav Neurosci* 128 6 (2014 Dec): 736–48.

Singh-Taylor, A., Korosi, A., Molet, J., et al. "Synaptic rewiring of stress-sensitive neurons by early-life experience: a mechanism for resilience?" *Neurobiol of Stress* 1 (2014): 109–15.

Yam, K.Y., Naninck, E.F., Schmidt, M.V., et al. "Early-life adversity programs emotional functions and the neuroendocrine stress system: the contribution of nutrition, metabolic hormones and epigenetic mechanisms." *Stress* 18 3 (2015): 328–42.

Chapter 4

Alesci, S., et al. "Major depression is associated with significant diurnal elevations in plasma interleukin-6 levels, a shift of its circadian rhythm, and loss of physiological complexity in its secretion: clinical implications." *J Clin Endocrinol Metab* 90 5 (2005): 2522–30.

Anacker, C., Zunszain, P.A., Carvalho, L.A., Pariante, C.M. "The glucocorticoid receptor: Pivot of depression and of antidepressant treatment?" *Psychoneuroendocrinology* 36 (2011): 415–25.

Bauer, M., Teixeira, A. "Annals of the New York Academy of Sciences special issue: neuroimmodulation in health and disease review inflammation in psychiatric disorders: what comes first?" *Ann NY Acad Sci* ISSN 0077-8923.

Bremner, J.D., et al. "Hippocampal volume reduction in major depression." *Am J Psychiatry* 157 1 (2000): 115–18.

Burke, H.M., Davis, M.C., Otte, C., Mohr, D.C. "Depression and cortisol responses to psychological stress: a meta-analysis." *Psychoneuroendocrinology* 30 (2005): 846–56.

Chen, Z.Y., Jing, D., Bath, K.G., et al. "Genetic variant BDNF (Val66Met) polymorphism alters anxiety-related behavior." *Science* 314 5796 (2006): 140–3.

Cohen, S., et al. "Chronic stress, glucocorticoid receptor resistance, inflammation, and disease risk." *Proc Natl Acad Sci USA* 109: 5995–9.

Duman, R.S., Monteggia, L.M. "A neurotrophic model for stress-related mood disorders." *Biol Psychiatry* 59 12 (2006): 1116–27.

Duric, V., McCarson, K.E. "Hippocampal neurokinin-1 receptor and brain-derived neurotrophic factor gene expression is decreased in rat models of pain and stress." *Neuroscience* 133 4 (2005): 999–1006.

Hannibal, K.E., Bishop, M.D. "Chronic stress, cortisol dysfunction, and pain: a psychoneuroendocrine rationale for stress management in pain rehabilitation." *Phys Ther* 94 12 (2014 Dec): 1816–25.

Heim, C., Ehlert, U., Hellhammer, D.H. "The potential role of hypocortisolism in the pathophysiology of stress-related bodily disorders." *Psychoneuroendocrinology* 25 (2000): 1–35.

Herbert J., Goodyer, I.M., Grossman, A.B., et al. "Do corticosteroids damage the brain?" *J. Neuroendocrinol* 18 (2006): 393–411.

Horowitz, M.A., Zunszain, P.A. "Neuroimmune and neuroendocrine abnormalities in depression: two sides of the same coin." *Ann NY Acad Sci* 1351 (2015 Sep): 68–79.

Juruena, M.F., Cleare, A.J., Papadopoulos, A.S., et al. "Different responses to dexamethasone and prednisolone in the same depressed patients." *Psychopharmacology (Berl)* 189 (2006): 225–35.

Kaymak, S.U., et al. "Hippocampus, glucocorticoids and neurocognitive functions in patients with first-episode major depressive disorders." *Eur Arch Psychiatry Clin Neurosci* 260 (2010): 217–23.

Miller, A.H., Maletic, V., Raison, C.L. "Inflammation and its discontents: the role of cytokines in the pathophysiology of major depression." *Biol Psychiatry* 65 9 (2009): 732–41.

Miller, G.E., et al. "A functional genomic fingerprint of chronic stress in humans: blunted glucocorticoid and increased NF-kappaB signaling." *Biol Psychiatry* 64 (2012): 266–72.

Mitoma, M., Yoshimura, R., Sugita, A., et al. "Stress at work alters serum brain-derived neurotrophic factor (BDNF) levels and plasma 3-methoxy-4-hydroxyphenylglycol (MHPG) levels in healthy volunteers: BDNF and MHPG as possible biological markers of mental stress?" *Prog Neuropsychopharmacol Biol Psychiatry* 32 3 (2008): 679–85.

Ongür, D., Drevets, W.C, Price, J.L. "Glial reduction in the subgenual prefrontal cortex in mood disorders." *Proc Natl Acad Sci USA* 95 (1998): 13290–5.

Pace, T.W., et al. "Increased stress-induced inflammatory responses in male patients with major depression and increased early life stress." *Am J Psychiatry* 163 9 (2006): 1630–3.

Pace, T.W., Hu, F., Miller, A.H. "Cytokine-effects on glucocorticoid receptor function: relevance to glucocorticoid resistance and the pathophysiology and treatment of major depression." *Brain Behav Immun* 21 (2007 Jan): 9–19.

Pariante, C.M. "Risk factors for development of depression and psychosis. Glucocorticoid receptors and pituitary implications for treatment with antidepressant and glucocorticoids." *Ann NY Acad Sci* 1179 (2009): 144–52.

Pariante, C.M., Miller, A.H. "Glucocorticoid receptors in major depression: relevance to pathophysiology and treatment." *Biol Psychiatry* 49 (2001): 391–404.

Post, R.M. "Kindling and sensitization as models for affective episode recurrence, cyclicity, and tolerance phenomena." *Neurosci Biobehav Rev* 31 6 (2007): 858–73.

Raison, C.L., Miller, A.H. "When not enough is too much: the role of insufficient glucocorticoid signaling in the pathophysiology of stress-related disorders." *Am J Psychiatry* 160 (2003 Sep): 1554–65.

Rajkowska, G., Miguel-Hidalgo, J.J. "Gliogenesis and glial pathology in depression." *CNS Neurol Disord Drug Targets* 6 (2007): 219–33.

Rajkowska, G., Miguel-Hidalgo, J.J, et al. "Morphometric evidence for neuronal and glial prefrontal cell pathology in major depression." *Biol Psychiatry* 45 (1999): 1085-98.

Schüle, C., Zill, P., Baghai, T.C., et al. "Brain-derived neurotrophic factor Val-66Met polymorphism and dexamethasone/CRH test results in depressed patients." *Psychoneuroendocrinology* 31 8 (2006): 1019–25.

Sheline, Y.I., et al. "Depression duration but not age predicts hippocampal volume loss in medically healthy women with recurrent major depression." *J Neurosci* 19 (1999): 5034–43.

Sheline, Y.I., et al. "Hippocampal atrophy in recurrent major depression." *Proc Natl Acad Sci USA* 93 (1996): 3908–13.

Sheline, Y.I., et al. "Untreated depression and hippocampal volume loss." *Am J Psychiatry* 160 (2003): 1516–8.

Si, X., et al. "Age-dependent reductions in the level of glial fibrillary acidic protein in the prefrontal cortex in major depression." *Neuropsychopharmacol* 29 (2004): 2088–96.

Tong, L., Balazs, R., Soiampornkul, R., et al. "Interleukin-1 beta impairs brain derived neurotrophic factor-induced signal transduction." *Neurobiol Aging* 29 9 (2008): 1380–93.

van Praag, H., et al. "Functional neurogenesis in the adult hippocampus." *Nature* 415 6875 (2002): 1030–4.

Videbech, P., Ravnkilde, B. "Hippocampal volume and depression: a meta-analysis of MRI studies." *Am J Psychiatry* 161 (2004): 1957–66.

Chapter 5

Akbaraly, T.N., Kivimäki, M., Brunner, E.J., et al. "Association between metabolic syndrome and depressive symptoms in middle-aged adults: results from the Whitehall II study." *Diabet Care* 32 (2009): 499–504.

Ali, S., Stone, M., Peters, J., et al. "The prevalence of co-morbid depression in adults with type 2 diabetes: a systematic review and meta-analysis." *Diabet Med* 23 11 (2006 Nov): 1165–73.

Anderson, R.J., Freedland, K.E., Clouse, R.E., Lustman, P.J. "The prevalence of comorbid depression in adults with diabetes: a meta-analysis." *Diabet Care* 24 6 (2001 Jun): 1069–78.

Aragonès, E., Piñol, J.L., Labad, A. "Depression and physical comorbidity in primary care." *J Psychosom Res* 63 2 (2007): 107–11.

Arsenault, B.J., Earnest, C.P., Després, J.P., et al. "Obesity, coffee consumption and CRP levels in postmenopausal overweight/obese women: importance of hormone replacement therapy use." *Eur J Clin Nutr* 63 (2009): 1419–24.

Bankier, B., Januzzi, J.L., Littman, A.B. "The high prevalence of multiple psychiatric disorders in stable outpatients with coronary heart disease." *Psychosom Med* 66 5 (2004): 645–50.

Barth, J., Schumacher, M., Herrmann-Lingen, C. "Depression as a risk factor for mortality in patients with coronary heart disease: a meta-analysis." *Psychosom Med* 66 (2004 Nov–Dec): 802–13.

Caneo, C., Marston, L., Bellón, J.Á., King, M. "Examining the relationship between physical illness and depression: is there a difference between inflammatory and non-inflammatory diseases? A cohort study." *Gen Hosp Psychiatry* 43 (2016): 71–7.

Colditz, G.A., Willett, W.C., Rotnitzky, A., Manson, J.E. "Weight gain as a risk factor for clinical diabetes mellitus in women." *Ann Intern Med* 122 (1995 Apr 1): 481–6.

de Groot, M., Anderson, R., et al. "Association of depression and diabetes complications: a meta-analysis." *Psychosom Med* 63 4 (2001 Jul–Aug): 619–30.

Dowlati, Y., Herrmann, N., Swardfager, W., et al. "Efficacy and tolerability of antidepressants for treatment of depression in coronary artery disease: a meta-analysis." *Can J Psychiatry* 55 2 (2010 Feb): 91–9.

Dowlati, Y., Herrmann, N., Swardfager, W., et al. "A meta-analysis of cytokines in major depression." *Biol Psychiatry* 67 (2010): 446–57.

Egede, L.E. "Diabetes, major depression, and functional disability among U.S. adults." *Diabet Care* 27 2 (2004 Feb): 421–8.

Egede, L.E. "Medical cost of depression and diabetes." In Katon, W., Maj, M., Sartorius, N., eds. *Depression and diabetes.* Hoboken, NJ: Wiley Blackwell, 2010: 63–79.

Everson-Rose, S.A., Lewis, T.T., Karavolos, K., et al. "Depressive symptoms and increased visceral fat in middle-aged women." *Psychosom Med* 71 (2009): 410–6.

Fangauf, S.V., Herbeck Belnap, B., Meyer, T., et al. "Associations of NT-proBNP and parameters of mental health in depressed coronary artery disease patients." *Psychoneuroendocrinology* 96 (2018 Oct): 188–94.

Flegal, K.M. "Trends in obesity among adults in the United States, 2005 to 2014." *JAMA* 27 2 (2016 Jun 7): 2284–91.

Frasure-Smith, N., Lespérance, F. "Depression and cardiac risk: present status and future directions." *Postgrad Med J* 86 1014 (2010 Apr): 193–6.

Hales, C.M, et al. "Prevalence of obesity among adults and youth: United States, 2015–2016." *NCHS Data Brief* 288 (2017 Oct). https://www.cdc.gov/nchs/data/databriefs/db288.pdf.

Hedley, A.A., Ogden, C.L., Johnson, C.L., et al. "Prevalence of overweight and obesity among US children, adolescents, and adults, 1999–2002." *JAMA* 291 (2004): 2847–50.

Holt, R.I., de Groot, M., Lucki, I., et al. "NIDDK international conference report on diabetes and depression: current understanding and future directions." *Diabet Care* 37 8 (2014 Aug): 2067–77.

Howren, M.B., Lamkin, D.M., Suls, J. "Associations of depression with C-reactive protein, IL-1, and IL-6: a metaanalysis." *Psychosom Med* 71 (2009): 171–86.

Hubert, H.B., Feinleib, M., McNamara, P.M., Castelli, W.P. "Obesity as an independent risk factor for cardiovascular disease: a 26-year follow-up of participants in the Framingham Heart Study." *Circulation* 67 (1983): 968–77.

Katon, W.J. "Clinical and health services relationships between major depression, depressive symptoms, and general medical illness." *Biol Psychiatry* 54 3 (2003): 216–26.

Katon, W.J. "Epidemiology and treatment of depression in patients with chronic medical illness." *Dialogues Clin Neurosci* 13 1 (2011): 7–23.

Khandaker, G.M., Pearson, R.M., Zammit, S., et al. "Association of serum interleukin 6 and C-reactive protein in childhood with depression and psychosis in young adult life: a population-based longitudinal study." *JAMA Psychiat* 71 10 (2014): 1121–8.

Kim, B.S., Lee, H.J., Shin, H.S., et al. "Presence and severity of coronary artery disease and changes in B-type natriuretic peptide levels in patients with a normal systolic function." *Transl Res* 148 4 (2006): 188–95.

Köhler, O., Benros, M.E., Nordentoft, M., et al. "Effect of anti-inflammatory treatment on depression, depressive symptoms, and adverse effects: a systematic review and meta-analysis of randomized clinical trials." *JAMA Psychiatry* 71 12 (2014): 1381–91.

Kroenke, K., Spitzer, R.L., Williams, J.B., et al. "Physical symptoms in primary care. Predictors of psychiatric disorders and functional impairment." *Arch Fam Med* 3 9 (1994): 774–9.

Ladwig, K.-H., Lederbogen, F., Albus, C., et al. "Position paper on the importance of psychosocial factors in cardiology: update 2013." *Ger Med Sci* 12 12 (2014 May 7): 1–24.

Lafortuna, C.L., Agosti, F., Proietti, M., Adorni, F., Sartorio, A. "The combined effect of adiposity, fat distribution and age on cardiovascular risk factors and motor disability in a cohort of obese women (aged 18–83)." *J Endocrinol Invest* 29 (2006): 905–12.

Lavie, C.J., Milani, R.V., Ventura, H.O. "Obesity and cardiovascular disease: risk factor, paradox, and impact of weight loss." *J Am Coll Cardiol* 53 (2009): 1925–32.

Lett, H.S., Blumenthal, J.A., Babyak, M.A., et al. "Depression as a risk factor for coronary artery disease: evidence, mechanisms, and treatment." *Psychosom Med* 66 (2004): 305–15.

Lichtman, J.H., Bigger Jr., J.T., Blumenthal, J.A., et al. "Depression and coronary heart disease: recommendations for screening, referral, and treatment: a science advisory from the American Heart Association Prevention Committee of the Council on Cardiovascular Nursing, Council on Clinical Cardiology, Council on Epidemiology and Prevention, and Interdisciplinary Council on Quality of Care and Outcomes Research: endorsed by the American Psychiatric Association." *Circulation* 118 17 (2008 Oct 21): 1768–75.

Lichtman, J.H., Froelicher, E.S., Blumenthal, J.A., et al. "Depression as a risk factor for poor prognosis among patients with acute coronary syndrome: systematic review and recommendations: a scientific statement from the American Heart Association." *Circulation* 129 12 (2014): 1350–69.

Lloyd, C.E., Roy, T., Nouwen, A., Chauhan, A.M. "Epidemiology of depression in diabetes: international and cross-cultural issues." *J Affect Disord* 142 Suppl (2012 Oct): S22–9.

MacMahon, K.M.A., Lip, G.Y.H. "Psychological factors in heart failure: a review of the literature." *Arch Intern Med* 162 5 (2002): 509–16.

Manson, J.E., Bassuk, S.S. "Obesity in the United States: a fresh look at its high toll." *JAMA* 289 (2003): 229–30.

Meijer, A., Conradi, H.J., Bos, E.H., et al. "Prognostic association of depression following myocardial infarction with mortality and cardiovascular events: a meta-analysis of 25 years of research." *Gen Hosp Psychiatry* 33 (2011): 203–16.

Meyer, T., Buss, U., Herrmann-Lingen, C. "Role of cardiac disease severity in the predictive value of anxiety for all-cause mortality." *Psychosom Med* 72 1 (2010): 9–15.

Meyer, T., Hussein, S., Lange, H.W., Herrmann-Lingen, C. "Anxiety is associated with a reduction in both mortality and major adverse cardiovascular events five years after coronary stenting." *Eur J Preventive Cardiol* 22 1 (2015): 75–82.

Milaneschi, Y., Corsi, A.M., Penninx, B.W., et al. "Interleukin-1 receptor antagonist and incident depressive symptoms over 6 years in older persons: the InCHIANTI study." *Biol Psychiatry* 65 11 2009): 973–8.

Mykletun, A., Bjerkeset, O., Dewey, M., et al. "Anxiety, depression, and cause-specific mortality: the HUNT study." *Psychosom Med* 69 4 (2007): 323–31.

Nakamura, H., Ito, H., Egami, Y., et al. "Waist circumference is the main determinant of elevated C-reactive protein in metabolic syndrome." *Diabetes Res Clin Pract* 79 (2008): 330–6.

Nguyen, N.T., Nguyen, X.M., Lane, J., Wang, P. "Relationship between obesity and diabetes in a US adult population: findings from the National Health and Nutrition Examination Survey, 1999–2006." *Obes Surg* 21 3 (2011 Mar): 351–5.

Nicholson, A., Kuper, H., Hemingway, H. "Depression as an aetiologic and prognostic factor in coronary heart disease: a meta-analysis of 6,362 events among 146,538 participants in 54 observational studies." *Eur Heart J* 27 (2006): 2763–74.

Ogden, C.L., Carroll, M.D., Kit, B.K., Flegal, K.M. "Prevalence of obesity in the United States, 2009–2010." *Natl Ctr Health Stat* 82 (2012 Jan): 1–8.

Park, J., Euhus, D.M., Scherer, P.E. "Paracrine and endocrine effects of adipose tissue on cancer development and progression." *Endocr Rev* 32 (2011): 550–70.

Park, M., Katon, W.J., Wolf, F.M. "Depression and risk of mortality in individuals with diabetes: a meta-analysis and systematic review." *Gen Hosp Psychiatry* 35 3 (2013 May–Jun): 217–25.

Pasco, J.A., Jacka, F.N., Williams, L.J., et al. "Clinical implications of the cytokine hypothesis of depression: the association between use of statins and aspirin and the risk of major depression." *Psychother Psychosom* (2010): 323–5.

Patten, S.B. "Long-term medical conditions and major depression in a Canadian population study at waves 1 and 2." *J Affect Disord* 63 (2001): 35–41.

Pratt, L.A., Brody, D.J. "Depression and obesity in the U.S. adult household population, 2005–2010." *NCHS Data Brief* 167 (2014 Oct): 1–8.

Purdy, J. "Chronic physical illness: a psychophysiological approach for chronic physical illness." *Yale J Biol Med* 86 1 (2013): 15–28.

Roest, A.M., Martens, E.J., Denollet, J., de Jonge, P. "Prognostic association of anxiety post myocardial infarction with mortality and new cardiac events: a meta-analysis." *Psychosom Med* 72 6 (2010): 563–9.

Rudisch, B., Nemeroff, C.B. "Epidemiology of comorbid coronary artery disease and depression." *Biol Psychiatry* 54 (2003): 227–40.

Rutledge, T., Redwine, L.S., Linke, S.E., Mills, P.J. "A meta-analysis of mental health treatments and cardiac rehabilitation for improving clinical outcomes and depression among patients with coronary heart disease." *Psychosom Med* 75 4 (2013 May): 335–49.

Semenkovich, K., Brown, M.E., Svrakic, D.M., Lustman, P.J. "Depression in type 2 diabetes mellitus: prevalence, impact, and treatment." *Drugs* 75 6 (2015 Apr): 577–87.

Siu, A.L., US Preventive Services Task Force (USPSTF), Bibbins-Domingo, K., Grossman, D.C., et al. "Screening for depression in adults: US Preventive Services Task Force recommendation statement." *JAMA* 315 4 (2016 Jan 26): 380–7.

Smith, D.J., Court, H., McLean, G., et al. "Depression and multimorbidity: a cross-sectional study of 1,751,841 patients in primary care." *J Clin Psychiatry* 75 11 (2014 Nov): 1202–8.

Smolderen, K.G., Buchanan, D.M., Gosch, K., et al. "Depression treatment and 1-year mortality after acute myocardial infarction: insights from the TRIUMPH registry (translational research investigating underlying disparities in acute myocardial infarction patients' health status)." *Circulation* 135 18 (2017 May 2): 1681–9.

Stegmann, M.E., Ormel, J., de Graaf, R., et al. "Functional disability as an explanation of the associations between chronic physical conditions and 12-month major depressive episode." *J Affect Disord* 124 1–2 (2010): 38–44.

Stenman, M., Holzmann, M.J., Sartipy, U. "Antidepressant use before coronary artery bypass surgery is associated with long-term mortality." *Int J Cardiol* 167 6 (2013 Sep 10): 2958–62.

Stenman, M., Holzmann, M.J., Sartipy, U. "Relation of major depression to survival after coronary artery bypass grafting." *Am J Cardiol* 114 5 (2014 Sep 1): 698–703.

Todaro, J.F., Shen, B.-J., Raffa, S.D., Tilkemeier, P.L., Niaura, R. "Prevalence of anxiety disorders in men and women with established coronary heart disease." *J Cardiopulm Rehabil Prev* 27 2 (2007 Mar–Apr): 86–91.

van Melle, J.P., de Jonge, P., Spijkerman, T.A., et al. "Prognostic association of depression following myocardial infarction with mortality and cardiovascular events: a meta-analysis." *Psychosom Med* 66 (2004): 814–22.

Watkins, L.L., Koch, G.G., Sherwood, A., et al. "Association of anxiety and depression with all-cause mortality in individuals with coronary heart disease." *J Am Heart Assoc* 2 2 (2013): e000068.

Wee, C.C., Mukamal, K.J., Huang, A., et al. "Obesity and C-reactive protein levels among White, Black, and Hispanic US adults." *Obesity* 16 (2008): 875–80.

Zhao, G., Ford, E.S., Li, C., et al. "Waist circumference, abdominal obesity, and depression among overweight and obese U.S. adults: National Health and Nutrition Examination Survey 2005–2006." *BMC Psychiatry* 11 (2011): 130.

Chapter 6

Abuidhail, J., Abujilban, S. "Characteristics of Jordanian depressed pregnant women: a comparison study." *J Psychiatr Ment Health Nurs* 21 (2014): 573–9.

Abujilban, S.K., Abuidhail, J., Al-Modallal, H., Hamaideh, S., Mosemli, O. "Predictors of antenatal depression among Jordanian pregnant women in their third trimester." *Health Care Women Int* 35 (2014): 200–15.

Andersson, L., Sundstrom-Poromaa, I., Wulff, M., Astrom, M., Bixo, M. "Depression and anxiety during pregnancy and six months postpartum: a followup study." *Acta Obstet Scand* 85 (2006): 937–44.

Baca, E., Garcia-Garcia, M., Porras-Chavarino, A. "Gender differences in treatment response to sertraline versus imipramine in patients with nonmelancholic depressive disorders." *Prog Neuropsychopharmacol Biol Psychiatry* 28 1 (2004 Jan): 57–65.

Berlanga, C., Flores-Ramos, M. "Different gender response to serotonergic and noradrenergic antidepressants. A comparative study of the efficacy of citalopram and reboxetine." *J Affect Disord* 95 1–3 (2006 Oct): 119–23.

Biaggi, A., Conroy, S., Pawlby, S., et al. "Identifying the women at risk of antenatal anxiety and depression: a systematic review." *J Affect Disord* 191 (2016): 62–77.

Blanco, C., Vesga-Lopez, O., Stewart, J.W., et al. "Epidemiology of major depression with atypical features: results from the National Epidemiologic Survey on Alcohol and Related Conditions (NESARC)." *J Clin Psychiatry* 73 (2012): 224–32.

Bottomley, K.L., Lancaster, S.J. "The association between depressive symptoms and smoking in pregnant adolescents." *Psychol Med* 13 (2008): 574–82.

Brittain, K., Myer, L., Koen, N., Koopowitz, S., et al. "Risk factors for antenatal depression and associations with infant birth outcomes: results from a South African birth cohort study." *Paediatr Perinat Epidemiol* 29 6 (2015): 505–14.

Burcusa, S.L., Iacono, W.G. "Risk for recurrence in depression." *Clin Psychol Rev* 27 (2007): 959–85.

Chaplin, T.M., Hong, K., Bergquist, K., Sinha, R. "Gender differences in response to emotional stress: an assessment across subjective, behavioral, and physiological domains and relations to alcohol craving." *Alcohol Clin Exp Res* 32 7 (2008 Jul): 1242–50.

Crawford, M.B., DeLisi, L.E. "Issues related to sex differences in antipsychotic treatment." *Curr Opin Psychiatry* 29 3 (2016): 211–7.

Cuijpers, P., Vogelzangs, N., Twisk, J., et al. "Is excess mortality higher in depressed men than in depressed women? A meta-analytic comparison." *J Affect Disord* 161 (2014): 47–54.

Eaton, N.R., Keyes, K.M., Krueger, R.F., et al. "An invariant dimensional liability model of gender differences in mental disorder prevalence: evidence from a national sample." *J Abnorm Psychol* 121 (2012): 282–8.

Fellenzer, J.L., Cibula, D.A. "Intendedness of pregnancy and other predictive factors for symptoms of prenatal depression in a population-based study." *Matern Child Health J* 18 (2014): 2426–36.

Gawlik, S., Muller, M., Hoffmann, L., et al. "Prevalence of paternal perinatal depressiveness and its link to partnership satisfaction and birth concerns." *Arch Womens Ment Health* 17 1 (2014 Feb): 49–56.

Gelaye, B., Kajeepeta, S., Williams, M.A. "Suicidal ideation in pregnancy: an epidemiologic review." *Arch Womens Ment Health* 19 5 (2016): 741–51.

Gentile, S. "Suicidal mothers." *J Inj Violence Res* 3 (2011): 90–7.

Georgakis, M.K., Thomopoulos, T.P., Diamantaras, A.A., et al. "Association of age at menopause and duration of reproductive period with depression after menopause: a systematic review and meta-analysis." *JAMA Psychiatry* 73 2 (2016 Feb): 139–49.

Glasser, S., Lerner-Geva, L. "Focus on fathers: paternal depression in the perinatal period." *Perspect Public Health* (2018 Jul 25): 1757913918790597.

Goldstein, J.M., Holsen, L., Handa, R., Tobet, S. "Fetal hormonal programming of sex differences in depression: linking women's mental health with sex differences in the brain across the lifespan." *Front Neurosci* 8 (2014): 247.

Hardeveld, F., Spijker, J., De Graaf, R., et al. "Prevalence and predictors of recurrence of major depressive disorder in the adult population." *Acta Psychiatr Scand* 122 (2010): 184–91.

Heim, C., Ehlert, U., Hellhammer, D.H. "The potential role of hypocortisolism in the pathophysiology of stress-related bodily disorders." *Psychoneuroendocrinology* 25 (2000): 1–35.

Howard, L.M., Molyneaux, E., Dennis, C.L., et al. "Non-psychotic mental disorders in the perinatal period." *Lancet* 384 (2014): 1775–88.
Hughes, J.F., Page, D.C. "The history of the Y chromosome in man." *Nat Genet* 48 6 (2016 May 27): 588–9.
Joyce, P.R., Mulder, R.T., Luty, S.E., et al. "A differential response to nortriptyline and fluoxetine in melancholic depression: the importance of age and gender." *Acta Psychiatr Scand* 108 1 (2003 Jul): 20–3.
Kiecolt-Glaser, J.K., Newton, T.L. "Marriage and health: his and hers." *Psychol Bull* 127 (2001): 472–503.
Kornstein, S.G., Schatzberg, A.F., Thase, M.E., et al. "Gender differences in treatment response to sertraline versus imipramine in chronic depression." *Am J Psychiatry* 157 9 (2000 Sep): 1445–52.
Kudielka, B.M., Kirschbaum, C. "Sex differences in HPA axis responses to stress: a review." *Biol Psychol* 69 1 (2005 Apr): 113–32.
Kuehner, C. "Gender differences in unipolar depression: an update of epidemiological findings and possible explanations." *Acta Psychiatr Scand* 108 (2003): 163–74.
Lamers, F., Vogelzangs, N., Merikangas, K.R., et al. "Evidence for a differential role of HPA-axis function, inflammation and metabolic syndrome in melancholic versus atypical depression." *Mol Psychiatry* 18 (2013): 692–9.
Lange, B., Mueller, J.K., Leweke, F.M., Bumb, J.M. "How gender affects the pharmacotherapeutic approach to treating psychosis—a systematic review." *Expert Opin Pharmacother* 18 4 (2017): 351–62.
Laursen, T.M., Musliner, K.L., Benros, M.E., et al. "Mortality and life expectancy in persons with severe unipolar depression." *J Affect Disord* 193 (2016): 203–7.
Lee, A.M., Lam, S.K., Lau, S.M., Chong, C.S., et al. "Prevalence, course, and risk factors for antenatal anxiety and depression." *Obstet Gynecol* 110 (2007): 1102–12.
Lindahl, V., Pearson, J.L., Colpe, L. "Prevalence of suicidality during pregnancy and the postpartum." *Arch Womens Ment Health* 8 2 (2005 Jun): 77–87.
Lusskin, S., Pundiak, T., Habib, S. "Perinatal depression: hiding in plain sight." *Can J Psychiatry* 52 (2007): 479–88.
Mackenzie, C.S., El-Gabalawy, R., Chou, K.L., Sareen, J. "Prevalence and predictors of persistent versus remitting mood, anxiety, and substance disorders in a national sample of older adults." *Am J Geriatr Psychiatry* 22 (2014): 854–65.
Marazziti, D., Baroni, S., Picchetti, M., et al. "Pharmacokinetics and pharmacodynamics of psychotropic drugs: effect of sex." *CNS Spectr* 18 3 (2013): 118–27.
Marcus, S.M., Flynn, H.A., Blow, F.C., Barry, K.L. "Depressive symptoms among pregnant women screened in obstetrics settings." *J Womens Health (Larchmt)* 12 (2003): 373–80.

Marcus, S.M., Kerber, K.B., Rush, A.J., et al. "Sex differences in depression symptoms in treatment-seeking adults: confirmatory analyses from the Sequenced Treatment Alternatives to Relieve Depression study." *Compr Psychiatry* 49 (2008): 238–46.

Martin, L.A., Neighbors, H.W., Griffith, D.M. "The experience of symptoms of depression in men vs women." *JAMA Psychiatry* 70 10 (2013 Oct): 1100–6.

Milner, A., Sveticic, J., De Leo, D. "Suicide in the absence of mental disorder? A review of psychological autopsy studies across countries." *Int J Soc Psychiatry* 59 (2013): 545–54.

Mohamad Yusuff, A.S., Tang, L., Binns, C.W., Lee, A.H. "Prevalence of antenatal depressive symptoms among women in Sabah, Malaysia." *J Matern Fetal Neonatal Med* (2015): 1–5.

Munk-Olsen, T., Laursen, T.M., Meltzer-Brody, S., et al. "Psychiatric disorders with postpartum onset: possible early manifestations of bipolar affective disorders." *Arch Gen Psychiatry* 69 (2012): 428–34.

Munk-Olsen, T., Laursen, T.M., Pedersen, C.B., et al. "New parents and mental disorders: a population-based register study." *JAMA* 296 21 (2006): 2582–9.

O'Hara, M.W., McCabe, J.E. "Postpartum depression: current status and future directions." *Ann Rev Clin Psychol* 9 (2013): 379–407.

Paulson, J.F., Bazemore, S.D. "Prenatal and postpartum depression in fathers and its association with maternal depression: a meta-analysis." *JAMA* 303 19 (2010): 1961–9.

Penninx, B.W., Nolen, W.A., Lamers, F., et al. "Two-year course of depressive and anxiety disorders: results from the Netherlands Study of Depression and Anxiety (NESDA)." *J Affect Disord* 133 (2011): 76–85.

Plant, D.T., Pariante, C.M., Sharp, D., Pawlby, S. "Maternal depression during pregnancy and offspring depression in adulthood: role of child maltreatment." *Br J Psychiatry* 207 (2015): 213–20.

Raisanen, S., Lehto, S.M., Nielsen, H.S., Gissler, M., Kramer, M.R., Heinonen, S. "Risk factors for and perinatal outcomes of major depression during pregnancy: a population-based analysis during 2002–2010 in Finland." *BMJ Open* 4 (2014): e004883.

Robertson-Blackmore, E., Putnam, F.W., Rubinow, D.R., Matthieu, M., Hunn, J.E., Putnam, K.T., Moynihan, J.A., O'Connor, T.G. "Antecedent trauma exposure and risk of depression in the perinatal period." *J Clin Psychiatry* 74 (2013): e942–8.

Ross, L.E., McLean, L.M. "Anxiety disorders during pregnancy and the postpartum period: a systematic review." *J Clin Psychiatry* 67 (2006): 1285–98.

Siegel, R.S., Brandon, A.R. "Adolescents, pregnancy, and mental health." *J Pediatr Adolesc Gynecol* 27 3 (2014): 138–50.

Silverstein, B., Edwards, T., Gamma, A., et al. "The role played by depression associated with somatic symptomatology in accounting for the gender

difference in the prevalence of depression." *Soc Psychiatry Psychiatr Epidemiol* 48 (2013): 257–63.
Spijker, J., de Graaf, R., Bijl, R.V., et al. "Determinants of persistence of major depressive episodes in the general population. Results from the Netherlands Mental Health Survey and Incidence Study (NEMESIS)." *J Affect Disord* 81 (2004): 231–40.
Sramek, J.J., Murphy, M.F., Cutler, N.R. "Sex differences in the psychopharmacological treatment of depression." *Dialogues Clin Neurosci* 18 4 (2016 Dec): 447–57.
Stein, A., Pearson, R.M., Goodman, S.H., et al. "Effects of perinatal mental disorders on the fetus and child." *Lancet* 384 (2014): 1800–19.
Stroud, L.R., Salovey, P., Epel, E.S. "Sex differences in stress responses: social rejection versus achievement stress." *Biol Psychiatry* 52 (2002): 318–27.
Thase, M.E. "Atypical depression: useful concept, but it's time to revise the DSM-IV criteria." *Neuropsychopharmacol* 34 (2009): 2633–41.
Verona, E., Kilmer, A. "Stress exposure and affective modulation of aggressive behavior in men and women." *J Abnorm Psychol* 116 2 (2007 May): 410–21.
Vesga-López, O., Blanco, C., Keyes, K., et al. "Psychiatric disorders in pregnant and postpartum women in the United States." *Arch Gen Psychiatry* 65 7 (2008): 805–15.
Vliegen, N., Casalin, S., Luyten, P. "The course of postpartum depression: a review of longitudinal studies." *Harv Rev Psychiatry* 22 (2014): 1–22.
Zagni, E., Simoni, L., Colombo, D. "Sex and gender differences in central nervous system-related disorders." *Neurosci J* (2016): 1–13.

Chapter 7

Kroenke, K., Spitzer, R.L., Williams, J.B. "The PHQ-9: validity of a brief depression severity measure." *J Gen Intern Med* 16 9 (2001 Sep): 606–13.

Chapters 9–12

Abdallah, C.G., Adams, T.G., Kelmendi, B., et al. "Ketamine's mechanism of action: a path to rapid-acting antidepressants." *Depress Anxiety* 33 8 (2016 Aug): 689–97.
Andrade, C. "Ketamine for depression, 1: clinical summary of issues related to efficacy, adverse effects, and mechanism of action." *J Clin Psychiatry* 78 4 (2017 Apr): e415–9.
Arroll, B., Elley, C.R., Fishman, T., Goodyear-Smith, F.A., et al. "Antidepressants versus placebo for depression in primary care." *Cochrane Database Syst Rev* 3 (2009 Jul 8): CD007954.

Berman, R.M., Thase, M.E., Trivedi, M.H., et al. "Long-term safety and tolerability of open-label aripiprazole augmentation of antidepressant therapy in major depressive disorder." *Neuropsychiatr Dis Treat* 7 (2011): 303–12.

Buysse, D.J. "Insomnia." *JAMA* 309 (2013): 706–16.

Changsu, H., Sheng-Min, W., et al. "Second-generation antipsychotics in the treatment of major depressive disorder: current evidence." *Expert Rev Neurother* 13 7 (2013): 851–70.

Citrome, L. "A review of the pharmacology, efficacy and tolerability of recently approved and upcoming oral antipsychotics: an evidence-based medicine approach." *CNS Drugs* 27 11 (2013): 879–911.

Daly, E.J., Singh, J.B., Fedgchin, M. "Efficacy and safety of intranasal esketamine adjunctive to oral antidepressant therapy in treatment-resistant depression." *JAMA Psychiatry* 75 2 (2018 Feb): 139–48.

Dodd, S., Mitchell, P.B., Bauer, M., et al. "Monitoring for antidepressant-associated adverse events in the treatment of patients with major depressive disorder: an international consensus statement." *World J Biol Psychiatry* 19 5 (2018 Aug): 330–48.

Fornaro, M., Anastasia, A., Novello, S., et al. "The emergence of loss of efficacy during antidepressant drug treatment for major depressive disorder: an integrative review of evidence, mechanisms, and clinical implications." *Pharmacol Res* 139 (2019 Jan): 494–502.

Geddes, J.R., Carney, S.M., Davies, C., et al. "Relapse prevention with antidepressant drug treatment in depressive disorders: a systematic review." *Lancet* 361 9358 (2003): 653–61.

Goddard, A.W., Brouette, T., Almai, A., et al. "Early coadministration of clonazepam with sertraline for panic disorder." *Arch Gen Psychiatry* 58 7 (2001): 681–6.

Gomez, A.F., Barthel, A.L., Hofmann, S.G. "Comparing the efficacy of benzodiazepines and serotonergic anti-depressants for adults with generalized anxiety disorder: a meta-analytic review." *Expert Opin Pharmacother* (2018): 883–94.

Gray, S.L., Eggen, A.E., Blough, D., et al. "Benzodiazepine use in older adults enrolled in a health maintenance organization." *Am J Geriatr Psychiatry* 11 (2003): 568–76.

Han, C., Wang, S.M., Kato, M., Lee, S.J., et al. "Second-generation antipsychotics in the treatment of major depressive disorder: current evidence." *Expert Rev Neurother* 13 7 (2013): 851–70.

Kennedy, S.H., Lam, R.W., McIntyre, R.S., et al. CANMAT Depression Work Group. "Canadian Network for Mood and Anxiety Treatments (CANMAT) 2016 Clinical Guidelines for the Management of Adults with Major Depressive Disorder: Section 3. Pharmacological Treatments." *Can J Psychiatry* 61 9 (2016 Sep): 540–60.

Komossa, K., Depping, A.M., Gaudchau, A., et al. "Second-generation antipsychotics for major depressive disorder and dysthymia." *Cochrane Database Syst Rev* 12 (2010 Dec 8): CD008121.

Lam, R.W., Kennedy, S.H., Parikh, S.V., et al. CANMAT Depression Work Group. "Canadian Network for Mood and Anxiety Treatments (CANMAT) 2016 Clinical Guidelines for the Management of Adults with Major Depressive Disorder: Introduction and Methods." *Can J Psychiatry* 61 9 (2016 Sep): 506–9.

Lam, R.W., McIntosh, D., Wang, J., et al. CANMAT Depression Work Group. "Canadian Network for Mood and Anxiety Treatments (CANMAT) 2016 Clinical Guidelines for the Management of Adults with Major Depressive Disorder: Section 1. Disease Burden and Principles of Care." *Can J Psychiatry* 61 9 (2016 Sep): 510–23.

Leucht, C., Huhn, M., Leucht, S. "Amitriptyline versus placebo for major depressive disorder." *Cochrane Database Syst Rev* 12 (2012 Dec 12): CD009138.

McIntyre, R.S., Rosenbluth, M., Ramasubbu, R., et al. Canadian Network for Mood and Anxiety Treatments (CANMAT) Task Force. "Managing medical and psychiatric comorbidity in individuals with major depressive disorder and bipolar disorder." *Ann Clin Psychiatry* 24 2 (2012 May): 163–9.

McLachlan, G. "Treatment resistant depression: what are the options?" *BMJ* 363 (2018 Dec 18): k5354.

Molero, P., Ramos-Quiroga, J.A., Martin-Santos, R., et al. "Antidepressant efficacy and tolerability of ketamine and esketamine." *CNS Drugs* 32 5 (2018 May): 411–20.

Morgenthaler, T., Kramer, M., Alessi, C., et al; American Academy of Sleep Medicine. "Practice parameters for the psychological and behavioral treatment of insomnia: an update. An American Academy of Sleep Medicine report." *Sleep* 29 (2006): 1415–9.

Nelson, J.C., Papakostas, G.I. "Atypical antipsychotic augmentation in major depressive disorder: a meta-analysis of placebo-controlled randomized trials." *Am J Psychiatry* 166 9 (2009 Sep): 980–91.

Papakostas, G.I. "Augmentation strategies in the treatment of major depressive disorder. Examining the evidence on augmentation with atypical antipsychotics." *CNS Spectr* 12 12 Suppl 22 (2007 Dec): 10–2.

Papakostas, G.I. "Limitations of contemporary antidepressants: tolerability." *J Clin Psychiatry* 68 Suppl 10 (2007): 11–7.

Papakostas, G.I., Fava, M., Thase, M.E. "Treatment of SSRI-resistant depression: a meta-analysis comparing within- versus across-class switches." *Biol Psychiatry* 63 7 (2008 Apr 1): 699–704.

Papakostas, G.I., Perlis, R.H., Seifert, C., Fava, M. "Antidepressant dose reduction and the risk of relapse in major depressive disorder." *Psychother Psychosom* 76 5 (2007): 266–70.

Papakostas, G.I., Shelton, R.C., Smith, J., Fava, M. "Augmentation of antidepressants with atypical antipsychotic medications for treatment-resistant major depressive disorder: a meta-analysis." *J Clin Psychiatry* 68 6 (2007 Jun): 826–31.

Reinhold, J.A., Rickels, K. "Pharmacological treatment for generalized anxiety disorder in adults: an update." *Expert Opin Pharmacother* 16 (2015): 1669–81.

Riemann, D., Baglioni, C., Bassetti, C., et al. "European guideline for the diagnosis and treatment of insomnia." *J Sleep Res* 26 (2017): 675–700.

Schatzberg, A.F., Haddad, P., Kaplan, E.M., et al. "Serotonin reuptake inhibitor discontinuation syndrome: a hypothetical definition. Discontinuation Consensus panel." *J Clin Psychiatry* 58 Suppl 7 (1997): 5–10.

Schutte-Rodin, S., Broch, L., Buysse, D., et al. "Clinical guideline for the evaluation and management of chronic insomnia in adults." *J Clin Sleep Med* 4 (2008): 487–504.

Seedat, S., Stein, M.B. "Double-blind, placebo-controlled assessment of combined clonazepam with paroxetine compared with paroxetine monotherapy for generalized social anxiety disorder." *J Clin Psychiatry* 65 (2004): 244–8.

Solomon, C.G., Winkelman, J.W. "Insomnia disorder." *N Engl J Med* 373 (2015): 1437–44.

Soumerai, S.B., Simoni-Wastila, L., Singer, C., et al. "Lack of relationship between long-term use of benzodiazepines and escalation to high dosages." *Psychiatr Serv* 54 (2003): 1006–11.

Spielmans, G.I., Berman, M.I., Linardatos, E., et al. "Adjunctive atypical antipsychotic treatment for major depressive disorder: a meta-analysis of depression, quality of life, and safety outcomes." *PLoS Med* 10 3 (2013): e1001403.

Spielmans, G.I., Kirsch, I. "Drug approval and drug effectiveness." *Annu Rev Clin Psychol* 10 (2014): 741–66.

Stein, M.B., Sareen, J. "Clinical practice. Generalized anxiety disorder." *N Engl J Med* 373 (2015): 2059–68.

Trivedi, M.H., Hollander, E., Nutt, D., Blier, P. "Clinical evidence and potential neurobiological underpinnings of unresolved symptoms of depression." *J Clin Psychiatry* 69 2 (2008 Feb): 246–58.

Trivedi, M.H., Rush, A.J., Wisniewski, S.R., et al. "Evaluation of outcomes with citalopram for depression using measurement-based care in STAR*D: implications for clinical practice." *Am J Psychiatry* 163 1 (2006 Jan): 28–40.

Undurraga, J., Baldessarini, R.J. "Randomized, placebo-controlled trials of antidepressants for acute major depression: thirty-year meta-analytic review." *Neuropsychopharmacol* 37 4 (2012): 851–64.

Vieta, E., Colom, F. "Therapeutic options in treatment-resistant depression." *Ann Med* 43 7 (2011 Nov): 512–30.

Willems, I.A.T., Gorgels, W.J.M.J., Oude Voshaar, R.C., et al. "Tolerance to benzodiazepines among long-term users in primary care." *Fam Pract* 30 (2013): 404–10.

Zhou, X., Michael, K.D., Liu, Y., et al. "Systematic review of management for treatment-resistant depression in adolescents." *BMC Psychiatry* 14 (2014 Nov 30): 340.

Chapter 13

Abbott, C.C., Jones, T., Lemke, N.T., et al. "Hippocampal structural and functional changes associated with electroconvulsive therapy response." *Transl Psychiatry* 4 (2014): e483.
Anderson, E.L.R., Reti, I.M. "ECT in pregnancy: a review of the literature from 1941 to 2007." *Psychosom Med* 71 2 (2009): 235–42.
Cho, C.H. "New mechanism for glutamate hypothesis in epilepsy." *Front Cell Neurosci* 7 (2013): 127–9.
Duthie, A.C., Perrin, J.S., Bennett, D.M., et al. "Anticonvulsant mechanisms of electroconvulsive therapy and relation to therapeutic efficacy." *J ECT* 31 3 (2015): 173–8.
Farrant, M., Nusser, Z. "Variations on an inhibitory theme: phasic and tonic activation of GABA(A) receptors." *Nat Rev Neurosci* 6 3 (2005): 215–29.
Fink, M., Kellner, C.H., McCall, W.V. "The role of ECT in suicide prevention." *J ECT* 30 1 (2014): 5–9.
Husain, M.M., Rush, A.J., Fink, M., et al. "Speed of response and remission in major depressive disorder with acute electroconvulsive therapy (ECT): a consortium for research in ECT (CORE) report." *J Clin Psychiatry* 65 4 (2004): 485–91.
Joshi, S.H., Espinoza, R.T., Pirnia, T., et al. "Structural plasticity of the hippocampus and amygdala induced by electroconvulsive therapy in major depression." *Biol Psychiatry* 79 4 (2016): 282–92.
Kellner, C.H., Fink, M., Knapp, R., et al. "Relief of expressed suicidal intent by ECT: a consortium for research in ECT study." *Am J Psychiatry* 162 5 (2005): 977–82.
Kellner, C.H., Knapp, R.G., Petrides, G., et al. "Continuation electroconvulsive therapy vs pharmacotherapy for relapse prevention in major depression: a multisite study from the consortium for research in electroconvulsive therapy (CORE)." *Arch Gen Psychiatry* 63 12 (2006): 1337–44.
Leiknes, K.A., Cooke, M.J., Jarosch-von Schweder, L., et al. "Electroconvulsive therapy during pregnancy: a systematic review of case studies." *Arch Womens Ment Health* 18 1 (2015): 1–39.
Liang, C.S., Chung, C.H., Ho, P.S., et al. "Superior anti-suicidal effects of electroconvulsive therapy in unipolar disorder and bipolar depression." *Bipolar Disord* 20 6 (2018 Sep): 539–46.
Luchini, F., Medda, P., Mariani, M.G., et al. "Electroconvulsive therapy in catatonic patients: efficacy and predictors of response." *World J Psychiatry* 5 2 (2015): 182–92.
McDonald, W.M. "Neuromodulation treatments for geriatric mood and cognitive disorders." *Am J Geriatr Psychiatry* 24 12 (2016): 1130–41.
McKay, M.S., Zakzanis, K.K. "The impact of treatment on HPA axis activity in unipolar major depression." *J Psychiatr Res* 44 3 (2010): 183–92.

Milev, R.V., Giacobbe, P., Kennedy, S.H., et al; CANMAT Depression Work Group. "Canadian Network for Mood and Anxiety Treatments (CANMAT) 2016 Clinical Guidelines for the Management of Adults with Major Depressive Disorder: Section 4. Neurostimulation Treatments." *Can J Psychiatry* 61 9 (2016 Sep): 561–75.

Obbels, J., Verwijk, E., Vansteelandt, K. "Long-term neurocognitive functioning after electroconvulsive therapy in patients with late-life depression." *Acta Psychiatr Scand* 138 (2018): 223–31.

Parikh, S.V., Quilty, L.C., Ravitz, P., et al; CANMAT Depression Work Group. "Canadian Network for Mood and Anxiety Treatments (CANMAT) 2016 Clinical Guidelines for the Management of Adults with Major Depressive Disorder: Section 2. Psychological Treatments." *Can J Psychiatry* 61 9 (2016 Sep): 524–39.

Petroff, O.A. "GABA and glutamate in the human brain." *Neuroscientist* 8 6 (2002): 562–73.

Prudic, J., Sackeim, H.A., Devanand, D.P. "Medication resistance and clinical response to electroconvulsive therapy." *Psychiatry Res* 31 3 (1990): 287–96.

Ravindran, A.V., Balneaves, L.G., Faulkner, G., et al; CANMAT Depression Work Group. "Canadian Network for Mood and Anxiety Treatments (CANMAT) 2016 Clinical Guidelines for the Management of Adults with Major Depressive Disorder: Section 5. Complementary and Alternative Medicine Treatments." *Can J Psychiatry* 61 9 (2016 Sep): 576–87.

Rotheneichner, P., Lange, S., O'Sullivan, A., et al. "Hippocampal neurogenesis and antidepressive therapy: shocking relations." *Neural Plast* (2014): 723915.

Saatcioglu, O., Tomruk, N.B. "The use of electroconvulsive therapy in pregnancy: a review." *Isr J Psychiatry Relat Sci* 48 1 (2011): 6–11.

Sarran, C., Albers, C., Sachon, P., Meesters, Y. "Meteorological analysis of symptom data for people with seasonal affective disorder." *Psychiatry Res* 257 (2017 Nov): 501–5.

Schloesser, R.J., Orvoen, S., Jimenez, D.V., et al. "Antidepressant-like effects of electroconvulsive seizures require adult neurogenesis in a neuroendocrine model of depression." *Brain Stimul* 8 5 (2015): 862–7.

Semkovska, M., McLoughlin, D.M. "Objective cognitive performance associated with electroconvulsive therapy for depression: a systematic review and meta-analysis." *Biol Psychiatry* 68 6 (2010): 568–77.

Torring, N., Sanghani, S.N., Petrides, G., et al. "The mortality rate of electroconvulsive therapy: a systematic review and pooled analysis." *Acta Psychiatr Scand* 135 5 (2017): 388–97.

UK ECT Review Group. "Efficacy and safety of electroconvulsive therapy in depressive disorders: a systematic review and meta-analysis." *Lancet* 361 9360 (2003): 799–808.

Wells, K., Scanlan, J.N., Gomez, L., et al. "Decision making and support available to individuals considering and undertaking electroconvulsive therapy (ECT): a qualitative, consumer-led study." *BMC Psychiatry* 18 (2018): 236.

Wirz-Justice, A., Graw, P., Kräuchi, K., et al. "'Natural' light treatment of seasonal affective disorder." *J Affect Disord* 37 2–3 (1996 Apr 12): 109–20.
Wittenauer Welsh, J., Janjua, A.U., Garlow, S.J., et al. "Use of expert consultation in a complex case of neuroleptic malignant syndrome requiring electroconvulsive therapy." *J Psychiatr Pract* 22 6 (2016): 484–9.
Zhang, J., Narr, K.L., Woods, R.P., et al. "Glutamate normalization with ECT treatment response in major depression." *Mol Psychiatry* 18 3 (2013): 268–70.

Chapter 14

Aso, E., Ozaita, A., Serra, M.À., Maldonado, R. "Genes differentially expressed in CB1 knockout mice: involvement in the depressive-like phenotype." *Eur Neuropsychopharmacol* 21 1 (2011 Jan): 11–22.
Aspis, I., Feingold, D., Weiser, M., et al. "Cannabis use and mental health-related quality of life among individuals with depressive disorders." *Psychiatry Res* 230 2 (2015 Dec 15): 341–9.
Bahorik, A.L., Campbell, C.I., Sterling, S.A., et al. "Adverse impact of marijuana use on clinical outcomes among psychiatry patients with depression and alcohol use disorder." *Psychiatry Res* 259 (2018 Jan): 316–22.
Bahorik, A.L., Cornelius, J.R., Bangalore, S.S., et al. "Brief report: The impact of alcohol and cannabis misuse on cognition among individuals with schizophrenia." *Schizophr Res Cogn* 1 3 (2014 Sep 1): 160–63.
Bahorik, A.L., Leibowitz, A., Sterling, S.A., et al. "Patterns of marijuana use among psychiatry patients with depression and its impact on recovery." *J Affect Disord* 213 (2017 Apr 15): 168–71.
Bahorik, A.L., Newhill, C.E., Eack, S.M. "Characterizing the longitudinal patterns of substance use among individuals diagnosed with serious mental illness after psychiatric hospitalization." *Addiction* 108 7 (2013 Jul): 1259–69.
Bahorik, A.L., Newhill, C.E., Eack, S.M. "Neurocognitive functioning of individuals with schizophrenia: using and not using drugs." *Schizophr Bull* 40 4 (2014 Jul): 856–67.
Bahorik, A.L., Satre, D.D., Kline-Simon, A.H., et al. "Alcohol, cannabis, and opioid use disorders, and disease burden in an integrated health care system." *J Addict Med* 11 1 (2017 Jan/Feb): 3–9.
Bahorik, A.L., Sterling, S.A., Campbell, C.I., et al. "Medical and non-medical marijuana use in depression: Longitudinal associations with suicidal ideation, everyday functioning, and psychiatry service utilization." *J Affect Disord* 241 (2018 Dec 1): 8–14.
Belendiuk, K.A., Baldini, L.L., Bonn-Miller, M.O. "Narrative review of the safety and efficacy of marijuana for the treatment of commonly state-approved medical and psychiatric disorders." *Addict Sci Clin Pract* 10 (2015 Apr 21): 10.

Blessing, E.M., Steenkamp, M.M., Manzanares, J., Marmar, C.R. "Cannabidiol as a potential treatment for anxiety disorders." *Neurotherapeutics* 12 4 (2015 Oct): 825–36.

Bonn-Miller, M.O., Babson, K.A., Vandrey, R. "Using cannabis to help you sleep: heightened frequency of medical cannabis use among those with PTSD." *Drug Alcohol Depend* 136 (2014 Mar 1): 162–5.

Bonn-Miller, M.O., Vujanovic, A.A., Boden, M.T., Gross, J.J. "Posttraumatic stress, difficulties in emotion regulation, and coping-oriented marijuana use." *Cogn Behav Ther* 40 1 (2011): 34–44.

Bonn-Miller, M.O., Vujanovic, A.A., Drescher, K.D. "Cannabis use among military veterans after residential treatment for posttraumatic stress disorder." *Psychol Addict Behav* 25 3 (2011 Sep): 485–91.

Booz, G.W. "Cannabidiol as an emergent therapeutic strategy for lessening the impact of inflammation on oxidative stress." *Free Radic Biol Med* 51 5 (2011 Sep 1): 1054–61.

Campbell, C.I., Bahorik, A.L., Kline-Simon, A.H., Satre, D.D. "The role of marijuana use disorder in predicting emergency department and inpatient encounters: a retrospective cohort study." *Drug Alcohol Depend* 178 (2017 Sep 1): 170–5.

Crippa, J.A., Guimarães, F.S., Campos, A.C., Zuardi, A.W. "Translational investigation of the therapeutic potential of cannabidiol (CBD): toward a new age." *Front Immunol* 9 (2018 Sep 21): 2009.

Crippa, J.A., Zuardi, A.W., Martín-Santos, R., et al. "Cannabis and anxiety: a critical review of the evidence." *Hum Psychopharmacol* 24 7 (2009 Oct): 515–23.

Degenhardt, L., Hall, W., Lynskey, M. "Exploring the association between cannabis use and depression." *Addiction* 98 11 (2003 Nov): 1493–504.

Farris, S.G., Zvolensky, M.J., Boden, M.T., Bonn-Miller, M.O. "Cannabis use expectancies mediate the relation between depressive symptoms and cannabis use among cannabis-dependent veterans." *J Addict Med* 8 2 (2014 Mar–Apr): 130–6.

Feingold, D., Weiser, M., Rehm, J., Lev-Ran, S. "The association between cannabis use and anxiety disorders: Results from a population-based representative sample." *Eur Neuropsychopharmacol* 26 3 (2016 Mar): 493–505.

Feingold, D., Weiser, M., Rehm, J., Lev-Ran, S. "The association between cannabis use and mood disorders: A longitudinal study." *J Affect Disord* 172 (2015 Feb 1): 211–8.

Gorzalka, B.B., Hill, M.N. "Putative role of endocannabinoid signaling in the etiology of depression and actions of antidepressants." *Prog Neuropsychopharmacol Biol Psychiatry* 35 7 (2011 Aug 15): 1575–85.

Kevorkian, S., Bonn-Miller, M.O., Belendiuk, K., et al. "Associations among trauma, posttraumatic stress disorder, cannabis use, and cannabis use disorder in a nationally representative epidemiologic sample." *Psychol Addict Behav* 29 3 (2015 Sep): 633–8.

Mechoulam, R., Parker, L.A. "The endocannabinoid system and the brain." *Annu Rev Psychol* 64 (2013): 21–47.

Nicholson, A.N., Turner, C., Stone, B.M., Robson, P.J. "Effect of Delta-9-tetrahydrocannabinol and cannabidiol on nocturnal sleep and early-morning behavior in young adults." *J Clin Psychopharmacol* 24 3 (2004 Jun): 305–13.

Trull, T.J., Wycoff, A.M., Lane, S.P., et al. "Cannabis and alcohol use, affect and impulsivity in psychiatric out-patients' daily lives." *Addiction* 111 11 (2016 Nov): 2052–9.

Turna, J., Patterson, B., Van Ameringen, M. "Is cannabis treatment for anxiety, mood, and related disorders ready for prime time?" *Depress Anxiety* 34 (2017): 1006–17.

Volkow, N.D., Compton, W.M., Weiss, S.R. "Adverse health effects of marijuana use." *N Engl J Med* 371 9 (2014 Aug 28): 879.

Chapter 15

Barnes, D.E., Yaffe, K. "The projected effect of risk factor reduction on Alzheimer's disease prevalence." *Lancet Neurol* 10 9 (2011): 819–28.

Brommelhoff, J.A., Gatz, M., Johansson, B., et al. "Depression as a risk factor or prodromal feature for dementia? Findings in a population-based sample of Swedish twins." *Psychol Aging* 24 2 (2009): 373–84.

Centers for Disease Control and Prevention. "Birth defects: data and statistics; global." 2017. Available at www.cdc.gov/features/birth-defects-day/index.html. Accessed November 26, 2017.

Centers for Disease Control and Prevention. CDC Wonder [database]: mortality query. Available at http://wonder.cdc.gov. Accessed April 24, 2015.

Cipriani, A., Zhou, X., Del Giovane, C. "Comparative efficacy and tolerability of antidepressants for major depressive disorder in children and adolescents: a network meta-analysis." *Lancet* 388 10047 (2016 Aug 27): 881–90.

Cougnard, A., Verdoux, H., Grolleau, A., Moride, Y., Begaud, B., Tournier, M. "Impact of antidepressants on the risk of suicide in patients with depression in real-life conditions: a decision analysis model." *Psychol Med* 39 8 (2009): 1307–15.

Coupland, C., Dhiman, P., Morriss, R., et al. "Antidepressant use and risk of adverse outcomes in older people: population based cohort study." *BMJ* 343 (2011): d4551.

Cox, G.R., Callahan, P., Churchill, R., et al. "Psychological therapies versus antidepressant medication, alone and in combination for depression in children and adolescents." *Cochrane Database Syst Rev* 11 (2012 Nov 14): CD008324.

Cox, G.R., Fisher, C.A., De Silva, S., et al. "Interventions for preventing relapse and recurrence of a depressive disorder in children and adolescents." *Cochrane Database Syst Rev* 11 (2012 Nov 14): CD007504.

Dubicka, B., Wilkinson, P.O. "Latest thinking on antidepressants in children and young people." *Arch Dis Child* 103 8 (2018 Aug): 720–1.

Finer, L.B., Zolna, M.R. "Declines in unintended pregnancy in the United States, 2008–2011." *N Engl J Med* 374 (2016): 843–52.

Gallagher, D., Kiss, A., Lanctot, K., Herrmann, N. "Depression and risk of Alzheimer dementia: a longitudinal analysis to determine predictors of increased risk among older adults with depression." *Am J Geriatr Psychiatry* 26 (2018): 819–27.

Gibbons, R.D., Hur, K., Bhaumik, D.K., Mann, J.J. "The relationships between antidepressant prescription rates and rate of early adolescent suicide." *Am J Psychiatry* 163 11 (2006): 1898–904.

Gould, M.S., Kleinman, M.H., Lake A.M., Forman, J., et al. "Newspaper coverage of suicide and initiation of suicide clusters in teenagers in the USA, 1988–96: a retrospective, population-based, case-control study." *Lancet Psych* 1 1 (2014): 34–43.

Gould, M.S., Greenberg, T., Velting, D.M., Shaffer, D. "Youth suicide risk and preventive interventions: a review of the past 10 years." *J Am Acad Child Adolesc Psychiatry* 42 4 (2003): 386–405.

Grunbaum J.A., Kann, L., Kinchen, S., et al; Centers for Disease Control and Prevention. "Youth risk behavior surveillance—United States, 2003." [Published corrections appear in *MMWR Morb Mortal Wkly Rep* 53 24 (2004): 536 and *MMWR Morb Mortal Wkly Rep* 54 24 (2005): 608.]

Hetrick, S.E., Cox, G.R., Witt, K.G., et al. "Cognitive behavioural therapy (CBT), third-wave CBT and interpersonal therapy (IPT) based interventions for preventing depression in children and adolescents." *Cochrane Database Syst Rev* 8 (2016 Aug 9): CD003380.

Hetrick, S.E., McKenzie, J.E., Cox, G.R., et al. "Newer generation antidepressants for depressive disorders in children and adolescents." *Cochrane Database Syst Rev* 11 (2012 Nov 14): CD004851.

Kok, R.M., Nolen, W.A., Heeren, T.J. "Efficacy of treatment in older depressed patients: a systematic review and meta-analysis of double-blind randomized controlled trials with antidepressants." *J Affect Disord* 141 (2012): 103–15.

MacQueen, G.M., Frey, B.N., Ismail, Z., et al; CANMAT Depression Work Group. "Canadian Network for Mood and Anxiety Treatments (CANMAT) 2016 Clinical Guidelines for the Management of Adults with Major Depressive Disorder: Section 6. Special Populations: Youth, Women, and the Elderly." *Can J Psychiatry* 61 9 (2016 Sep): 588–603.

March, J., Silva, S., Petrycki, S., et al; Treatment for Adolescents with Depression Study (TADS) Team. "Fluoxetine, cognitive-behavioral therapy, and their combination for adolescents with depression: Treatment for

Adolescents with Depression Study (TADS) randomized controlled trial." *JAMA* 292 7 (2004 Aug 18): 807–20.
Mitchell, A.J., Subramaniam, H. "Prognosis of depression in old age compared to middle age: a systematic review of comparative studies." *Am J Psychiatry* 162 (2005): 1588–601.
Moon, B., Kim, S., Park, Y.H., et al: "Depressive symptoms are associated with progression to dementia in patients with amyloid-positive mild cognitive impairment." *J Alzheimers Dis* 58 4 (2017): 1255–64.
National Institute of Mental Health. "Recommendations for reporting on suicide." Available at www.nimh.nih.gov/health/topics/suicide-prevention/recommendations-for-reporting-on-suicide.shtml. Accessed July 27, 2015.
Olfson, M., Shaffer, D., Marcus, S.C., Greenberg, T. "Relationship between antidepressant medication treatment and suicide in adolescents." *Arch Gen Psychiatry* 60 10 (2003): 978–82.
Simon, G.E., Savarino, J. "Suicide attempts among patients starting depression treatment with medications or psychotherapy." *Am J Psychiatry* 164 7 (2007 Jul): 1029–34.
Simon, G.E., Savarino, J., Operskalski, B., Wang, P. "Suicide risk during antidepressant treatment." *Am J Psychiatry* 163 1 (2006): 41–7.
Spira, A.P., Rebok, G.W., Stone, K.L., et al. "Depressive symptoms in oldest-old women: risk of mild cognitive impairment and dementia." *Am J Geriatr Psychiatry* 20 12 (2012): 1006–15.
Vilalta-Franch, J., Lopez-Pousa, S., Llinas-Regla, J., et al. "Depression subtypes and 5-year risk of dementia and Alzheimer disease in patients aged 70 years." *Int J Geriatr Psychiatry* 28 4 (2013): 341–50.

Chapter 16

American Foundation for Suicide Prevention. "Suicide statistics." afsp.org/about-suicide/suicide-statistics/.
Asarnow, J.R., Baraff, L.J., Berk, M., et al. "Pediatric emergency department suicidal patients: two-site evaluation of suicide ideators, single attempters, and repeat attempters." *J Am Acad Child Adolesc Psychiatry* 47 8 (2008 Aug): 958–66.
Asarnow, J.R., Baraff, L.J., Berk, M., et al. "Suicide ideation, plan, and attempt in the Mexican adolescent mental health survey." *J Am Acad Child Adolesc Psychiatry* 47 1 (2008 Jan): 41–52.
Bridge, J.A., Horowitz, L.M., Fontanella, C.A., et al. "Prioritizing research to reduce youth suicide and suicidal behavior." *Am J Prev Med* 47 3 Suppl 2 (2014 Sep): S229–34.
Brodsky, B.S., Spruch-Feiner, A., Stanley, B. "The zero suicide model: applying evidence-based suicide prevention practices to clinical care." *Front Psychiatry* 9 (2018 Feb 23): 33.

Daniel, S.S., Goldston, D.B., Erkanli, A., et al. "Prospective study of major loss life events and risk for suicidal thoughts and behaviors among adolescents and young adults." *Suicide Life Threat Behav* 47 4 (2017 Aug): 436–49.

Fleischmann, A., Arensman, E., Berman, A., et al. "Overview evidence on interventions for population suicide with an eye to identifying best-supported strategies for LMICs." *Glob Ment Health (Camb)* 3 (2016 Feb 12): e5.

Glenn, C.R., Franklin, J.C., Nock, M.K. "Evidence-based psychosocial treatments for self-injurious thoughts and behaviors in youth." *J Clin Child Adolesc Psychol* 44 1 (2015): 1–29.

Harrod, C.S., Goss, C.W., Stallones, L., DiGuiseppi, C. "Interventions for primary prevention of suicide in university and other post-secondary educational settings." *Cochrane Database Syst Rev* 10 (2014 Oct 29): CD009439.

Goldston, D., Erkanli, A., Daniel, S., et al. "Developmental trajectories of suicidal thoughts and behaviors from adolescence through adulthood." *J Am Acad Child Adolesc Psychiatry* 55 5 (2016 May): 400–7.

Hawton, K., Witt, K.G., Taylor Salisbury, T.L., et al. "Interventions for self-harm in children and adolescents." *Cochrane Database Syst Rev* 12 (2015 Dec 21): CD012013.

Hawton, K., Witt, K.G., Taylor Salisbury, T.L., et al. "Pharmacological interventions for self-harm in adults." *Cochrane Database Syst Rev* 7 (2015 Jul 6): CD011777.

Hawton, K., Witt, K.G., Taylor Salisbury, T.L., et al. "Psychosocial interventions for self-harm in adults." *Cochrane Database Syst Rev* 5 (2016 May 12): CD012189.

Labouliere, C.D., Vasan, P., Kramer, A., et al. "'Zero suicide'—a model for reducing suicide in United States behavioral healthcare." *Suicidologi* 23 1 (2018): 22–30.

Mortier, P., Kiekens, G., Auerbach, R.P., et al. "A risk algorithm for the persistence of suicidal thoughts and behaviors during college." *J Clin Psychiatry* 78 7 (2017 Jul): e828–36.

Niederkrotenthaler, T., Reidenberg, D.J., Till, B., Gould, M.S. "Increasing help-seeking and referrals for individuals at risk for suicide by decreasing stigma: the role of mass media." *Am J Prev Med* 47 3 Suppl 2 (2014 Sep): S235–43.

Nock, M.K., Green, J.G., Hwang, I., et al. "Prevalence, correlates, and treatment of lifetime suicidal behavior among adolescents: results from the National Comorbidity Survey Replication Adolescent Supplement." *JAMA Psychiatry* 70 3 (2013 Mar): 300–10.

O'Connor, R.C., Rasmussen, S., Hawton, K. "Distinguishing adolescents who think about self-harm from those who engage in self-harm." *Br J Psychiatry* 200 4 (2012 Apr): 330–5.

Public Health Agency of Canada. "Suicide in Canada: infographic." June 16, 2016. canada.ca/en/public-health/services/publications/healthy-living/suicide-canada-infographic.html.

Shah, A. "The relationship between suicide rates and age: an analysis of multinational data from the World Health Organization." *Int Psychogeriatr* 19 (2007): 1141–52.

Taliaferro, L.A., Muehlenkamp, J.J. "Factors associated with current versus lifetime self-injury among high school and college students." *Suicide Life Threat Behav* 45 1 (2015 Feb): 84–97.

Taliaferro, L.A., Muehlenkamp, J.J. "Risk factors associated with self-injurious behavior among a national sample of undergraduate college students." *J Am Coll Health* 63 1 (2015): 40–8.

Taliaferro, L.A., Muehlenkamp, J.J. "Risk and protective factors that distinguish adolescents who attempt suicide from those who only consider suicide in the past year." *Suicide Life Threat Behav* 44 1 (2014 Feb): 6–22.

U.S. Surgeon General and the National Action Alliance for Suicide Prevention. *Goals and objectives for action: a report of the U.S. Surgeon General and of the National Action.* Alliance for Suicide Prevention. surgeongeneral.gov/library/reports/national-strategy-suicide-prevention/index.html.

World Health Organization. "Distribution of suicide rates (per 100,000) by gender and age," Geneva. who.int/mental_health/prevention/suicide/suicide_rates_charte/en/index.html.

Index

Note: F or T before a page number indicates a figure or table.

About the Author

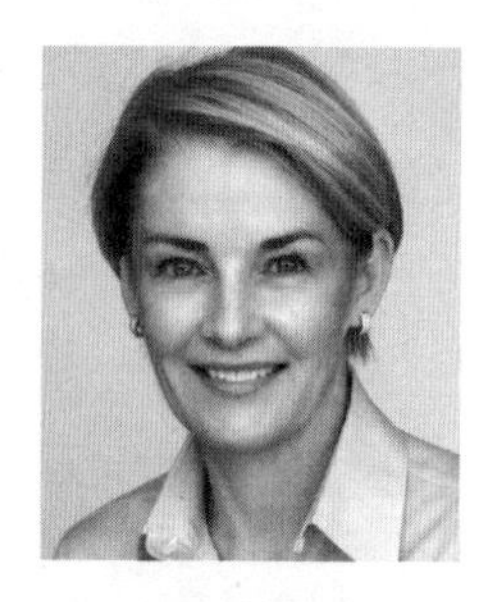

DR. DIANE MCINTOSH graduated from Dalhousie University with an undergraduate degree in pharmacy before completing medical school and residency training in psychiatry. She is a clinical assistant professor at the University of British Columbia and has a community psychiatry practice, with a particular interest in the neurobiology of mood and anxiety disorders and ADHD. She is extensively involved in continuing medical education programs to colleagues nationally and internationally, including her own educational program, PsychedUp CME (psychedupcme.com). She is the cofounder of SwitchRx (switchrx.ca), the online psychiatric medication switching tool. Most recently, she co-founded wedomatter .org, which advocates for more compassionate care for psychiatric patients and their families.

drdianemcintosh.com